AF840662

DERMATOLOGY - LABORATORY AND CLINICAL RESEARCH

BIOLOGICAL AND NON-BIOLOGICAL THERAPY IN PEMPHIGUS

AN UPDATED THERAPEUTIC GUIDE

DERMATOLOGY - LABORATORY AND CLINICAL RESEARCH

Additional books in this series can be found on Nova's website under the Series tab.

Additional e-books in this series can be found on Nova's website under the eBooks tab.

DERMATOLOGY - LABORATORY AND CLINICAL RESEARCH

BIOLOGICAL AND NON-BIOLOGICAL THERAPY IN PEMPHIGUS

AN UPDATED THERAPEUTIC GUIDE

ANDRÉS TIRADO-SÁNCHEZ

NOVA BIOMEDICAL
New York

Copyright © 2016 by Nova Science Publishers, Inc.

All rights reserved. No part of this book may be reproduced, stored in a retrieval system or transmitted in any form or by any means: electronic, electrostatic, magnetic, tape, mechanical photocopying, recording or otherwise without the written permission of the Publisher.

We have partnered with Copyright Clearance Center to make it easy for you to obtain permissions to reuse content from this publication. Simply navigate to this publication's page on Nova's website and locate the "Get Permission" button below the title description. This button is linked directly to the title's permission page on copyright.com. Alternatively, you can visit copyright.com and search by title, ISBN, or ISSN.

For further questions about using the service on copyright.com, please contact:
Copyright Clearance Center
Phone: +1-(978) 750-8400 Fax: +1-(978) 750-4470 E-mail: info@copyright.com.

NOTICE TO THE READER

The Publisher has taken reasonable care in the preparation of this book, but makes no expressed or implied warranty of any kind and assumes no responsibility for any errors or omissions. No liability is assumed for incidental or consequential damages in connection with or arising out of information contained in this book. The Publisher shall not be liable for any special, consequential, or exemplary damages resulting, in whole or in part, from the readers' use of, or reliance upon, this material. Any parts of this book based on government reports are so indicated and copyright is claimed for those parts to the extent applicable to compilations of such works.

Independent verification should be sought for any data, advice or recommendations contained in this book. In addition, no responsibility is assumed by the publisher for any injury and/or damage to persons or property arising from any methods, products, instructions, ideas or otherwise contained in this publication.

This publication is designed to provide accurate and authoritative information with regard to the subject matter covered herein. It is sold with the clear understanding that the Publisher is not engaged in rendering legal or any other professional services. If legal or any other expert assistance is required, the services of a competent person should be sought. FROM A DECLARATION OF PARTICIPANTS JOINTLY ADOPTED BY A COMMITTEE OF THE AMERICAN BAR ASSOCIATION AND A COMMITTEE OF PUBLISHERS.

Additional color graphics may be available in the e-book version of this book.

Library of Congress Cataloging-in-Publication Data

ISBN: 978-1-63484-662-2
Library of Congress Control Number: 2016936842

Published by Nova Science Publishers, Inc. † New York

To my beloved wife Jesica…
To my sons Ricardo and Joel...
Thank you for your support and patience.

To my dear mom...
Thank you for your advice and encouragement.

To my patients...
This book is for you; thank you for letting me learn from you.

CONTENTS

ABSTRACT

The main objective in treating pemphigus vulgaris is to control the disease, prevent relapses, and avoid adverse events associated with the prolonged use of steroids and immunosuppressive agents. Finding the most effective steroid-sparing agent has formed much of the focus of recent research. Systemic corticosteroids remain the gold standard for pemphigus vulgaris.

In this book, the reader through direct images, tables and text will have a complete view of this group of life-threating diseases; this is of interest not only to dermatologists, but for all those health professionals whom at some point in their lives have tried or at least had the opportunity to see a patient with these diseases. This book is obviously also intended for those who have experienced first hand pemphigus vulgaris.

This book is also a suitable medium for understanding the pemphigus group. Residents and researchers in dermatology and close disciplines can use the book as a quick reference guide when dealing with these patients. This book will help both dermatologists and non-dermatology physicians for treating each disease practically. Each chapter reviews the current literature of treatments for each disease, rates disease severity, and provides guidelines for the use of available medications. This book will help guide clinicians in carrying out suitable treatments based on the severity.

Finally, in this book, we aim to provide a quick study guide for students and a reference for physicians who practice treating these types of patients. The author hopes the reader enjoys reading this book as much as he did composing it.

Keywords: pemphigus, pathogenesis, diagnosis,treatment, glucocorticoids, rituximab, biological treatment

PREFACE

The first edition of the book "Biological and Non-Biological Therapy in Pemphigus: An Updated Therapeutic Guide," has been done with the aim of introducing the clinician, especially those with expertise in Dermatology, to the wide world of pemphigus. The ideas discussed are anything but complex, simplifying the proper interaction with the content, always upholding an open position about the different theories and points of view directed to explain this dramatic, yet disturbing disease.

To simplify the study of this group of diseases, the book is divided into eight sections: the first one cover general aspects of the skin, in a normal view, and gradually and almost slightly with the pathological view. In the second part of the book, essential aspects of the etiopathogenesis of pemphigus are addressed. In part three, epidemiological aspects of the disease, its global distribution and possible explanations for this geographical distribution are extended; in the fourth section, clinical characteristics of pemphigus and its different types are explained in detail; in the fifth part, concisely address the main diagnostic resources available for histological and immunological diagnosis of the disease; in Part 6 and 7 of the book, the available schemes of conventional treatment (non-biological, mainly corticosteroids, the gold standard treatment for pemphigus vulgaris) and emerging (biological, mainly rituximab, the still unreachable paradise) treatment alternatives are properly addressed in detail. In the last part of the book (part 8), newly issues as additional therapy, especially pain and infection are reviewed; also, the instruments for monitoring not only the severity of the disease and therefore the response to treatment, but important aspects such as quality of life are also described.

The patients with the disease who visited our hospital are thanked for giving us their trust and sharing their knowledge on symptoms and treatment outcome. I hope this book gives the reader the knowledge and passes on the experience gained in two decades managing pemphigus.

Andrés Tirado-Sánchez
Winter 2016

PART 1. PHYSIOLOGICAL AND PATHOLOGICAL BACKGROUND

Chapter 1

THE BIOLOGY OF THE EPIDERMIS: THE BASICS

During the first weeks of fetal life, the embryonic epidermis is composed only of a single layer of close cells and undifferentiated progressively acquire the features of keratinocytes.

Adult epidermis consists of three types of cells: keratinocytes, melanocytes and dendritic cells (Langerhans cells); the former have direct connections with close keratinocytes by desmosomes, and compounds containing keratin intermediate filaments of low molecular weight.

1.1. THE KERATINOCYTE, THE MAIN CELL OF THE EPIDERMIS

The main cell of the epidermis is the keratinocyte or squamous cell. It originates from the ectoderm and its specific function is to produce keratin, a protein complex that not only filamentous form the surface covering of the epidermis (stratum corneum), but is the structural protein of hair and nails. Multiple genes have been identified in different keratin, distinguishing two subfamilies: the acidic and basic keratins. Thus, the products of a basic keratin gene and another acid combine to give rise to different types of keratin found in the various tissues and vary depending on the type and degree of the differentiation [1].

The epidermis can be divided into the following layers, starting with the innermost: basal layer, spinous layer, granular layer and stratum corneum. These names reflect the different aspect that acquires as keratinocyte be differentiating reaching morphology keratinized cell.

Part of the basal cells proliferate and differentiate gradually as they move through the entire thickness of the epidermis. As a cell passes upwardly through the epidermis it changes its morphological appearance and get more flattened core [2].

Similarly there is a regional variation in thickness of the anatomical layers of the skin; depending on location, we can remark variations in the thickness of the different layers of the epidermis. Thus, we find at the palms and soles, the maximum thickness of the corneum and granular layers, while almost nonexistent in the most delicate skin of the flexor surface of forearms and abdomen. By contrast, basal layer has the thickness matching to a single cell, regardless of location [3].

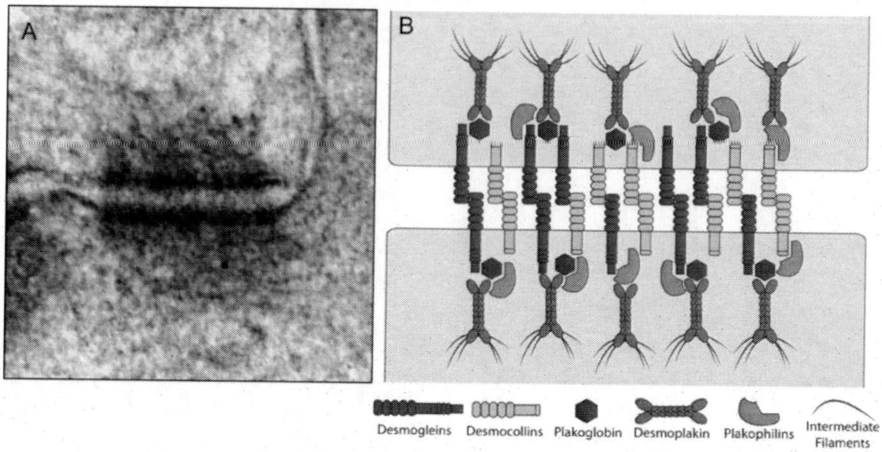

Figure 1. Desmosome structure. (A) Electron microscopy of a young desmosome, which lacks a dense midline, connecting two adjacent cells in a keratinocyte monolayer. (B) Schematic representation of desmosomal structure. Desmogleins (Dsg) and desmocollins (Dsc) constitute the extracellular link between cells, and are responsible for the appearance of the dense midline; they form homo- and heterodimers, whose intracellular tails bind the Armadillo family proteins plakoglobin (Pg) and the plakophilins (Pkp), which serve to link cadherins to the plakin protein desmoplakin (Dsp), which in turn tethers desmosomes to the intermediate filament network. Reproduced with permission of John Wiley and Sons from Ref. 711.

During keratinization or keratinized cell transformation, the keratinocyte through a first phase synthesis, followed by a phase of degradation. In the first phase, the keratinocyte collects within the cytoplasm intermediate filaments comprised of a fibro protein, keratin, provided with a pattern of helical folding alpha. These tonofilaments are grouped in bundles that converge and limit at the plasma membrane, forming binding specialized complexes, called desmosomes (Figure 1). The degradative phase of keratinization is characterized by disappearing cell organelles and to consolidate all its contents, resulting in a mixture of formless material and filament wrapped by a cell membrane thickening [3].

Intercellular space separates plasma membranes of close cells. Histochemical studies with electron microscopy have shown the glycoprotein and lipids space and lamellar granules, are located mainly at the contact between the granular and corneal layers [1].

Granulosa keratinocytes area also filamentous keratin system, called keratohyalin granules, are particles composed of shapeless material with a high content of sulphurous containing proteins. This material, called profilaggrin, is the forerunner of filaggrin, which receives this name because is thought to be responsible for promoting the aggregation of keratin filaments. Filaggrin change-over takes place in the granular layer, forming the electron-interfilamentous protein matrix of mature epidermal keratin [1, 3].

Organelles called Odland corpuscles, also called granules keratinosomes membrane are located intracellularly in keratinocytes of the upper layers, pouring its contents into the extracellular space in the conjunction between granular and corneal layers. All this provides a barrier against water loss and, with filaggrin control cohesion between cells in the stratum corneum [3].

Keratinocytes play a role in immune function of the skin by taking part in the communication, and control of cell systems which help in inducing immune responses. Similarly, they secrete cytokines and inflammatory mediators and may also express surface molecules such as ICAM-1 molecules or major histocompatibility complex class II; this shows that keratinocytes actively respond to immune effectors' signals [1].

1.2. BIOLOGICAL INTERACTIONS OF KERATINOCYTES

The epidermis has a structural membrane that protects inner homeostasis, where keratinocyte performs an orchestrated process of proliferation and differentiation through differential expression of structural proteins, surface molecules and enzymes.

In recent years, it has become obvious the epidermis is a complex multicellular organ, in which a sophisticated cross talk between its cells, the environment and the body's metabolism takes place to ensure its many essential roles. While the air-liquid and the liquid-liquid barriers of the epidermis form potent measures for separating the inside from the outside environment, epidermal keratinocytes also have an immunostimulatory role to build up the defence system in cooperation with epidermal immune cells, like dendritic cells [1-3]. The epidermidis, however, not just a protective measure against harmful external influences and maintenance of the inner homeostasis but is also a true sensory organ important for perception and transmission of environmental and internal signals including touch or electromagnetic stimulation. New control mechanisms for the proliferation and differentiation process have emerged, including epigenetic control [4-6]; molecular changes affecting barrier functions [7, 8]; genetic signals associated with an antigen-specific Ig response in retriever breeds [9, 10]. It has also become clear the keratinocyte expresses a multitude of surface adhesion molecules that fulfill receptor functions carrying signals into the cells and going out, which is of relevance in autoimmune diseases like pemphigus vulgaris [6, 11-14]. Finally, the capacity of the epidermis to self-renew in a cyclical manner throughout the lifetime has revealed the presence of tissue stem cells on basal stratum [15]. The capacity of epidermal keratinocytes for self-renewal has also provided the basis for establishing long-term keratinocyte cultures, which at first contributed to the modeling and study of the proliferation and differentiation process *in vitro* [16, 17], and will also provide a source of multipotent stem cells for developments in regenerative medicine. The recently explained self-organizing principle of tissue, which has been revealed through a specialized culture of embryonic and induced pluripotent stem cells [18] now, provides the starting point for the next generation of regenerative medicine, which is expected to involve all organs and their tissue-resident stem cells, in particular the easily accessible skin and its appendages. This information revealed the great complexity and active role of the skin in balanced homeostasis.

Chapter 2

The Immune System in Normal Skin and in Pemphigus Skin

The skin is one of the largest organs of the human body and provides primary defense against invading pathogens and several injuring causes. It traduces various functions such as control of the body temperature and receiving sensory information from the environment, and as a barrier organ, preserves immunological homeostasis.

The skin is a complex immunological network structured by several cellular components and soluble mediators secreted by resident and migratory cells, to launch both local and systemic immune response and to activate the immune system in severe cutaneous infections.

2.1. Skin Immunity: The Normal Way

Various residing immune and nonimmune cells which take part in a cutaneous immune reaction, like epidermal Langerhans cells, dermal dendritic cells, and keratinocytes, function as nonprofessional antigen-presenting cells and as cellular source of proinflammatory cytokines such as IL-1, IL-18, type I interferons, and TNFα. There is a growing body of evidence referring to the immunological functions of the skin, represented by the skin immune system, and the skin-associated lymphoid tissue, also called, SALT, important for the immune surveillance of the skin [19-21].

Nonimmune cells and resident immune cells of the skin mediate both innate and adaptive immune responses [22]. The first line of defense or innate immunity comprises the keratinocytes, macrophages, mast cells, as well as vascular and lymphoid endothelial cells. Various antigen-presenting cells involving epidermal Langerhans cells, inflammatory epidermal dendritic cells, are key players to link both innate and adaptive immunity in the skin [23-25].

Granulocytes, natural killer cells, and natural killer T cells, are typically recruited to the skin and are involved in the control of certain pathogens and in up-regulating the inflammatory response. In non-pathological frames, B lymphocytes are not a constituent of the skin but are detected during skin infection and inflammatory conditions. In contrast, T lymphocytes are often seen as a part of the skin in normal and inflamed frames, mainly in the form of memory cells [21, 22, 26].

Keratinocytes form the epithelial component of skin, and epithelia are regarded as a structural part of the innate immune system. In a process of differentiation, keratinocytes divide and gradually transform themselves into corneal cells forming the stratum corneum, which consists of protein-filled corneal envelops (keratin, filaggrin, and others) and a lipid-rich extracellular matrix. The corneal layer forms a first-line physical barrier that protects the body from invading pathogens, antigens, and allergens.

In addition, keratinocytes are a major source of antimicrobial peptides including cathelicidin and β-defensins. Also, keratinocytes express pattern recognition receptors, including Toll-like receptors, functioning as initiators of innate immune responses. Keratinocytes not only serve as a proinflammatory component of innate immune defenses, but also have some features of the adaptive immunity system, as they may act as antigen-presenting cells, produce downregulating factors such as IL-1 receptor antagonist, and α-MSH (α-melanocyte-stimulating hormone) [27], and can promote type 1 T-helper cell responses in the skin through production of IL-23 [28] or may steer the outcome towards a type 2 T-cell response by production of the cytokine thymic stromal lymphopoietin [29].

Various humoral and cellular elements together form the immune system. The general concept is that *Pattern Recognition Receptor* or called PRR, which can be regarded as any receptor recognizing *Pathogen-Associated Molecular Patterns* or so-called PAMPs and capable of triggering antimicrobial function in leukocytes, are present on cell membranes or found within the cell. The pathogen-associated molecular patterns are defined as highly conserved structures of common pathogens that are essential for microbe survival and include, for example, components of bacterial cell walls such as lipopolysaccharide, lipoteichoic acid and peptidoglycan fungal cell-wall component zymosan, and viral double-stranded RNA [30]. Apart from the prototypic Toll-like receptors, the group of pattern recognition receptors also encompasses several other gene families such as Caterpillers [31], nucleotide-binding oligomerization domains 1 and 2, and the family of C-type lectins that binds to unique branching and positioning of sugar residues on a given molecule and includes soluble proteins, such as the collectin mannose-binding lectin, and transmembrane proteins, such as Langerin, dendritic cell-SIGN, and Dectin-1 [32].

Binding of pathogen-associated molecular patterns to pattern recognition receptors, of which variable combinations can be detected on many cells including keratinocytes and dendritic cells [33], begins signal transduction pathways that lead to the production of antimicrobial peptides, cytokines (many of them, such as TNFα, are proinflammatory), and chemokines [34]. Several of these cytokines up-regulate adhesion molecules, and with chemokines, enhance recruitment of effector leukocytes [35]. At first, these effector leukocytes may include phagocytes, such as granulocytes and macrophages, and cytotoxic cells, such as killer cells. Later, adaptive immunity related cells such as cytotoxic T-cells, memory T-cells, and regulatory T-cells may be recruited and lead to adaptive immune responses as well as to tapering down inflammation.

Of note is that in diseases that are traditionally seen as mainly T-cell mediated, innate immune responses may be dysfunctional, that is innate immunity is clearly defective in atopic dermatitis [36], while all elements of innate immunity are activated or up-regulated in psoriasis [37].

In vivo evidence for the presence of acquired immunity in the immune system is represented by the concept of immune surveillance. When acquired immunity mechanisms are inhibited, as occurs in iatrogenic immunosuppression in transplant patients and in patients with HIV-induced T-cell loss, malignancies occur more often. Viral and tumor escape mechanisms are enhanced by reduced immune responses, and oncogenic viruses related to tumors as well as other malignancies arise uncontrolled. Compared with the physiology of acquired immunity responses in normal human skin, the pathology that results from ill-directed acquired immune responses in human skin is more familiar and more extensively studied. Allergic contact dermatitis is a standard example of acquired, T-cell–mediated immunity that goes beyond its original function, leading to exaggerated responses on hapten challenge, clinically revealing it self-in developing localized, highly pruritic allergic contact eczema. Misdirected autoantibodies form another well-known example of cutaneous pathology induced by acquired immunity. The autoimmune bullous diseases including pemphigus, pemphigoid, linear IgA disease, and acquired epidermolysis bullosa are clear examples.

2.2. Pemphigus Immunity: The Abnormal Way

Pemphigus is a group of rare acquired organ-specific, autoimmune diseases, pathogenetically characterized by autoantibodies directed against adhesion molecules of the skin and/or mucous membranes [38-40]. These autoantibodies trigger a cascade of events which finally result in either loss of adhesion of epidermal keratinocytes, resulting in split formation and clinically seeming flaccid blisters and often painful erosions [41-42]. Based on clinical characteristics and histopathological analysis, pemphigus clinical forms can be categorized into several subgroups, and they can be classified into further details by their target autoantigens and the circulating autoantibody profile using techniques such as immunoblotting, immunofluorescence analysis, ELISA, and flow cytometry. Also, some studies revealed basic mechanisms into autoimmune process leading to loss of self-tolerance to identify autoantigens involved in these disorders [43-46].

Pemphigus is considered as a model of an autoantibody-mediated autoimmune disorder, since the passive transfer of patients' IgG is enough to induce a blistering phenotype in neonatal mice (passive transfer model) [47]. Clinically, neonatal pemphigus, that is, the transient development of blisters in neonates whose mothers suffer from active pemphigus, is explained by the placental transmission of maternal autoantibodies [48]. The desmosomal cadherins desmoglein 1 and 3 are well-defined target antigens in pemphigus [39]; however, IgG autoantibodies against various non-desmosomal autoantigens, e.g., acetylcholine receptors, annexins, non-desmosomal adhesion molecules, as well as intracellular targets such as mitochondrial parts [49-51]. The pathogenic relevance of the non-desmosomal autoantibodies is not completely determined [51]. Except for IgA pemphigus, circulating autoantibodies are of the IgG isotype of which IgG4 correlates well with disease activity [52-53]. Different theories of acantholysis have been proposed, including steric hindrance of desmosomal desmoglein interactions, binding to non-desmosomal desmoglein proteins resulting in reduced recruitment of non-desmosomal desmoglein to the desmosomes, endocytosis of autoantibody-desmoglein complexes, activation of various signaling pathways, and induction of apoptosis (apoptolysis) are still being under investigation [54-9]. Pemphigus can be divided into several subtypes of which pemphigus vulgaris and pemphigus foliaceus constitute the major types [60]. Other rare variants include paraneoplastic pemphigus, characterized by severe mucosal involvement and bronchiolitis obliterans and often associated with underlying lymphoproliferative malignancies. The clinical hallmarks of IgA pemphigus are annular vesicles and pustules, crusty erosions, and erythematous plaques [61].

2.3. Autoimmunity and Autoimmune Disease: Chaos and Distortion of Normal Immunity

The term autoimmunity refers to the specific memory-type immune reactions, directed against one or more self-epitopes. Under most conditions, autoimmunity is determined by immunoglobulins that react with either unknown or well-defined human antigens. It is supposed producing these autoantibodies needs prior activation of potentially auto reactive B cells by memory T-cells. These T cells must not only recognize a closely related peptide structure. Also, these T cells can stimulate B cells only when primed by activated antigen presenting cells.

Autoimmunity is a frequent event. Most likely, any individual raises immune reactions against many self-antigens. This autoimmunity leads only rarely to overt autoimmune disease. Therefore, developing autoimmune disease needs trespassing of many added security levels, beyond autoimmune reactivity [62]. Examples are antinuclear antibodies, which are found in even more than 50% of the female population older than 50 years. Compared with this frequency, antinuclear antibodies-associated autoimmune diseases are rare and affect less than 2% [63]. Only few autoimmune diseases progress continuously during short waves of disease activity and between these waves have long periods of quiescence.

These auto reactive T and B cells do normally not disappear during these periods of quiescence, therefore, a series of control mechanisms protect from autoimmune disease. Precursor T cells develop within the bone marrow and reach the thymus through the blood. These immature forerunner cells undergo a series of activation and maturation events that eventually result in a forerunner population that expresses a T-cell receptor and both, CD4 and CD8 molecules. The T-cell receptor expresses two independent immunoglobulin-like chains, the α- and the β-chain. The β-chain is expressed with a pre-α-chain; the definite T-cell receptor α-chain replaces the pre-α-chain before developing the $CD4^+$ $CD8^+$, double positive status. In normal conditions, T cells express only one pair of T-cell receptor α /β-chains. This resulting replacement of the pre-α-chain by a definite T-cell receptor-α-chain however, may lead to the occurrence of T cells which express two receptors, one single β-chain and independent α-chains. Thus, one T cell may have two, independent specificities [64-65]. Once the double positive status is achieved, T-cells interact with thymus MHC molecules.

This interaction of the double positive cells, which are highly sensitive to death signals, will decide their further outcome as most of the double positive cells die during this selection process. T-cells with rather high affinity for peptide loaded and possible also empty MHC molecules die through induction of apoptosis. T cells that express a T-cell receptor with an affinity that is too low for recognizing peptide loaded MHC molecules die. Only a few T cells, less than 10%, survives this selection and leaves the thymus as a single positive T cell, expressing either CD4 or CD8 and a T-cell receptor [66-8]. During thymic selection, T-cell receptor structures with high affinity for self-may not only lead to deletion; another mode is temporary suppression of the T-cell receptor. If a T cell with two distinct T-cell receptor α-chains then receives at the same time a survival signal by the second receptor, this cell may become positively selected and result in a peripheral T cell population with two distinct T-cell receptor; one corresponding to an auto-reactive receptor.

2.4. Tolerance (Central and Peripheral): The "Know Yourself" Principle

The acquired immune system must operate in balance between aggressive defense against potentially harmful invading pathogens and the tolerance of self-antigens and non-harmful organisms. Further, once a defensive immune response is initiated, mechanisms must come into effect to temper and eventually terminate that response to block the damage to host tissues resulting from continuing and uncontrolled activation. Experiments described by Billingham et al. in 1953, show that fetal exposure to antigenically different cells in fetal chicks and mice resulted in acquisition of enduring postnatal immune tolerance to tissues of the mismatched antigenic background. They showed that fetal exposure to foreign antigen lead to the absence of cells that would mount such an immune response, suggesting that elimination of such cells during development was the major mechanisms for establishing immunetolerance [69].

The thymus and the apoptosis and paralysis occurring during the development of B cells recognizing plentiful antigens in the periphery, delete about 90% of self-reactive T and B cells. This phenomenon is termed as *central tolerance*. However, roughly 10% of these cells survive [67, 70]. However, not all antigens are presented in thymus, bone marrow or peripheral blood. In one individual, all cells express the same MHC class I and a large spectrum of common minor antigens. However, each cell also expresses its own set of antigens that is related to its function and localization.

Thus, the mature immune system encounters a larger spectrum of antigens in the periphery than in the thymus. Tolerance against these antigens requires a multitude of mechanisms which are collected under the term *peripheral tolerance* [71-2]. *Central tolerance* is mainly based on deletion of potentially auto reactive T cells [73].

2.5. How Peripheral and Central Tolerance Work?

One mechanism of peripheral tolerance may be deletion; this is mainly associated with the sudden appearance of a large number of antigens. This mechanism has been demonstrated for antigens that were presented in large numbers, thus during infection or following injection of super antigens [74-5]. Whether this mechanism applies also under physiological conditions is not clear. But it may become relevant during tissue destruction, when large quantities of self-antigens are presented, thus in skin burning, viral infections of skin, muscle or other organs or following stroke. However, this phenomenon has not yet been analyzed in detail. Another mechanism is suppression of T-cell receptor expression, which has been shown with pregnant mice expressing a transgenic T-cell receptor that recognizes the foreign MHC class I molecule-expressed by the father and the fetus. The level of this transgenic T-cell receptor is high before and after pregnancy, but low during pregnancy. These T cells are also functionally silenced. During pregnancy, pregnant female mice become even tolerant of otherwise highly immunogenic tumor cells expressing this same antigen [76]. Thus, suppression of a T-cell receptor expression is closely associated with the occurrence of peripheral tolerance and may contribute to it. However, there are other mechanisms that significantly contribute to peripheral tolerance [76-7].

In an experiment performed on mice that simultaneously express a peptide antigen of the lymphocytic choriomeningitis virus by the endocrine pancreas and T cells with a T-cell receptor transgenic for the lymphocytic choriomeningitis virus peptide [78-9]. These animals have autoreactive $CD8^+$ T cells that are functionally normal, express normal levels of the T-cell receptor and kill peptide-loaded targets *in vitro* to the same extend as transgenic T cells from control animals. Nevertheless, these animals do not develop autoimmune disease, which means that, besides the target organ, expressing an endogenous potentially immunogenic peptide and normal levels of T-cell receptor, other signals are needed for inducting autoimmune disease. Such a situation may be the effect of "ignorance" of the target by the auto reactive T-cells [80]. This may be the result of missing adhesion molecules or the absence of co-stimulatory signals [78]. However, it may also be because of expression of auto antigens at immunologically privileged sites, expressing apoptosis inducing molecules capable of killing activated T-cells or secondary to local silencing of activated T-cells that recognize target tissues without co-stimulatory molecules.

Reactivity and mode of action are not only given by the T-cell receptor and the spectrum of co-stimulatory T cells expressed by T cells. Most importantly, T cell functions are determined by the cytokines they produce. Naive T cells produce only interleukin (IL-) 2 when stimulated by peptides and professional antigen presenting cells [81]. Afterwards, T cells develop towards memory cells that are theoretically capable of producing a large spectrum of cytokines. It is now settled that T-cells normally do not-secrete a random pattern of cytokines, but distinguish into phenotypes that produce distinctive sets of cytokines associated with well-defined functional phenotypes [82-4].

T cells that produce mainly IL-2 and interferon-γ (IFN-γ) are associated with inflammatory, cell mediated immune responses. When expressing the CD4 molecule they are named Th1, when expressing the CD8 molecule, they are named Tc1 cells and induce type 1 immune responses. These types of immune responses are required for the control of several infections (bacteria, virus, fungi, and parasites). However, when directed against autoantigens, they may cause autoinflammatory and autoimmune diseases [72, 83, 85-9]. These diseases are normally well localized to one single organ or a group of organs that share a common antigen. These T-cells do not only induce direct tissue effects (for example psoriasis), they also induce B cells to produce complement binding antibodies, which may strengthen local inflammation and tissue destruction, as it is the case in patients with pemphigoid or pemphigus [90]. The most important counterpart of "type 1" immune responses are "type 2" responses. They are induced by $CD4^+$ T cells capable of producing IL-4 and IL-13. These two cytokines suppress multiple pro-inflammatory effector roles by macrophages, such as production of TNFα. Th2 cells are first known by their capacity to switch the immunoglobulin isotype of human B cells towards IgE and probably also IgG4 [91]. Thus, Th2 cells do not extinct immune responses. They may even induce autoimmune responses and probably also autoimmune disease, such as pemphigus, which is associated with autoantibodies of the IgG4 isotype and little local inflammation [92-3]. However, when directed against epitopes that are associated with type 1-mediated inflammatory autoimmune disease, type 2 immune responses may exert anti-inflammatory, protective effects. Treating Th1 mediated diseases with Th2 cells or the cytokine IL-4 that most potently induces Th2 and suppresses Th1 has been showed in animal models of organ specific autoimmune disease and skin inflammation [83, 89, 94]. Most importantly, however, this therapeutic strategy was also effective in humans suffering from psoriasis, a Th1 mediated auto inflammatory syndrome of the skin [95].

Th17 cell, a newly subset of Th cells and associated immune mechanisms, is defined by main production of IL-17. Following the description of Th17 cells, it was found that some of the autoimmune diseases that were believed to be type 1-mediated, in fact, are at least in part driven by Th17 cells (i.e., multiple sclerosis, and the experimental allergic encephalitis) [96]. Th17 mediated immune responses are often associated with infiltrates of polymorphonuclear leukocytes. Today Th17 cells are believed to mediate many of the hallmarks of several diseases like psoriasis and pemphigus [97].

Another dimension of immune control is the different types of regulatory T-cells (Treg cells) that mediate immune tolerance and thus are counter regulators of autoimmunity. Cell mediated as well as cytokine mediated control of immune-responses by Treg cells have been described. In contrast to all other phenotypes, these Treg cells seem to have the capacity of turning immune responses off. This regulatory effect may be important in treating autoimmune diseases, since Treg are capable of silencing several types of immune responses including Th1, Th17, and Th2 dominated immune responses [98-99]. Referring to the historic attribution given to $CD8^+$ T-cells, suppressor T-cells experience a time of renaissance. These $CD4^+$ T-cells are capable to suppress auto aggressive immune reactions and were found to express CD25, GITR, CTLA-4, and most importantly a specific transcription factor, fork head box p3 (Foxp3) [100]. Foxp3 is not only a marker for these Treg, it is of functional importance for the suppressive mode of action of Treg [101-2]. As a result, patients deficient in the Foxp3 transcription factor develop a multiorgan autoimmune disease [103]. Treg cells are difficult to induce and grow to expand *in vitro* and probably also *in vivo*, but finding Foxp3 and increasingly clarifying the underlying mechanisms of Treg development will help to answer the questions about the significance these cells may play in the therapy of autoimmune disease.

Central immune tolerance is orchestrated by the culling of auto reactive T-cell precursors during differentiation in the thymus. Stochastic somatic rearrangement of T-cell receptor genes in developing immature thymocytes results in a staggering diversity of potential T-cell antigen specificities, many of which have potential to react against self-MHC or important structural, developmental, and functional proteins (e.g., insulin or collagen). To prevent these auto reactive cells from developing to maturity and causing damage, immature thymocytes traffic through the thymus medulla where they meet self-antigen and other cross-presented antigens of self-MHC. Those cells and their T-cell receptors bind avidly to self-antigen and MHC and transmit a strong signal through their T-cell receptor then undergo apoptosis, leading to deletion of potentially auto reactive T-cells. This process, known as clonal deletion, is also complemented by other mechanisms of removing auto reactive clones, including clonal diversion, T-cell receptor editing, and induction of anergy [104]. These first-line mechanisms to prevent anti-self immune reactions and autoimmune disease are important but not perfect, and auto reactive T-cells can and do escape the thymus, as is evident in autoimmune diseases that are driven by these cells. That periodic escape of auto reactive clones from thymus negative selection is likely the rule rather than the exception, even without clinical autoimmune disease. This is proved by experiments in which tissue-specific transgenic expression of co-stimulatory molecules and cytokines can result in antigen-specific immune attack of those tissues, meaning that mature lymphocytes escape clonal deletion and are capable of mediating reactions against self-antigen [105]. To deal with these rogue cells, a secondary line of defense exists in the form of active peripheral tolerance that is enforced by populations of regulatory cells with the ability to suppress potentially harmful autoimmune responses. The most extensively studied, and best understood, of these is the $CD4^+$ $CD25^+$ $FoxP3^+$ Treg. Tregs play an important role in immunity both preventing autoimmunity by inhibiting anti-self responses and also acting to suppress defensive immune responses at a proper stage to prevent host tissue damage. It is important to consider the role of Tregs in setting up and upholding peripheral tolerance to understand their participation in the immune process. The early discovery of Tregs came from experiments in which specific populations of $CD4^+$ cells that also highly express the high affinity IL-2 receptor α-chain, CD25, were found to be protective in mouse models of autoimmunity [106-9]. It was later shown the transcription factor FoxP3 was not only a specific marker for $CD4^+$ $CD25^+$ Tregs, but was also important for their development, maintenance of phenotype, and function [110-5].

The mechanisms by which Tregs function to suppress immune responses have been intensively studied, and there seem to be diverse Treg responses that come into play depending on the context of activation and the environment in which they are managing [116-7]. Specifically, the mechanisms of Treg-mediated suppression seem to be determined at least in part by whether they are preserving immune quiescence to prevent immune activation in the physiological homeostatic steady state or are responding to dampen an active inflammatory response [118]. The mechanisms used by Tregs to suppress immune responses include: transmission of inhibitory signals by cell-cell surface interactions or secreted cytokines, decreasing conventional T cell activation or fitness by limiting growth factors like IL-2 or essential amino acids, direct target-cell cytotoxicity, and/or modulation of antigen presenting cell function [116-8]. Like other αβT-cell receptor-utilizing T cells, Tregs have a diverse T-cell receptor repertoire and can respond to a wide range of antigens. It is though they do not seem to have an absolute requirement for recognition of specific self-antigens to mediate suppression, clonal Treg pools responding against a specific antigen recognized by their T-cell receptors seem to be more effective suppressors than polyclonal populations mediating nonspecific suppression [119-22].

Tregs play an important role in preserving peripheral tolerance and immune homeostasis. Inadequate or dysfunctional Treg responses are thought to contribute to the pathogenesis of several diseases resulting from broken self-tolerance, including the pemphigus group. Not only are Tregs a dominant mediator of peripheral self-tolerance, they also appear to be important in modulating the innate and acquired immune responses to foreign antigen [123-6]. Most circulating Tregs distinguish from T-cell forerunners in the thymus, and are then phenotypically and functionally distinct compared with conventional $FoxP3^-$ $CD4^+$ T-cells [127]. These "thymic" or "natural" Tregs play an important role in maintenance of tolerance to self-antigen, and to other antigens presented in the thymus. Tregs can also, however, be generated under specific circumstances from FoxP3−$CD4^+$ conventional T cells after thymic egress [128-31]. These cells have been called "peripheral" or "induced" Treg (iTreg), and may play a role more in the tempering of responses to antigens not encountered in the thymus, including pathogen-related antigens. Differentiation or change-over of conventional Tregs into iTregs is dependent on several factors, including the strength of antigen signal, specific signals from antigen presenting cells, and the nature of the local cytokine milieu. In particular, activation of T cells under the influence of transforming growth factor-β (TGF-β) and IL-2 can induce naïve $CD4^+$ T cells to induce FoxP3 expression and adopt a regulatory phenotype [132-3].

Occasionally, broken or incomplete tolerance (for example autoimmune diseases) represents the failure of a tolerogenic fetal T-cell population. Though these considerations remain theoretical, advancing investigations will lead to further insights into the process of normal human fetal immune development and its influence of on how our immune systems learn to interact with us, and the environment in which we exist.

2.6. Dendritic Cells and T Cells: Moderators of Autoimmunity

All organs are drained by dendritic cells. These cells are normally considered as potent stimulators of T-cells that prime at first for IFN-γ Producing $CD4^+$ and $CD8^+$ T-cells [134-6]. They are indispensable in regulating the delicate balance between immunity and tolerance [137]. By interacting with other cells of the immune system through cell-cell contact or the production of cytokines, dendritic cells induce a right answer to a specific antigen. Dendritic cells can also prevent (auto) immunity by inducing apoptosis of autoreactive T-cells in the thymus on the one hand (that is, central tolerance), and by induction of anergy, deletion, or tolerance through cooperation with regulatory T-cells (Treg) in the periphery on the other hand (that is, peripheral tolerance). Thus, it has been hypothesized that defects in the number, phenotype, and/or function of dendritic cells cause the development of autoimmune diseases. Further, dendritic cell-based antigen-specific modulation of the unwanted responses is evaluated for therapeutic approaches in recent years and may have several advantages in contrast to standard treatments which can induce various complications and have serious side effects. Indeed, considering the key role of dendritic cells in inducting and activating both effector T-cells and Treg, dendritic cells can be used to suppress or redirect immune responses in an antigen-specific manner [137].

Dendritic cell acquire this capacity following antigen uptake while they migrate to the draining lymph nodes. This capacity in activating and stimulating T cells to become efficient effector cells, capable of mediating inflammatory immune responses and of inducing immunoglobulin production by B cells, requires a certain activation status by these antigen presenting cells [135].

Thus these cells co-express adhesion molecules that allow adherence of naive and activated T-cells. They express a panel of co-stimulatory molecules that are required for the activation of specifically binding T cells and, in addition, they produce cytokines. Both, the sum of cell bound signals and of antigen presenting cell-derived cytokines results not only in the stimulation and maturation of the specific T-cells but also settles their differentiation. Thus, the maturation process that dendritic cell undergo during their migration from the periphery to the draining lymph node will eventually settle, whether the primary activation of T-cells may lead Th1, Th2, Th17, Th22 or inducible Treg cells [138-41].

When residing in peripheral organs, dendritic cells are continuously processing many antigens delivered by the local milieu. At this stage, dendritic cells have little migratory and antigen presenting capacity. Few immature and quiescent dendritic cell that migrate from peripheral organs to the draining lymph node are not capable of activating T-cells to become auto aggressive. They seem either to contribute to the phenomenon of "ignorance" or to promote the differentiation of naive but potentially auto reactive T-cells towards an immunosuppressive Treg phenotype [62, 142]. In contrast, dendritic cells start to mature and to leave their residing site after a correct stimulus, such as the pathogen associated molecular pattern derived from infectious agents (bacterial DNA), bind to Toll-like receptors that are increasingly recognized as most relevant activators of dendritic cells. Obviously, this is driven by more than just one pathogen-associated molecular pattern, however the impact of combinative innate immune sensing is not already known [143]. These innate signals transform antigen presenting cell not only from a cell capable of attracting naive and memory T cells into lymph nodes, but to determine the differentiation of antigen presenting cell towards different dendritic cell phenotypes that are capable to coordinate Th1, Th2, Th17, Th22 or Treg cells. Therefore, dendritic cells and their capacity to direct the functional phenotype of the future immune response, directed against either self-or foreign antigens, is one central element of immune control [134, 138-9]. These regulatory mechanisms underlying dendritic cell-induced immune responses, present during the early activation of dendritic cell, order dendritic cell to produce IL-12 and pathogen-associated molecular patterns tend to promote Th1 development leading to a proper anti-infectious immunity. However, some pathogen-associated molecular patterns and other signals lead to an inappropriate Th2 immunity in response to microbes. These Th2 reactions can be switched to effective Th1 reactions, a mechanism that may also regulate autoimmunity. Paradoxically, IL-4 is a potent factor driving this switch, because IL-4 orders activated dendritic cells to produce IL-12 and promotes Th1 cell development [94]. Immune responses in general develop by the successive activation of dendritic cells and then T cells. Thus, the contrasting effects of IL-4 on immune responses with the opposing functional phenotypes are a result from IL-4 signaling in early dendritic cells activation leading to a Th1 phenotype and on IL-4 induced T cell differentiation inducing Th2 cells during a later stage. So far, how Th17 cells and Th2 cells are regulated and influence each other is not exactly known, however, it seems as if Th2 cytokines modulate dendritic cell in a way that these dendritic cells cannot support Th17 differentiation and maintenance [144]. Besides Toll-like receptors signaling, there is a multitude of other recognition pathways that include the lectins and other cytosolic pathogen recognition receptors such as the retinoic acid – inducible gene I (RIG-I), (like receptors (RLRs) and the nucleotide-binding domain and leucine-rich repeat) containing receptors (NLRs) [143, 145]. Other levels of innate recognition and control of inflammation include the inflammasome providing rapid IL-1 levels [146] and recognition of apoptotic cell material [147]. In this context, it is interesting that complex cellular communication pathways support recognition and inflammation. Thus, activated NK cells can also prime dendritic cell to produce IL-12 and to induce CD8 T cell memory responses, a mechanism that may be also underlying an activation of autoreactive lymphocytes [148]. Activation of self-reactive T and B cells autoimmune diseases require the presence of autoreactive T cells and, in the case of immunoglobulin-mediated diseases, of autoreactive B cells. In view of the potent and large number of regulatory mechanisms that protect against autoimmune disease, activation of autoreactive T and B cells is thought to require a series of destabilizing events. One important aspect is the activation and reactivation of potentially auto reactive T-cells [149]. However, induction of autoreactive T cells or B cells alone does not induce or predispose for autoimmune diseases, as occurs in individuals, genetically predisposed of developing autoimmune diabetes, in those patients, the relative risk of becoming diabetes increases significantly if their T cells respond vigorously against endogenous antigens from pancreatic islet cells. In contrast, individuals from the same population are largely protected against autoimmune diabetes, when they exert high immunoglobulin titers but weak T cell responses against the same antigens [150]. This further underlines that "reactivity" does not equal autoimmune disease. One of the fundamental questions that are still unanswered yields with the primary event leading to the induction of autoreactivity. Some data suggest that, in the presence of a proper genetic background, minimal events such as normal tissue necrosis may be sufficient for inducting, perhaps even potentially harmful, autoreactivity [151-2]. Most data suggest that a series of tolerance inducing mechanisms normally inhibits T and B cells to react against many autoantigens [153]. Therefore, stimuli that induce reactivity against these auto antigens have to overcome the diverse tolerance-inducing barriers. Epidemiologic data suggest that the realization of autoimmune diseases is often preceded by infectious diseases and attention was given to the events by which infections may abolish the status of tolerance [154-5]. At least three mechanisms are thought to contribute to this phenomenon: (1) reactivation of tolerant T and B cells, (2) induction of autoreactive T cells by molecular mimicry and (3) variation of the cytokine pattern during the course of infectious diseases.

2.7. T and B Cell Tolerance Disrupted: Let the Game Begins

Experiments with transgenic or non-transgenic mice animals have shown that, in principle, tolerant T and B cells can be reactivated by infectious agents. Infections are capable of restoring in silenced T cells the capacity to produce cytokines [89, 149]. Similarly, reactivity and immunoglobulin production by B cells that were silenced either by exogenous or transgenic endogenous antigens can be restored with mitogens, including bacteria derived lipopolisacchrides [156-7]. Even though these experiments have shown that infectious agents can abolish solid T and B cell tolerance, there are little data showing that this reactivation of tolerant T and B cells can also lead to autoimmune disease. One first example suggesting such a situation is given by double transgenic mice that bear a T-cell receptor recognizing a transgenic self-antigen expressed by hepatocytes. Injection of bacterial DNA motifs that activate dendritic cell and promote dendritic cell-development also induced transient liver damage, as evidenced by an increase of transaminases. However, this phenomenon was short-lived and no data are available proving that autoimmune disease can be the direct consequence of polyclonal T-cell activation [158].

Therefore, these data suggest that immunizations against antigens that are structurally related to self-antigens are essential for the induction of autoimmunity. This aspect is especially significant since molecular mimicry does not require molecular identity [159, 160]. Various examples suggest that this may be of relevance for autoimmune diseases of the skin. Thus, the first eruption of the juvenile psoriasis is preceded by streptococcal infections in most patients [161] and lichen planus is associated in a large number of patients with an acute or chronic liver disease [162]. In some patients lichen planus may even be provoked by active or even passive vaccination against hepatitis [163-4]. Despite the experimental prove for both, reactivation of tolerant T-cells and for molecular mimicry, the exact role of infections in the pathogenesis of autoimmune diseases is unknown. One important alternative would be the direct infection and molecular change through infectious disease [165-7]. In the skin a very similar phenomenon is visible during fungal infections. The border, the clinically manifest eczema, reflects the immune reaction against a large load of fungi. Inside the inflammatory margin, the eczema and the fungal load are significantly milder. In fast growing fungi, the eczema may present as a polycyclic disease. A third level where infections could directly interfere with auto reactive T-cells is the pattern of cytokines that T-cells produce. Thus, infection with the nematode *Nippostrongylus brasiliensis* cannot only restore reactivity in silenced $CD4^+$ T-cells but also induce IL-4 production by these silenced T-cells [168].

2.8. B Cells and Immunoglobulins: The Aggressive Expansion. Act I

Developing B cells that express immunoglobulin receptors with high affinity for self-components also undergo negative selection, and are removed in the bone marrow through one of two central tolerance mechanisms: (1) deletion or (2) receptor editing [169]. Receptor editing is a central tolerance mechanism by which the genes encoding the immunoglobulin receptors on developing high affinity self-reactive B cells undergo recombination, such the newly edited receptors lack high affinity reactivity for self-components. However, B cells expressing immunoglobulin receptors with low affinity for self-components can escape deletion and receptor editing, and enter the peripheral circulation and lymphoid organs. An increased part of auto reactive B cells has been reported in type 1 diabetes and other autoimmune conditions, as well as in healthy individuals who have the *PTPN22* autoimmune susceptibility gene [170]. Auto reactive B cells gather without Tregs in the IPEX autoimmunity syndrome [171], suggesting that tolerance in the T and B cell compartments is interrelated.

B cells with low affinity receptors for self-components undergo B cell anergy, resulting in down-regulation of surface IgM [172]. Anergic B cells display a high degree of auto reactivity, account for many mature naïve B cells and seem to be abnormally activated in systemic lupus erythematosus [173]. B cell anergy is thought to result from chronic antigen-receptor occupancy [174], which could occur in the presence of self-components that bind low affinity B cell antigen receptors. Defective control of B cell receptor signaling has been implicated as a mechanism by which B cell anergy fails in autoimmunity [175]. The B cell activating factor (BAFF; also known as B lymphocyte stimulator or BLyS), family of cytokines contributes to B cell tolerance by regulating B cell development, selection and homeostasis [176]. Immature B cells can be more or less reliant for survival on BAFF, depending on the antigen-binding strength of their immunoglobulin receptor. By this mechanism, B cells expressing low affinity receptors for self-components can be inappropriately preserved by the excess levels of BAFF present in autoimmune conditions such as systemic lupus erythematosus [171]. BAFF could also influence homeostasis and tolerance in mature B cells, which can up regulate BAFF receptors in response to stimulation by Toll-like receptors [177]. Toll-like receptors and B cell immunoglobulin antigen receptors control activation of B cells through integrated signaling pathways, and Toll-like receptors have been linked to autoimmunity [178]. It has been suggested that B cell activation by the

Toll-like receptors pathway could allow preexisting low affinity autoreactive B cells to become effectors, and BAFF might be involved in this process [176]. Probably the best example for an immunoglobulin-mediated disease is pemphigus vugaris. It is associated with little inflammation and seems to be directly mediated by binding auto reactive immunoglobulins to the desmogleins that guarantee the adhesion between keratinocytes [179]. Indeed, transfer of patient sera and monoclonal antibodies directed against desmoglein 3 into the skin of newborn mice can directly induce acantholysis [180]. This critical role for a direct binding of immunoglobulins to desmoglein structures is further supported by the observation that in patients with pemphigus vugaris the disease activity correlates closely with the serum levels of the autoantibodies [181]. Such a close association is unusual for other autoimmune diseases, including lupus erythematosus or bullous pemphigoid. For comparisons, bullous pemphigoid is of special interest. It is also an immunoglobulin mediated bullous skin disease. In sharp contrast to pemphigus vulgaris, the clinical manifestation of bullous pemphigoid does not only require deposition of autoantigens but also an inflammatory milieu that causes detachment of the basement membrane [182-3]. Thus, transfer of specific sera or immunoglobulins under the skin of newborn nude mice alone is not plenty for inducting blisters. It requires, in addition, activation of the complement cascade and inflammation, involving the recruitment of granulocytes [184].

2.9. Tissue Damage, Th1 and Th17 Cells: The Aggressive Expansion. Act II

Th1 and Th17 cells seem to be associated with two distinct types of tissue damage. One type of tissue damage is rather characterized by a sterile inflammation (Th1), the other with the strong collection of polymorphonuclear granulocytes (Th17). Sterile Th1/Tc1 responses are found in lichen planus, most patients with multiple sclerosis or autoimmune diabetes. They are associated with activated macrophages, which seem to be the effector cells of these immune responses. Like macrophages that are stimulated *in vitro* in the presence of IFN-γ, they produce large amounts of TNFα, oxygen radicals, NO and other mediators of inflammation [185]. Activated $CD8^+$ T cells (Tc1) with potent killer functions seem also to be involved [186]. In concert, these mediators can cause severe tissue destruction that ultimately results in compensatory scar formation. Because of the capacity of the skin to regenerate even severe tissue damage, lichen planus heals under most conditions without scaring. However, persistent alopecia, onychodystrophy or even scars of the normal skin are potential complications. Under other conditions, Th17 cells dominate autoimmune diseases, which are associated with a strong infiltrate of polymorphonuclear lymphocytes. Such a constellation characterizes psoriasis, rheumatoid arthritis and most types of inflammatory bowel disease, especially Crohn's disease [141]. In addition, targeting the p40 subunit of both IL-12 and IL-23 also demonstrated to be an effective therapy for psoriasis pointing out that induction of Th1 cells (IL-12) or induction and maintenance of Th17 cells (IL-23) together with some inherent effector roles of these two cytokines are important for the immune pathogenesis of psoriasis [187]. In this context, IL-17 and IL-17-induced cytokines regulate PMN infiltration and in addition, mast cells triggered by Th cells lead to strong PMN recruitment through their mediators: TNFα, which induces the expression of intravascular adhesion molecules [188-9], and the IL-8, which is the most important chemokine attracting PMN [188]. The communication pathways between Th1 and Th17 cells and mast cells still need to be characterized in further studies [190].

2.10. Th2 T Cells and T-B Cell Interactions: The Aggressive Expansion. Act III

Many autoimmune diseases are mediated by immunoglobulins. These humoral diseases can be divided into two major categories: (1) Immunoglobulins can induce damage through direct binding of their target-antigen. This is the situation in most of the bullous autoimmune diseases of the skin, especially pemphigus vulgaris. Alternatively (2) immunoglobulins bind to circulating antigens and cause damage through deposition along basement membranes or in vessels. The former situation is given in lupus erythematosus [63], the latter at sites of vasculitis. As the pattern of immune responses initiated by immunoglobulins strictly depends on the immunoglobulin isotype, the diseases caused by immunoglobulins depend not only on the antigen they recognize. The clinical spectrum of diseases initiated by autoantibodies ranges from urticaria, through cytopathic tissue damage leading to cytopenia, inflammatory tissue destruction following the deposition of immunoglobulins and complexes at membranes that lead to severe necrosis, because of acute vascular infarction. Here again, T cells play a central regulatory role. Under most conditions, B cells start only to produce autoantibodies, when stimulated by antigen-specific T cells. During this stimulation, T cells release a distinct pattern of cytokines controlling the immunoglobulin switch in the responding B cells. Cytokines of the Th2-family, IL-4 and IL-13 induce the isotype switch towards IgE and isotypes that do not have the ability to bind complement, IgG1 in mice and in humans probably IgG4. Th1 cells that are thought to organize the defense against intracellular pathogens and viruses induce preferentially complement-binding isotypes. We can observe this interaction and response in pemphigus vulgaris, where patients have frequently IgG4 antibodies against desmoglein 3 and strongest Th2 responses against this same autoantigen.

2.11. The Autoimmune Disease: The Conclusion

The mechanisms that lead from autoimmunity to an inflammatory disease or conversely are still unclear. Production and release of TNFα seems to be important for this step, since its blockade is one of the most effective therapeutic alternative to control autoimmunity, nevertheless the exact role of this cytokine is far from being elucidated [191]. Auto reactive T-cells are not only associated with autoimmune diseases but can directly cause the disease. Analysis from mice with non-obese diabetes revealed that both, $CD4^+$ and $CD8^+$ T-cells are required for inducting both, chronic inflammation (like psoriasis) and autoimmune disease (like pemphigus) [192].

A comparison of various models for organ-specific, inflammatory autoimmune disease revealed that organ specific inflammatory autoimmune diseases are primarily induced by T cells of the proinflammatory Th1 and Th17 phenotype. It is assumed that both, $CD4^+$ and $CD8^+$ T cells and also Th1 and Th17 cells are involved under most conditions, but the exact role of $CD8^+$ T cells is not clear. The best studied example investigating the exact role of Th1 and Th17 cells in autoimmunity is a model for multiple sclerosis, the experimental allergic encephalitis: In this model both Th1 and Th17 cells are capable to mediate autoimmune disease although with different strength and different pathology [96]. These investigations and the functional characterization were performed in the past for Th1 cells for models of autoimmune diseases in small animals and for the analysis of autoimmune responses in humans with organ-specific autoimmune disease such as autoimmune diabetes [87], multiple sclerosis [193, 194] or psoriasis [195, 196]. Analysis in regard to Th17 pathology are as performed for experimental allergic encephalitis [96], still ongoing, but immune responses associated with infiltrates of polymorphonuclear leukocytes such as psoriasis seem to be mediated by Th17 [22].

2.12. Achieving Induction of Functional Tolerance: The Solution

The therapeutic strategies available reflect a combination of corticosteroids and immunosuppressive agents, most of them acting on both T and B cells. Corticosteroids are used with the primary goal to reduce the acute inflammation and to limit tissue damage. They are also efficient therapies to suppress T and B cell responses, although not selectively, but long-term side effects are important, and even increase the mortality rate. Therefore, therapies normally combine corticosteroids with immunosuppressive agents to reduce immune responses to a level that optimally inhibits harmful immune reactions but still allows normal defense against infectious agents. Such therapies settle a helpful and fragile balance in most of the autoimmune diseases. Especially the late result is still poorly controlled and acute relapses and chronic infections may lead to new complications such as atherosclerosis, mainly on immunosuppressed subjects.

These novel strategies are based on the next three principles: (1) efficient blockade of the effector roles of immune responses; (2) absorbing harmful immunoglobulin fractions; or (3) correction of aberrant T-cell responses. The greatest achievement is currently obtained by blocking immune functions with anti-TNF-antibodies. This seems to be more efficient and better tolerated than any of the previously described immunosuppressive agents [197]. However, therapies based on anti-TNF-antibodies inhibit any immune response and therefore harbor a series of risks for patients with acute or chronic infections (viral infections, tuberculosis). Among autoimmune skin diseases, psoriasis has been shown to improve under anti-TNF-therapies [198]. This is an important fact and we know today that this therapeutic approach can be worthwhile for our patients with psoriasis, psoriatic arthritis, and acrodermatitis continua of Hallopeau. In addition, neutralizing TNFα may be a promising approach for acute diseases associated with inflammatory tissue destruction such as aphtous ulcers or pyoderma gangrenosum. In addition, antibodies to the p40 subunit of both IL-12 and IL-23 are now available (ustekinumab) and were successfully used in psoriasis [187] possibly targeting Th1 and Th17 mediated autoimmune disease; this therapy seems to be unsuccessful in pemphigus vulgaris, as we previously tested [199]. However, we have to keep in mind that other highly effective, less invasive (or aggressive), and less expensive therapies are available. Absorbency of harmful immunoglobulins is a logical approach that was developed from plasmapheresis. One problem is that it acts rather late in the immune response and B cells continue to produce pathogenic immunoglobulins, and thus is a temporary treatment. These therapies against T cell activation may affect either antigen presenting cells, co-stimulation or the T cells directly. Today, strategies modulating the co-stimulation of T cells mediated through CD28/CTLA4 or LFA-2/LFA-3 seem to be an approach to alter autoreactive T cell responses [200-1]. Another possibility would be to correct harmful cytokine production by specific T cells.

Three mechanisms are mentioned as novel therapy approaches: (1) induction of regulatory T-cells or called Treg, capable of inhibiting immune responses in an antigen-specific fashion; (2) deviation of harmful Th1 or Th17 responses into a protective Th2 or Treg responses; and (3) to perpetuate and to settle an anti-inflammatory Th2-memory, once they are initiated [202]. Indeed, a first study performed with psoriasis patients showed that IL-4 therapy is a highly effective treatment strategy for autoimmune diseases [95]. The third reflects the opposite, the redirection of harmful Th2 responses into a Th1-phenotype or Th17 phenotype, an approach that may be of interest in IgE-mediated diseases.

These antigen-specific T-cell based approaches are at an early clinical experimental phase and not suitable for acute interventions, nevertheless, the first studies showed that it is a promising approach [95]. For future development, these vaccination approaches are of special interest as they evade a series of major problems associated with all other therapies; two important aspects are: (1) these therapies are specific for the targeted antigen structure and should therefore not interfere with the other physiologically required immune responses [83]. The other is that they (2) target the site where T cell responses are translated from the innate to the adaptive immune response and therefore, they should provide long-lasting protection.

PART 2. ETHIOPATHOGENESIS OF PEMPHIGUS

Chapter 3

DESMOSOME PROTEIN TARGETS IN PEMPHIGUS

There are several types of pemphigus, each with unique clinical, histological, and immunological hallmarks. When different desmosome proteins are the target of the autoimmune response, different clinical and histological features are often seen.

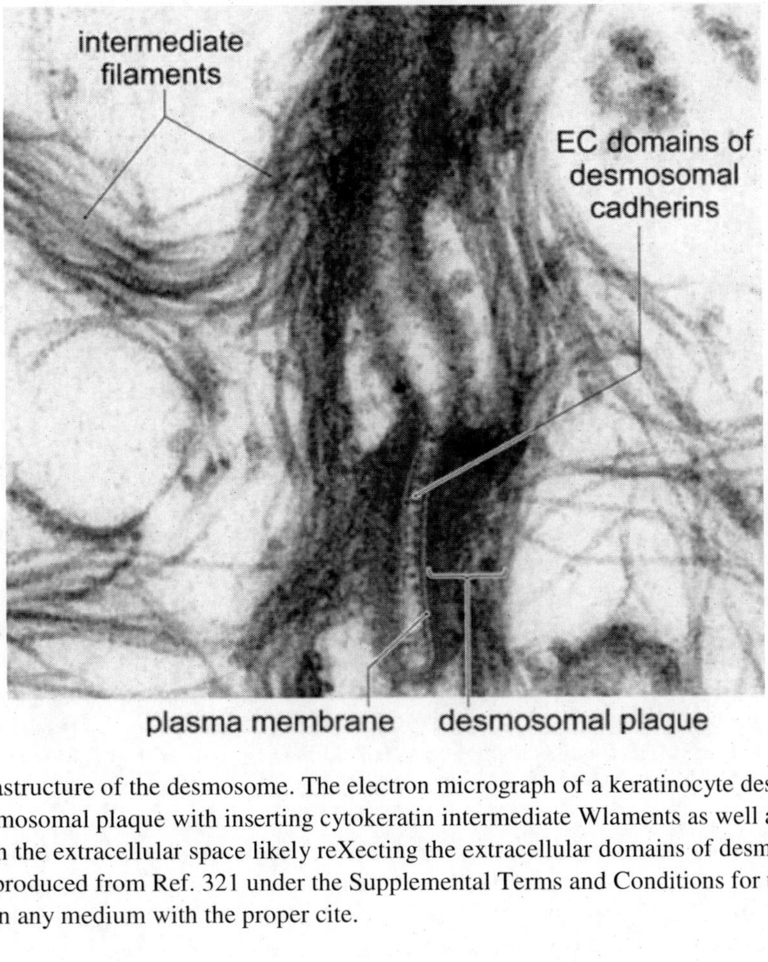

Figure 2. Ultrastructure of the desmosome. The electron micrograph of a keratinocyte desmosome shows the desmosomal plaque with inserting cytokeratin intermediate Wlaments as well as some fuzzy material within the extracellular space likely reXecting the extracellular domains of desmosomal cadherins. Reproduced from Ref. 321 under the Supplemental Terms and Conditions for unrestricted reproduction in any medium with the proper cite.

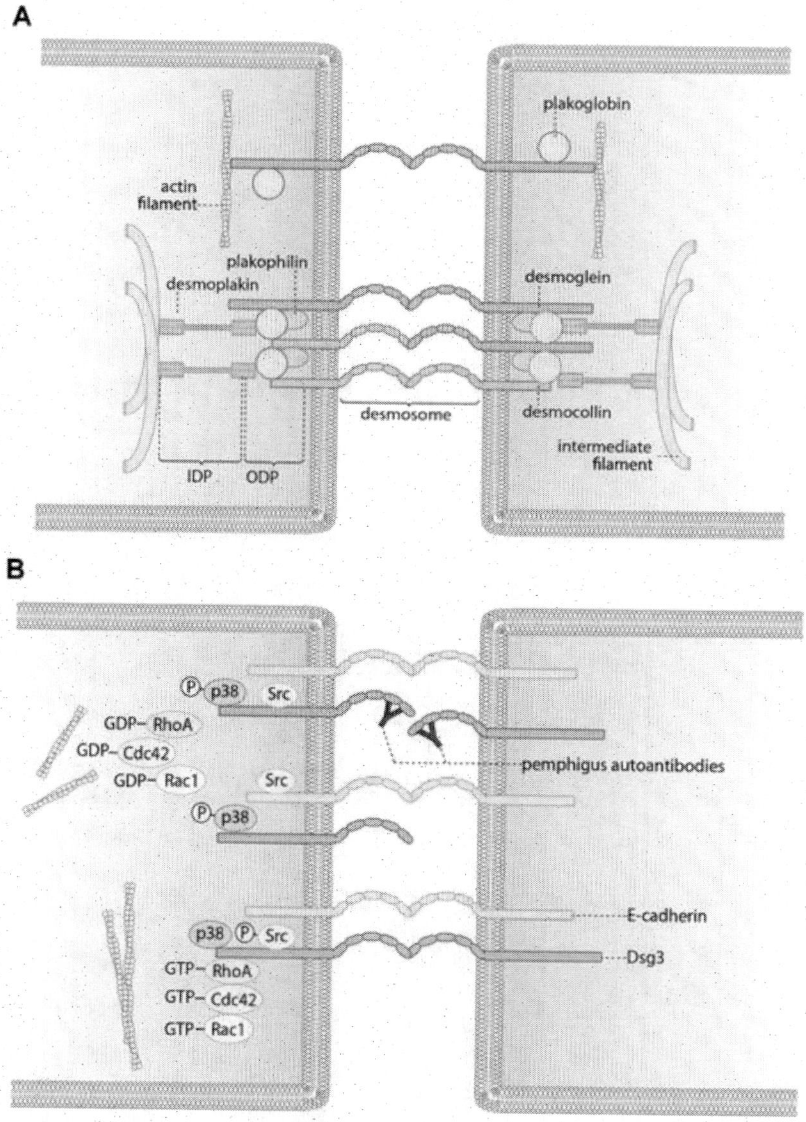

Figure 3. Molecular model of the desmosome and extradesmosomal adhesive signaling complexes. (A) The desmosomal cadherins desmoglein (violet) and desmocollin (pink) undergo homophilic and heterophilic binding of partner molecules on the same (*cis*) as well as on the neighboring cell (*trans*). The cytoplasmic domains are largely embedded in the outer dense plaque (ODP) where they are associated with plakoglobin (yellow) and plakophilin (orange). In the inner dense plaque (IDP), desmoplakin (green) links these adaptor molecules to the intermediate filament cytoskeleton (blue). Outside of desmosomes, desmosomal cadherin molecules exist that can bind actin filaments. (B) Extradesmosomal Dsg3 (violet) builds a signaling scaffold in a complex with E-cadherin (green) and Pg (yellow) and is coupled to actin filaments. The signaling molecules p38MAPK and Src both localize to that complex. In contrast to Src, which is phosphorylated in an adhesion-dependent manner, p38MAPK is phosphorylated when the interaction of Dsg3 is perturbed, that is, following pemphigus autoantibody binding. Enhanced expression of Dsg3 leads to activation of Rho-GTPases, their translocation to EDASCs, and reorganization of the cortical actin belt. Reproduced with permission of John Wiley and Sons from Waschke J, Spindler V. Desmosomes and extradesmosomes adhesive signaling contacts in pemphigus. Med Res Rev 2014; 34(6): 1127-45.

There are two major intercellular junctions that mediate cell-cell adhesion in the epidermis: (1) desmosomes and (2) adherens junctions. (Figure 2) Keratinocytes express trans membrane glycoproteins called desmogleins and desmocollins that form desmosomes, whereas E-cadherin forms adherens junctions. (Figure 3) Antibodies that mediate the disease are the IgG isotype and are directed against the ectodomain of desmosomal cadherins. Binding of these autoantibodies causes loss of epithelial cell-cell adhesion throught a process called "acantholysis," leading to blister formation within the epidermis [203].

Pemphigus autoantibodies are pathogenic when passively transferred into neonatal Balb/c mice, producing blisters at the injection site, thus resembling or simulating the "natural" human disease. Since several decades ago, the immunological targets for pemphigus autoantibodies have been characterized by immunoprecipitation and immunoblotting. With cloning techniques and cDNA libraries, isolating cDNA for pemphigus antigens showed that desmogleins are indeed the most important target antigens in the pemphigus group. Although current research is enlightening potential key steps in the pathogenesis of the disease, the causes and mechanisms that launch the disease are still controversial. ¿How the blister develops in pemphigus?; Several investigators have proposed different mechanisms to explain the induction of keratinocyte detachment on binding of pemphigus IgG autoantibodies. There are two major theories on how pemphigus autoantibodies cause blistering: (1) binding of pemphigus IgG directly interferes with desmosomal adhesion (steric hindrance); and (2) pemphigus IgG induces intracellular signaling that leads to loss of keratinocyte adhesion. Increasing evidence supports both theories as contributors to pemphigus pathogenesis [204]. Also, blocking of the autoantibody-induced direct interference of desmosomal adhesion and restraint of autoantibody-induced intracellular signaling reduce epidermal blistering *in vitro* and *in vivo*. Therefore, neither theory alone is enough to explain the disruption of keratinocyte adhesion induced by pemphigus autoantibodies, being the most accepted theory related to a multiple-hit hypothesis [49].

3.1. Intercellular Junctions and Adhesion Mediators

Intercellular junctions in the epidermis allow keratinocytes to adhere to one another and keep the integrity of the epithelium. As previously mention, morphological and biochemical studies have defined two major types of intercellular junctions in epithelial cells:(1) adherens junctions and (2) desmosomes [203-4]. These intercellular junctions are composed of a superfamily of calcium-dependent adherent proteins, called cadherins, which play an important role in regulating intercellular adhesion [205]. The cadherin superfamily is characterized by multiple "cadherin repeat" sequences of about 110 amino acids in their extracellular domains and are comprised of two major groups: *classical* (E-, P-, N-cadherin) and *desmosomal cadherins* (desmogleins and desmocollins). *Classical cadherins* are expressed in the adherens junctions and share high structural and sequence homology with the extracellular domains of *desmosomal cadherins* that are expressed in the desmosomes. All cadherins are type 1 transmembrane glycoproteins presenting five tandem cadherin repeats (EC1–EC5) of about 110 amino acids containing calcium-binding sites and a cell-adhesion recognition site in their extracellular domains [206-8].

The cell-adhesion recognition site is a tripeptide motif within the EC1 (the most amino-terminal repeat). In *classical cadherins,* this motif is HAV (histidine, alanine, valine), whereas in *desmosomal cadherins* the motif may be RAL (arginine, alanine, leucine), YAT (tyrosine, alanine, threonine), FAT (phenylalanine, alanine, threonine), or YAS (tyrosine, alanine, serine) [209]. *Classical cadherins* are ultimately linked to the actin cytoskeleton via α-and β-catenin [210-1], and *desmosomal cadherins* are linked to the intermediate keratin filaments through plakoglobin, plakophilin I, and desmoplakins I and II [212-3]. E-cadherin and P-cadherin are classical cadherins expressed in the epidermis. The first one is expressed in all layers of the epidermis, whereas the second one is limited to the basal cell layer [214].

3.2. The Desmosome: Structure and Function

Giulio Bizzozero (1864) made the first observation of the *desmosome*. He observed them as small dense nodules and called them "nodes of Bizzozero." The term *desmosome* emerged later with Joseph Shaffer in 1920, from the Greek words "desmo" (bond) and"soma" (body) [215]. Since then, using techniques such as electron microscopy, it has been possible to reveal its complex structure and organization.

Desmosomes are the most important intercellular adhering junctions in keratinocytes that provide strength for the epidermis. These junctions are connected directly with desmosomal cadherin proteins on the cell surface and anchor keratin intermediate filaments to their inner cytoplasmic surface to generate an intracellular keratin intermediate filaments-skeletal scaffold through several associate proteins [215].

The desmosome consists of two morphologically well-defined zones: (1) the extracellular core region (desmosomal core) and (2) the intracellular dense plaque region (desmosomal plaque) (Figure 2) [215]. With techniques such as genetic cloning and immunohistochemistry, the parts of the desmosome have been cloned, their organization within the organelle has been mapped, and their ability to interact with one another has been defined [216].

Despite these critical roles in upholding epidermal adhesion and integrity, desmosomes are not static. Rather, they are dynamic units that undergo regular remodeling. Two cell-cell adhesion states, stable hyperadhesion (Ca^{2+}-independent) and weak adhesion (Ca^{2+}-dependent) conditions, which are mutually reversible, are recognized. In pemphigus vulgaris, an autoimmune bullous disease caused by anti-desmoglein 3 antibodies, binding of these antibodies to desmoglein 3 causes the specific depletion of desmoglein 3 from desmosomes, linked to acantholysis in the epidermis [216-7].

There are three major units in the desmosome: (1) *desmosomal cadherins* (desmogleins and desmocollins); (2) *the armadillo family members* (plakoglobin and plakophilins); and (3) the *plakin family* (desmoplakins). All three units link to each other, and eventually to the intermediate keratin filaments, to maintain cell-cell adhesion [216-7].

3.3. Desmosomal Cadherins

Desmosomes were originally isolated from cow nose epidermis, making its chemical characterization possible [217]. High levels of glycosylated proteins were found to be the main part of the desmosomes, and they were postulated to mediate cell-cell adhesion [216-7]. Antibodies against a particular desmosomal glycoprotein were developed and used to screen a cDNA library. Thus, the first desmosomal cadherin was cloned, sequenced, and named desmoglein; the name arose from the Greek *glein*, which means glue [218]. Since then, the *desmosomal cadherin* family has been progressively expanded [219]. The *desmosomal cadherin* group consists of seven different proteins: four desmoglein isoforms (desmoglein1, 2, 3, and 4) and three desmocollin isoforms (Dsc1, 2, and 3), all encoded by separate genes located on chromosome 18 in humans [220].

Desmoglein 1 and desmocollin 1 are the major desmosomal cadherins in the skin where they are expressed throughout the epidermis, but most prominently in the upper layers. Desmoglein 3 and desmocollin 3 expression is strongest in the lower epidermis (suprabasal) and decreased toward the upper layers. Desmoglein1 and 3 and desmocollin 1 and 3 are mostly restricted to the stratified epithelia (subcorneal). Desmoglein 2 is expressed in simple epithelia and myocardia, whereas desmoglein 4 is mostly expressed in hair follicles. Desmocollins and desmogleins are always found as a pair in the desmosomes; however, the precise nature of their interaction is not known. Several studies point out that *desmosomal cadherins* contain a cell-adhesion recognition site within their N-terminal EC1 extracellular domain and that this site is critical for maintenance of desmosomal adhesion [206]. The cell-adhesion recognition site sequence for desmoglein1 and desmocollin 1 are RAL and YAT, respectively [208]. Peptides stemmed from these sequences were able to block the hemophilic adhesion mediated by desmoglein 1 and desmocollin 1 on incubation [207-8]. Based on predictions from the C-cadherin crystal structure, recent cryoelectron microscopy studies in human epidermis showed *cis* and *transinteractions* of the EC1 domains, possibly by insertion of the tryptophan in position 2 into the hydrophobic pocket of the cell-adhesion recognition site [221]. However, they also found some *cis* interactions of the extracellular four to five domains, and it has been suggested that *desmosomal cadherins* may show periodically zipper-like arrangements similar to classical cadherins [222]. *Classical cadherins* form homodimers in order to mediate adhesion. In contrast, *desmosomal cadherins* undergo both homophilic and heterophilic *trans* interactions. Using extracellular one to two fragments of desmoglein 2, desmocollin 2, or desmoglein 3; it was shown that homophilic interactions occur *in vitro*. 223-4 In addition, Waschke et al. [225], have estimated the strength of interaction between purified desmoglein 1 ectodomains by means of atomic force microscopy and showed that desmoglein 1 could form homodimers and that the molecular binding properties of this homophilic adhesion may be comparable to other cadherins. Thus, mutation of key amino acid residues such as tryptophanin position 2 and alanine at position 80 that are involved in adhesion mediated by classical cadherins abolished hemophilic adhesion of desmosomal cadherins [226]. Recent studies using a similar atomic force microscopy approach have shown desmocollin 3 homophilic binding and heterophilic interaction with desmoglein 1, but not with desmoglein 3 [227]. Heterophilic binding of desmoglein 2 with desmocollin 1 or 2 has also been demonstrated [224, 228]. Also, these heterophilic interactions also form in a calcium-dependent manner.

As previously stated, adherent junctions are Ca^{2+}-dependent cell-cell junctions mediated by E-cadherin that forms intercellular bridges at their extracellular N terminal. E-cadherin binds several associated proteins such as plakoglobin or β- and α-catenin at specific sites of their intracellular C-terminal domains, which, in turn, interacts with actin microfilaments [229]. As we previously stated, E-cadherin and P-cadherin are classical cadherins expressed in the epidermis. E-cadherin is expressed in all layers of the epidermis, whereas P-cadherin is limited to the basal cell layer [214].

3.4. The Armadillo Proteins

In the desmosomal plaque, the armadillo proteins plakoglobin and plakophilin associate with the cytoplasmic domains of desmosomal cadherins.

3.4.1. Plakoglobin

Originally defined in *Drosophila*, plakoglobin is also called γ-catenin and is encoded by a gene in chromosome 17 [230]. Its counterpart is β-catenin, expressed in adherens junctions. Similar to β-catenin, is capable of taking part in cell adhesion [231-2]. The central arm region of plakoglobin shares 65% aminoacid identity with β-catenin that associates with adherens junctions. Plakoglobin can substitute β-catenin in adherens junctions because both bind E-cadherin with similar affinity. However, plakoglobin has higher affinity for desmogleins which would explain to exclude β-catenin from desmosomes [233]. The arm domain of plakoglobin associates with both the intracellular domain of desmosomal cadherins and the N-terminus of desmoplakin [234-6]. Thus, plakoglobin is a critical linker in desmosomal adhesion.

3.4.2. Plakophilins

Plakophilins are members of another subfamily of the armadillo proteins. Three desmosomal Plakophilins (1, 2, and 3) have been described, and the genes encoding them are located on chromosomes 1, 12, and 11, respectively [237]. PKP1 and PKP2 have 2 isoforms (α and β) that result from alternative splicing [238-9]. There is a fourth plakophilin: PKP4, also known as p0071, which is related to δ-catenin [240]. Plakophilins (1–4) have been shown to bind directly to the intracellular domain of desmosomal cadherins. This is mediated by their amino-terminal head domain, and the roles for their armadillo repeats remain unknown. Plakophilins can also bind plakoglobin to promote clustering of desmosomal cadherins through lateral stabilizing, which increases desmosome strength [234].

3.4.3. Plakins

Another family of proteins responsible for cell-cell adhesion are the plakins, which are linkers between the cytoskeleton and cell-cell or cell-matrix interactions [241]. Desmoplakin is an essential part of the desmosomal plaque which is recruited by the armadillo proteins in order to link the intermediate filament network with the desmosomal junctional complex. Desmoplakin is encoded on chromosome and has 2 variants (DP-1 and DP-2) [242-3]. The amino-terminal domain of desmoplakin binds the other desmosomal plaque proteins (plakoglobin and plakophilin), its central coiled-coil rod domain mediates dimerization, and its carboxyterminal tail is the linker for intermediate filaments [234, 244]. Other members such as plectin, envoplakin, and periplakin are also found in desmosomes; however, their roles are still unclear. Inactivating plectin, which is present in desmosomes and hemidesmosomes, can affect cell-cell adhesion in mice and humans [245-6]. In addition, when using desmoplakin-deficient mice, skin blistering was observed and the desmosomes were not anchored to the intermediate filaments [247].

Epidermal growth factor receptor activation signaling may play important roles in the cross-talk between adherent junctions and desmosomes. In this regard, tyrosine phosphorylation of β-catenin and/or plakoglobin caused their dissociation from E-cadherin, leading to a decrease in desmoplakin from desmosomes and in cell-cell contacts in keratinocytes [248]. Moreover, introduction of a phosphorylation-deficient plakoglobin mutant into Plakoglobin-null cells prevented the epidermal growth factor receptor-dependent loss of desmoplakin from junctions [249]. Therefore, it is interesting that pemphigus vulgaris-IgG binding and/or desmoglein 3 depletion may interfere with this cross-talk through activation of a variety of intracellular signaling pathways, resulting in injured control of desmosome remodeling. In the next section we review some specific aspects of these interactions.

3.5. Interacting Dermosome Proteins with Autoantibodies = Pemphigus

The pemphigus group of diseases consists of many disease variants, each with unique clinical, histological, and immunologic features [250]. These disease variants include pemphigus vulgaris, pemphigus foliaceus, endemic pemphigus foliaceus (also known as *fogo selvagem)*, paraneoplastic pemphigus, and IgA pemphigus.

Pemphigus vulgaris typically presents with erosions limited to the mucosal (oropharyngeal and/or genital) tissue, classified as mucosal pemphigus vulgaris. In most patients the disease progresses to involve the cornified cutaneous surface as well with blisters and/or erosions over the trunk and extremities (classified as mucocutaneous pemphigus vulgaris). Histologically, pemphigus vulgaris presents a suprabasilar split with acantholysis. While mucosal pemphigus vulgaris patients classically harbor autoantibodies to desmoglein 3 alone, mucocutaneous pemphigus vulgaris patients show autoantibodies to both desmoglein 3 and 1 [250-2]. Desmoglein 3 and 1 affinity-purified autoantibodies from mucocutaneous pemphigus vulgaris patients are enough to induce suprabasilar acantholysis on passive transfer in the neonatal mouse model, by showing pathogenicity [47, 253-4]. In pemphigus vulgaris, desmoglein 3 is the best characterized major autoantigen [255-6]. Depending on their clinical phenotype, most pemphigus vulgaris patients display circulating IgG1 and IgG4 antibodies against desmoglein 3 or both desmoglein 1 and 3 proteins. 257-8]. The so-called desmoglein compensation theory aims at correlating the clinical phenotype (mucosal, mucocutaneous) with the autoantibody profile, i.e., whether only anti-desmoglein 3-IgG or in combination with anti-desmoglein 1-IgG is present [259]. In contrast to subepidermal blistering autoimmune diseases, such as bullous pemphigoid, in pemphigus vulgaris, histopathology of lesional skin shows a sparse infiltration of inflammatory cells; in early skin lesions, an eosinophilic infiltrate might be seen (eosinophilic spongiosis). Considering the pathogenic relevance of IgG autoantibodies in pemphigus vulgaris, autoreactive CD4$^+$ T cells and B cells are considered as crucial immune cells in this disease [181, 260-3]. Although direct experimental evidence is missing, it seems likely the activation of autoreactive CD4$^+$ T and B cells takes place in skin draining lymph nodes. Autorreactive, desmoglein 3-specific CD4$^+$ T cells have been isolated and functionally characterized from peripheral blood of pemphigus vulgaris patients [62, 93, 181, 264-6]. The desmoglein 3-specific activation of these autoreactive T cell clones is dependent on the HLA-class II haplotype that is prevalent in pemphigus vulgaris patients, i.e., HLADRB1*0402, HLA-DQB1*0503 [267-8]. Therapeutic depletion of B-cells using the anti-CD20 monoclonal antibody (rituximab) leads to a dramatic decline of circulating anti-desmoglein 3-IgG followed by a significant clinical improvement in pemphigus vulgaris patients [262, 269-72], suggesting that autoantibody-secreting plasma cells in pemphigus vulgaris are rather short-lived compared to plasma cells releasing pathogen-reactive IgG [273-4].

Pemphigus foliaceus presents clinically with superficial blisters or erosions over the trunk and extremities. In many patients, the blisters rupture spontaneously prior to presentation, and the clinical exam reveals only superficial crusting and erosions. There is no mucosal involvement in pemphigus foliaceus. Histologically, it shows a subcorneal split with acantholysis. Patients with pemphigus foliaceus classically harbor autoantibodies to desmoglein 1 alone [250-1]. Similar to pemphigus vulgaris, to settle desmoglein 1 as the target autoantigen was defined by affinity-purified desmoglein1-specific autoantibodies in the neonatal passive transfer model [203]. Pemphigus foliaceus is histologically characterized by the loss of keratinocyte adhesion in the subcorneal layer of the epidermis, resulting in superficial blister formation. Early skin lesions might reveal eosinophilic and neutrophilic spongiosis [275]. Pemphigus foliaceus patients present circulating autoantibodies, mainly of the IgG1 and IgG4 subclasses, against the desmosomal glycoprotein desmoglein 1 [39, 52, 62]. Anti-desmoglein 1-IgG4 has been shown to be associated with active pemphigus foliaceus disease [276]. Clinically, superficial blisters and scaly, crusted erosions develop in the seborrheic areas, i.e., face, scalp, and trunk, while the mucous membranes are typically not involved [277-8]. Desmoglein 1-reactive CD4$^+$ T cell responses in peripheral blood of patients with the endemic form of pemphigus foliaceus, *fogo selvagem*, have been identified [279]. In this study, memory CD4$^+$ Th2 cells responded to the extracellular domain of the desmoglein 1 protein in an HLA-DR-restricted manner [279]. Gebhardt et al., [280], showed that both pemphigus foliaceus patients and HLA-DR/–DQ-matched healthy individuals present Th1 and Th2 responses to the recombinant ectodomain of desmoglein 1, suggesting the presence of CD4$^+$ autoreactive T cells in peripheral blood is not restricted to pemphigus foliaceus and pemphigus vulgaris patients, respectively [266, 280].

Fogo selvagem is an endemic form of pemphigus foliaceus, in which patients develop mainly IgG4 autoantibodies specific for desmoglein 1 [281-2]. Moreover, in acute disease, the patients produce auto antibodies directed against NH2-terminal epitopes in the extracellular domain 1 (EC1) and EC2, whereas patients at preclinical stages predominantly show reactivity with COOH-terminal epitopes [283]. Recently, Qian et al., [284] provided evidence that salivary gland antigens of the sandfly, specifically the LJM11 salivary protein, is recognized by anti-desmoglein 1-IgG of these patients. The cross-reactivity with LJM11 salivary protein in genetically susceptible individuals might represent an environmental trigger to launch this autoimmune disease.

The endemic nature of this disease makes it an ideal population to study the fine aspects of genetic susceptibility and environmental triggers of disease [285]. Autoantibodies to desmoglein 1, mainly those of the IgG4 subclass, are a serologic indicator of disease in this patient population [282]. E-cadherin has also been shown to be a potential antigenic target in *fogo selvagem* [285]. A recent serological analysis reveals that *fogo selvagem* patients and many healthy controls living in endemic areas also harbor autoantibodies to other desmoglein and desmocollin family members, in addition to the anti-desmoglein 1 antibody previously reported.

Originally, pemphigus erythematosus (also known as Senear-Usher syndrome or seborrheic pemphigus) was described as a clinical subtype of pemphigus foliaceus presenting characteristics of lupus erythematosus. Although several cases of pemphigus erythematosus have been described, the criteria for making the diagnosis of pemphigus erythematosus are controversial and not well-defined yet. Pemphigus erythematosus patients present with erosions on the seborrheic areas and erythema in the malar region. Immunoserologically, pemphigus erythematosus patients show circulating IgG autoantibodies that are reactive with desmoglein 1, as in pemphigus foliaceus [284]. However, the autoantibody profile in pemphigus erythematosus seems to be more diverse, since another autoantibodies reactive with components of the hemidesmosome, such as the BP230 antigen and plakins, have been described [62].

Paraneoplastic pemphigus is a unique pemphigus variant that presents with extensive mucositis and polymorphic cutaneous lesions in the clinical setting of malignancy. The cutaneous involvement is variable including erosions, widespread blisters, erythema multiforme-like lesions, and lichenoid expression, whereas mucous membranes display severe and extensive mucositis and hemorrhagic erosions and crusts [286]. This rare pemphigus subtype is considered as an autoimmune multiorgan syndrome associated with an underlying neoplasia, mostly hematological disorders such as non-Hodgkin lymphoma, chronic lymphocytic leukemia, Castleman disease, or non-hematological malignancies, such as adenocarcinomas [287-8]. The autoantibody response in paraneoplastic pemphigus is more diverse compared to pemphigus vulgaris and pemphigus foliaceus, including IgG against desmoplakin, envoplakin, periplakin, plectin, and the recently identified 170-kDa antigen, the protease inhibitor α-2 macroglobulin-like-1 [289]. In contrast to the above mentioned pemphigus subtypes, in paraneoplastic pemphigus; histopathological findings might be as diverse as the clinical expression. Intraepidermal suprabasilar split formation is usually present as well as mononuclear infiltrates and intense interface dermatitis with vacuolar degeneration of the basal keratinocytes, respectively [288]. Also, histology reveals intraepidermal clefting with acantholysis, but also shows a dense lichenoid infiltrate with interface dermatitis and necrotic keratinocytes [289-90]. Patients with paraneoplastic pemphigus harbor autoantibodies to desmoglein1 and 3, which are thought to be responsible for the acantholysis as removal of the desmoglein 3-specific antibodies from paraneoplastic pemphigus sera abrogates the pathogenicity in the neonatal passive transfer model [291]. These patients also have autoantibodies to the plakin family of proteins, which are thought to be responsible for the dyskeratosis/necrotic keratinocytes [287, 290]. Interestingly, patients with erythema multiforme, a condition classically felt to be a non-immunologically mediated reaction pattern, can have a falsely positive indirect immunofluorescence on the classic paraneoplastic pemphigus rat bladder substrate. There are recent reports of patients with erythema multiforme harboring anti-desmoplakin antibodies, though the pathogenicity of these autoantibodies has not yet been established [292-3]. The pathogenicity studies are currently lacking. So far, there are no descriptions of isolated anti-desmoplakin (except on paraneoplastic pemphigus and erythema multiforme) or anti-plakoglobin-mediated cutaneous disease.

IgA pemphigus is characterized by tissue-bound IgA autoantibody deposits on the cell surface of epidermal keratinocytes [294-5]. Depending on clinical manifestations, histopathological findings, and immunofluorescence staining patterns, the two subtypes of IgA pemphigus, (1) the subcorneal pustular dermatosis and (2) the intraepithelial neutrophilic IgA dermatosis, can be distinguished [295]. Annular erythematous plaques, erythema with peripheral subcorneal pustules mainly in the intertrigines (the so called *subcorneal pustular IgA pemphigus*) and erythematous papules, vesicles, erosions, and crusts (also known as *intraepithelial neutrophilic IgA pemphigus*) represent typical clinical findings in IgA pemphigus patients. Circulating IgA autoantibodies that are reactive with desmosomal cadherins have been identified in these patients [296]. In subcorneal pustular IgA pemphigus, autoantibodies targeting the desmosomal proteins desmocollin 1, 2, and 3 have been described [297-8]. In intraepithelial neutrophilic IgA pemphigus, autoantibodies directed against the classical autoantigens in pemphigus, i.e., desmoglein 1 and 3, have also been identified [296, 299-301]. Desmocollin 1 has been shown to be the target antigen in the intraepithelial neutrophilic-type of IgA pemphigus, whereas the target antigen in the subcorneal pustular IgA pemphigus is likely a non-desmosomal antigen as shown by immunoelectron microscopy studies [296]. However, there is no distinct autoantibody profile depending on the subtype of IgA pemphigus. Recently, a case of subcorneal pustular IgA pemphigus displaying IgA autoantibodies against desmocollin 2 and 3 as well as BP180-reactive IgA autoantibodies, suggestive of linear IgA dermatosis has been reported [302]. The prevalence of IgA autoantibodies in contrast to the major subtypes of pemphigus, pemphigus vulgaris and pemphigus foliaceus, which are characterized by tissue-bound and circulating IgG autoantibodies, remains unclear in IgA blistering diseases.

IgA pemphigus is distinguished by the presence of autoantibodies of the IgA subclass present on direct immunofluorescence in a classical intercellular space staining pattern. Histologically, IgA pemphigus can be of the intraepidermal neutrophilic variant or can be of the subcorneal pustular dermatosis variant [303].

Finally, pemphigus herpetiformis is another rare but distinct variant of pemphigus with clinical characteristics resembling dermatitis herpetiformis, such as pruritic annular erythemas with peripheral vesicles and annular-shaped papular lesions [41, 304-5]. In most pemphigus herpetiformis patients, circulating anti-desmoglein 1- IgG autoantibodies and in fewer cases anti-desmoglein 3-IgG have been detected [306]. Patients with pemphigus herpetiformis-like, atypical pemphigus who developed autoantibodies against non-desmoglein desmosomal targets, such as desmocollin 1 [307] and 3, have been reported [308-9]. In a large immune-serological study [310], showed that sera of 15 pemphigus herpetiformis patients reacted mainly with desmoglein 1-and 3-epitopes located in the NH2-terminal regions of these autoantigens. So far there is no sound explanation for this atypical expression and the autoantibody profile in pemphigus herpetiformis compared with the classical pemphigus subtypes.

3.6. Effects of Autoantibodies in the Desmosome

Pemphigus foliaceus and pemphigus vulgaris are the most studied variants of pemphigus. There is an association of susceptibility to pemphigus with certain HLA-DR and HLA-DQ alleles [311]. However, the exact mechanism by which pemphigus autoantibodies induce loss of epidermal cell adhesion directly or indirectly has not been precisely determined, nevertheless, they have been proposed the following: (1) direct interference (steric hindrance), (2) activation of transmembrane signaling that downregulates cell-cell adhesion, (3) proteinase activation (plasminogen activator), and (4) desmoglein internalization. (Figure 4) There are two major theories that are mostly accepted but still in discussion: (a) direct interference of desmoglein *trans* interaction by pemphigus autoantibodies (steric hindrance); and (b) activation of transmembrane signaling pathways and/or apoptosis by pemphigus autoantibodies that indirectly results in acantholysis.

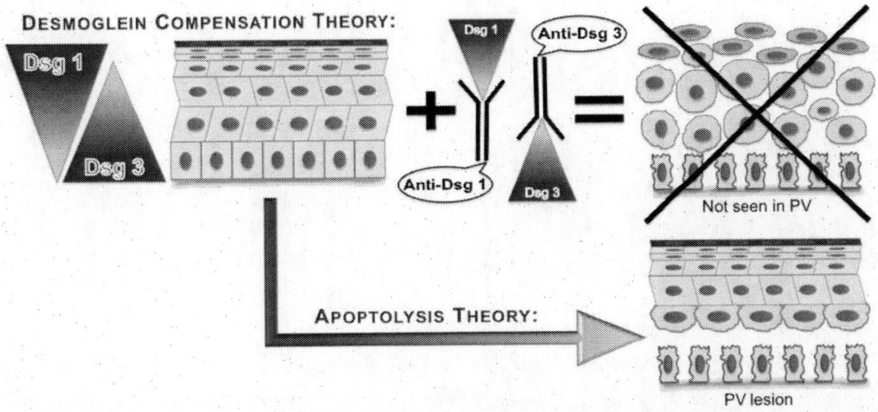

Figure 4. The hypothetical appearance of epidermis in the skin of pemphigus vulgaris patients that produce both desmoglein 1 and 3 antibodies based on the postulates of desmoglein compensation hypothesis versus real appearance of lesional epidermis in pemphigus vulgaris patients. Reproduced from Ref. 12 under the Supplemental Terms and Conditions for unrestricted reproduction in any medium with the proper cite.

3.7. Direct Interference of Desmogleins by Pemphigus Autoantibodies

Increasing evidence from several epitope mapping studies points out that pathogenic pemphigus auto antibodies target the amino-terminal end of desmoglein 1 and/or 3 ectodomains [276, 312-3]. Data based on the structure of classical cadherins suggest that this N-terminal region harbors the adhesive interface of desmosomal cadherins [222, 314]. In addition, the pathogenicity of pemphigus IgG autoantibodies has been consistently showed by passive transfer studies in neonatal mice [47, 314]. Moreover, not only the whole IgG molecule but also the F(ab)2 and F(ab) fragments were found to be pathogenic, independently of complement or plasminogen activator [259, 315-7], suggesting that due to their lack of ability to cross-link cell-surface molecules, possibly they interfere directly with adhesion.

Furthermore, monoclonal antibodies (like AK23) derived from a pemphigus vulgaris mouse model that binds the functionally N-terminal adhesive interface of desmoglein 3 induced pemphigus vulgaris lesions in mice, whereas monoclonal antibodies recognizing other regions of desmoglein 3 ectodomain did not cause lesions in mice [318]. It has been shown that pemphigus vulgaris-IgG and AK23 monoclonal antibody directly inhibit desmoglein 3 homophilic binding under cell-free conditions, suggesting that direct inhibition of desmoglein 3 binding occurs in pemphigus vulgaris [277, 319]. Direct blocking of desmoglein 1 binding was not observed by atomic force microscopy; however, keratinocyte dissociation and loss of desmoglein 1- and 3-coated microspheres to cultured keratinocytes were observed when using laser tweezer trapping [320], indicating that acantholysis may not be solely dependent on direct interference of desmoglein 1-desmoglein 1 binding by pemphigus autoantibodies. In studies using peptides against the desmoglein adhesive interface as well as tandem peptides (obtained by dimerization of two of the initial peptides) added evidence that direct inhibition of desmosomal proteins contributes to acantholysis when the tandem peptide prevented acantholysis induced by pemphigus vulgaris-IgG, yet this is not the case when using pemphigus foliaceus-IgG. Thus, some investigators proposed that pemphigus vulgaris and foliaceus acantholysis may involve different mechanisms [319-21].

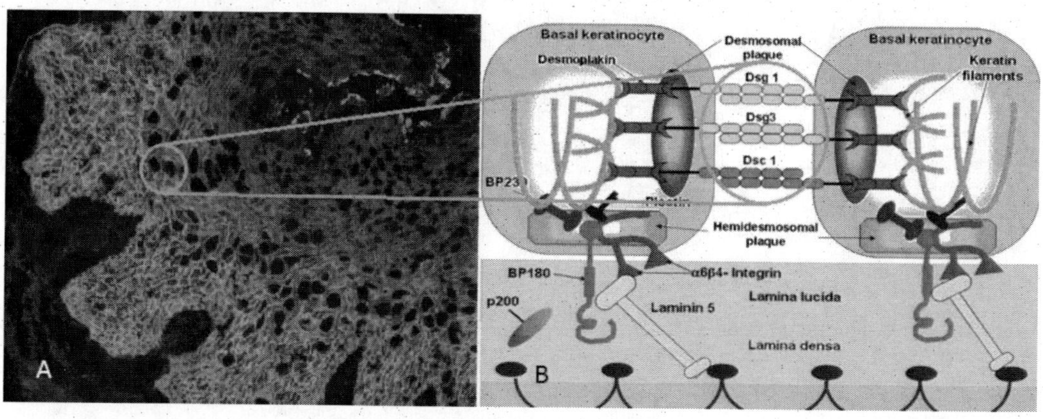

Figure 5. Specificity and binding patterns of antibodies in pemphigus. (A) Serological tests used for the diagnosis of pemphigus. Circulating autoantibodies show an intercellular binding pattern by indirect immunofluorescence microscopy on monkey esophagus (magnification, 3200). (B) Schematic diagram of the desmosome and the dermal-epidermal junction. Here are represented only structural proteins that function as autoantigens in autoimmune bullous skin diseases. Neighbouring keratinocytes are associated via the extracellular portions of desmosomal cadherins. As examples, homophilic interactions between desmoglein 1, desmoglein 3 and desmocollin 1 are depicted. Their intracellular portions bind to desmosomal plaque proteins that mediate the interaction of desmosomes with keratin filaments. Keratin filaments also bind to bullous pemphigoid antigen 230 (BP230) and plectin, the main intracellular constituents of the hemidesmosomes. BP230 and plectin function as ligands for transmembrane hemidesomosomal proteins, type XVII collagen (BP180) and $\alpha_6\beta_4$ integrin. These may connect the hemidesmosomes to laminin 5, which in addition to type IV collagen, is a major component of the lamina densa. Laminin 5 is a known ligand for type VII collagen, the major constituent of the anchoring fibrils, which connect lamina densa to the collagen bundles of the upper dermis. Reproduced with permission of John Wiley and Sons from Mihai S, Sitaru C. Immunopathology and molecular diagnosis of autoimmune bullous diseases. J Cell Mol Med 2007; 11: 462-81.

3.8. Signaling Pathways and Apoptosis by Pemphigus Autoantibodies

The direct interference of desmoglein *transinteractions* by pemphigus auto antibodies has been shown to be not enough to disrupt keratinocyte adhesion [225]; thus, more cellular events may be needed to cause blistering. (Figure 5) Previous *in vitro* studies show that pemphigus vulgaris-IgG induces different events in cultured keratinocytes including a transient increase in intracellular calcium and inositol 1,4,5-triphosphate [322], activation of protein kinase C, and phosphorylation of desmoglein 3, which may lead to internalization of desmoglein 3 from cell surface, therefore depleting desmoglein 3 from desmosomes [323-8]. Thus, activation of intracellular signaling within the target keratinocyte induced by binding of pemphigus IgG has been proposed to contribute to the loss of cell-cell adhesion. The p38 MAPK signaling pathway is a critical participator in the regulation of cellular and humoral autoimmune responses [329-30]. Usually started by cellular stress or inflammatory cytokines, its main task is to orchestrate cytokine gene expression including TNFα and IFNγ by transcriptional and posttranscriptional mechanisms such as stabilization of mRNA transcripts [331-2]. P38 MAPK is also important for cell survival, proliferation, differentiation, and apoptosis [333]. An increasing number of studies have provided data demonstrating the significant role of this cascade in the pathogenesis of several immune-mediated diseases, including rheumatoid arthritis, Sjögren's syndrome, systemic lupus erythematosus, autoimmune hepatitis, and psoriasis [334] Defects in p38 MAPK pathway can explain the increased expression of proinflammatory cytokines. For instance, there is increased TNFα protein expression, but similar mRNA levels, in lesional compared with non-lesional psoriatic skin, showing that TNFα expression in psoriatic skin is regulated posttranscriptionally by p38 MAPK, and therefore p38 signaling pathway can be targeted therapeutically [335].

p38 MAPK can be studied in experimental models and clinical material such as peripheral blood mononuclear cells or PBMC and pathological tissue from patients with autoimmune diseases [336]. The conventional techniques for p38 detection include Western blotting, immunoprecipitation, and confocal immunofluorescence microscopy that detects the active p38 kinase translocated to the cell nucleus. However, these applications need large populations of homogenous cells, and the data gained are not fully quantitative. Extended culturing of primary cells is also compulsory to increase cell densities. Extensive culturing periods, often in the presence of IL-2 and other growth factors, can affect or bias signaling analyses that depend on interaction of cell receptors and phosphorylation of intracellular proteins.

Given the key role p38 MAPK signaling pathway plays in inflammatory responses through producing cytokines and inflammatory mediators, its inhibition is considered to be a promising target for chronic inflammatory diseases.

Previous studies have shown that phosphorylation of p38-MAPK and heat shock protein 25 (the murine homolog of human heat shock protein 27, or HSP27) occurs rapidly after exposure of keratinocytes to pemphigus IgG and in the skin of mice treated with pathogenic IgG [337]. Also, phosphorylation of both p38-MAPK and HSP27 has been observed in the perilesional epidermis of pemphigus patients [338]. Furthermore, p38-MAPK inhibitors block both histological and gross blister formation in the pemphigus foliaceus passive transfer model [339], suggesting that activation of p38-MAPK is an early and important step in pemphigus foliaceus-IgG-induced acantholysis. p38-MAPK signaling has been implicated in other cellular responses such as desmosome assembly and disassembly, cytoskeleton reorganization, changes of the cell cycle, and apoptosis [340-1].

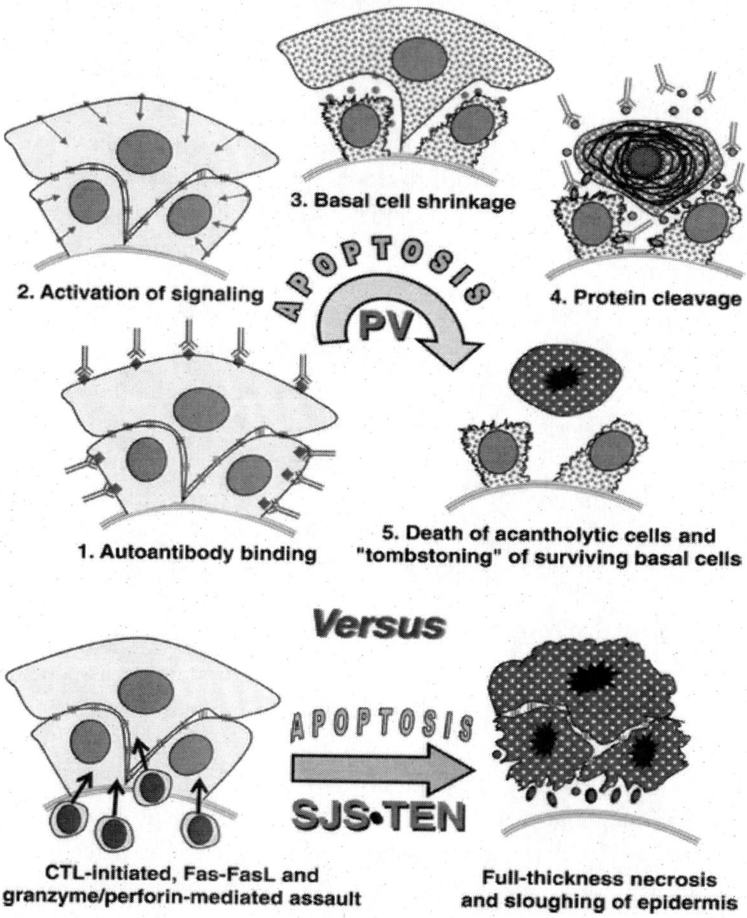

Figure 6. Epidermal apoptolysis versus apoptosis: Hypothetical sequences of pathologic events. Apoptolysis in pemphigus is triggered by binding of autoantibodies to the PV antigens capable of transducing apoptolytic signals from the keratinocyte plasma membrane (Step 1). Downstream signalling from ligated antigens elevates intracellular calcium and launches the cell death cascades (Step 2). Collapse and retraction of the tonofilaments cleaved by executioner caspases and dissociation of interdesmosomal adhesion complexes caused by phosphorylation of adhesion molecules result in basal cell shrinkage, while most of desmosomes remain intact (Step 3). This is a crossing step of the apoptotic lines and pemphigus acantholytic lines. Massive cleavage of cellular proteins by activated cell death enzymes leads to collapse of the cytoskeleton and tearing off desmosomes from the cell membrane with subsequent production of scavenging (i.e., secondary) autoantibodies mainly to shed adhesion molecules (Step 4). Suprabasal acantholytic cells die, manifested by nuclear fragmentation and TUNEL positivity, thus allowing suprabasal blister formation and rendering a ''tombstone'' appearance to surviving basal cells (Step 5). In marked contrast, a uniform apoptosis of both basal and suprabasal keratinocytes leads to full thickness necrosis and sloughing of the entire epidermis in SJS/TEN. Abbreviations: CTL, cytotoxic T lymphocytes; FasL, Fas Ligand; PV, pemphigus vulgaris; SJS/TEN, Stevens-Johnson syndrome/toxic epidermal necrolysis. Reproduced with permission of John Wiley and Sons from Grando SA, Bystryn JC, Chernyavsky AI. Apoptolysis: a novel mechanism of skin blistering in pemphigus vulgaris linking the apoptotic pathways to basal cell shrinkage and suprabasal acantholysis. Exp Dermatol 2009; 18: 764-70.

There is evidence that p38-MAPK is involved in keratinocyte apoptosis [342-3], and that DNA fragmentation and caspase activation are both induced in the epidermis of pemphigus foliaceus-IgG-treated mice [344]. Keratinocyte-derived and local production of apoptotic inducers such as nitric oxide synthase [345-6], Fas/Fas ligand (the last one have been increased in serum of patients with pemphigus) [347], and inhibitor Bcl-2 have also been detected in lesional skin of pemphigus foliaceus patients [345-6], Also, a biphasic activation of p38-MAPK after binding pemphigus IgG has been recently demonstrated where the first activation peak is linked to acantholysis and the second peak coincided with apoptosis, suggesting that apoptosis occurs downstream to acantholysis in pemphigus (Figure 6) [342]. Interestingly, other studies suggest that apoptosis occurs before acantholysis develops [348]; and, the apoptotic signaling could precede acantholysis without apoptotic cell death [349]. More important, caspase inhibitors have been shown to block pemphigus serum-induced keratinocyte apoptosis. Thus, it is not clear which precedes the other, but there is evidence that both are involved in pemphigus pathogenesis. Another signaling pathway suggested to be involved is through plakoglobin [350]; on the basis of keratinocytes from plakoglobin-deficient mice were resistant to keratinocyte dissociation induced by pemphigus vulgaris-IgG, suggesting also that direct restraint of desmoglein binding may not be enough to cause acantholysis and that plakoglobin could be part of a complex responsible for transferring the signal upon autoantibody binding from outside into the keratinocyte (called *outside-in* signaling) [12]. In addition, it has been shown that plakoglobin is involved in c-Myc repression, and c-Myc was also shown to be elevated in keratinocytes exposed to pemphigus auto antibodies [11, 351]. Nonetheless, the role of c-Myc signaling in pemphigus acantholysis remains unclear.

Although the mechanisms linking pemphigus IgG binding to acantholysis are not completely understood and widely accepted by the experts, much progress has been made in characterizing target pathways that may further help to enlighten the primary event that drives pemphigus acantholysis. Future experiments are needed to identify other pathways or complete the ones that are already under investigation. However, research on the involvement of non-desmosomal components may provide more answers. For example, early studies have shown that on binding of pemphigus autoantibodies to the epidermal cell surface, the first structural change observed was widening of the intercellular spaces between desmosomes where E-cadherin mediates cell adhesion. Only later did desmosomes begin to split in halves with resulting complete cell separation [352-3]. This interplay of direct interference and signaling mechanisms in pemphigus pathogenesis are nowadays unclear, and underscores the complexity and diversity of pemphigus acantholysis. Current and future studies toward to identify the primary component(s) of the molecular mechanism of acantholysis will advance our understanding on pemphigus pathogenesis and therefore provide targets for developing preventative and novel therapeutic strategies for pemphigus.

3.9. Plectin

Plectin also be recognized by autoantibodies in autoimmune, bullous skin diseases. Paraneoplastic pemphigus, a rare form of pemphigus with an underlying neoplasm, is characterized by a unique immune response against plakin family proteins, and plectin was specifically identified among these [354-5]. In 11 of 282 (3.9%) patients with subepidermal blistering diseases, an immunoblot staining pattern identical to that of anti-plectin monoclonal antibody HD121 was found [356]. Also, Laffitte et al., [357] could show IgG anti-plectin antibodies in a 5-month-old child with bullous pemphigoid. A case of epidermolysis bullosa acquisita with related IgA antibodies to plectin was described [358]. Epitope mapping of the plectin molecule showed the central coiled-coil rod domain is an immunodominant *hot spot*. Most patients with anti-plectin antibodies also had antibodies to other pemphigoid antigens. Therefore, the anti-plectin antibodies can be considered to be a bystander effect in various autoimmune, bullous diseases. Most likely they have evolved through epitope-spreading [356].

Chapter 4

APOPTOSIS AND ACANTHOLYSIS IN PEMPHIGUS: THE CONCEPT OF APOPTOLYSIS

Pemphigus involves a group of blistering diseases of the skin and mucous membranes, characterized by defects in adhesion (and therefore called acantholysis), that typically target and functionally disrupt specific cell-cell or cell-substrate adhesion components. In pemphigus, mainly humoral-mediated immune responses functionally disrupt targeted components of the adhesive structures.

Pemphigus foliaceus presents clinically as superficial erosions and crusts of the skin; the pathology of pemphigus foliaceus demonstrates acantholysis within the more superficial layers of the epidermis. In contrast, pemphigus vulgaris presents clinically as flaccid vesicles and erosions with histology demonstrating suprabasilar acantholysis [359]. As the name implies, clinical lesions are restricted to mucosa in mucosal pemphigus vulgaris; whereas, lesions of both mucosa and skin are present in mucocutaneous pemphigus vulgaris. Because of a yet unknown cause, autoantibodies are produced and bind to a number of desmosomal proteins and possibly other non-desmosomal keratinocyte antigens.

While the autoimmune nature of the disease is clear and the pathogenicity of the autoantibodies is widely accepted, pathophysiologic mechanisms by which the antibodies cause blistering are under active investigation.

Clues to the etiology of pemphigus as a humoral-mediated autoimmune disease were provided by Beutner et al., [360-1] who performed direct immunofluorescence of pemphigus patient skin biopsies and demonstrated the presence of immunoglobulins bound to epidermal keratinocytes. In subsequent studies by Anhalt et al., [47] IgG fractions purified from pemphigus patient sera were passively transferred to neonatal mice and induced end organ damage, i.e., blistering of the skin; analogous to what was observed in the human disease [47, 353]. Clinically, test animals treated with pemphigus vulgaris IgG formed flaccid blisters; histology demonstrated suprabasilar acantholysis, and by direct immunofluorescence, human IgG was demonstrated to be bound to the surface of the epidermal keratinocytes. The passive transfer model served not only to demonstrate that the humoral immune response was indeed pathogenic but also provided an experimental model by which to study the mechanism of pemphigus autoantibody-induced loss of adhesion. Amagai et al., [353, 256] and Eyre et al., [362] subsequently utilized patient purified IgG to screen cDNA libraries for the target antigens in pemphigus vulgaris and pemphigus foliaceus, identifying desmoglein 3 and 1, respectively.

4.1. Acantholysis

Identifying anti-desmoglein antibodies as the pathogenic agents suggested several mechanisms for blister induction in pemphigus including: (1) activation of complement and proteolytic activity by cell-bound IgG [316, 363-4]; (2) steric hindrance (direct antibody-mediated interference with the adhesive role of the desmoglein transmembrane cell adhesion proteins) [365]; and (3) activation of transmembrane signaling by desmoglein-bound IgG [322, 324, 339, 366-70]. Binding of pemphigus antibody to desmoglein 3 is sufficient to trigger disease, however, several additional mechanism explained have been added.

In the passive transfer model, the epidermal cell-cell detachment induced by pemphigus vulgaris autoantibodies is neither Fc [371], complement [316] nor plasminogen activator dependent [259]. Monovalent pemphigus vulgaris and pemphigus foliaceus IgG Fab' and anti-desmoglein single-chain variable region fragments, which are incapable of cross-linking desmosome cadherins, are pathogenic [317, 372]. The humoral autoimmune response in both pemphigus vulgaris and pemphigus foliaceus is polyclonal. Pathogenic and non-pathogenic autoantibodies have been described, and pathogenic antibodies are directed against the N-terminal EC1/2 domains of the extracellular portion of the desmoglein 3 and 1 polypeptides; whereas, non-pathogenic antibodies are directed against other regions of the polypeptide [313, 312]. Pathogenic monoclonal antibodies also bind EC1/2 of the desmoglein 3 ectodomain [318]. Collectively, these observations suggest that pathogenic pemphigus autoantibodies act as competitive inhibitors for N-terminal at the EC1/2 domains of desmoglein.

Culturing keratinocytes in the presence of pemphigus vulgaris sera led to various intracellular events that suggested activation of trans membrane signaling. For example, in 1995, Seishima et al., [322] reported that pemphigus IgG stimulated rapid, transient increases in keratinocyte intracellular calcium and inositol triphosphate. Later studies by this group associated signaling by phospholipase C [366] and proteinkinase C [326, 367] in pemphigus IgG-mediated blistering.

Changes in cell-cell adhesion often result in changes in the keratinocyte biology. Reasoning that such changes would likely be transmitted across the desmosome-adhesive junctions themselves, analogous to what had been observed for integrin cell-substrate adhesion molecules and for adherens junctions, possibly changes in desmosome-mediated adhesion similarly triggered cellular signaling events. Based on this explanation, a biochemical screen was at first designed to explore the consequences of disrupting desmosome adhesion, using pemphigus vulgaris IgG as a desmosome-specific reagent because it targets desmoglein [339]. The immunologic response in mucosal pemphigus vulgaris is characterized by antibodies to desmoglein 3, whereas mucocutaneous pemphigus vulgaris is characterized by antibodies to desmoglein 1 as well as 3. In these early series of experiments, IgG purified from mucosal pemphigus vulgaris patient sera was used, allowing signaling downstream of IgG binding to desmoglein 3 to be investigated. Following series of experiments extended these investigations to desmoglein 1-specific IgG and to IgG purified from mucocutaneous sera, containing desmoglein 1- and 3-specific IgG. Phosphorylation of serine, threonine, and tyrosine residues of proteins is a common regulatory post-translational variation that is central to many signaling pathways. This led to identifying the small HSP27, as a protein whose phosphorylation was altered in cells treated with pemphigus vulgaris IgG. Using antibodies to both HSP27 and its phosphorylated isoforms, the identity of HSP 27 was confirmed as keratinocytes treated with pemphigus vulgaris IgG showed increased amounts of phospho-HSP27 when tested by immunoblot of cell extracts using HSP27 and phospho-HSP27-specific antibodies [339].

HSP27 is a small-molecular-weight chaperone that oligomerizes into large multimeric structures to facilitate protein refolding when cells are physiologically stressed, for example, when cells are exposed to the thermal stress of a "heat shock." In addition to this role as a chaperone, HSP27 functions in signaling, where it is downstream of p38 mitogen-activated protein kinase (p38-MAPK, p38). Activation of p38 leads to p38-mediated phosphorylation and activation of mitogen-activated protein kinase 2 (MAPK-AP2, MK2), which in turn phosphorylates HSP27 [373]. Phosphorylation of HSP27 results in dissociation of large oligomeric HSP27 into smaller multimeric structures [374]. These smaller phosphorylated HSP27 tetramers have been suggested to function in signal transduction and to regulate the cytoskeleton including both actin and intermediate filaments [375-83]. Thus, the observation that pemphigus vulgaris IgG induced the rapid phosphorylation of HSP27, occurring within minutes of exposure of keratinocytes to pemphigus vulgaris IgG, led to several predictions that could be tested experimentally. Namely, (1) treatment of keratinocytes with pemphigus vulgaris IgG should lead to phosphorylation of p38 and dissociation of HSP27 from large oligomers to smaller tetramers, and (2) inhibition of p38 should prevent the phosphorylation of HSP27 and block its dissociation from large oligomers to the smaller tetrameric structures [339].

During the process of acantholysis, where keratinocytes lose adhesion between adjacent cells, keratin intermediate filaments and actin undergo reorganization [368]. Besides its effect on HSP27, p38 may also directly phosphorylate and regulate keratin intermediate filament structure. The role of HSP27 in regulating the cytoskeleton suggested that activation of p38-MK2-HSP27 signaling could have a role in mediating pemphigus vulgaris IgG-induced changes in the target keratinocytes that contributed to the loss of cell-cell adhesion. It is possible that inhibitors of p38 would block pemphigus vulgaris IgG-induced keratin intermediate filament and actin reorganization in pemphigus vulgaris IgG-treated cell cultures. Consistent with this, p38 inhibitors blocked pemphigus vulgaris IgG-induced retraction of keratin intermediate filaments as well as actin reorganization (basal cell contraction disrupted) [339]. These observations suggested that activation of the signaling pathway was not a consequence of pemphigus vulgaris IgG induced loss of adhesion, but part of the mechanism by which pemphigus vulgaris IgG induced loss of adhesion. If activation of p38 contributed to the mechanism by which pemphigus vulgaris IgG induced loss of adhesion, then inhibition of p38 should block blistering.

The previous theory was then tested using the pemphigus vulgaris passive transfer mouse model [384]. Wild-type mice were treated with pemphigus vulgaris IgG or normal human IgG as a control. Using immunofluorescence microscopy of skin biopsies as well as immunoblot of skin extracts, increased phosphorylation of p38 and HSP27 was noted in epidermal keratinocytes from pemphigus vulgaris IgG-treated mice. Active p38 inhibitors blocked blistering in pemphigus vulgaris IgG-treated mice. When analyzed by direct immunofluorescence, pemphigus vulgaris IgG was observed bound to the keratinocytes of pemphigus vulgaris IgG-treated murine skin in the inhibitor-treated mice pointing out the p38 inhibitors did not block binding of pemphigus vulgaris IgG to the skin, but inhibited the ability of pemphigus vulgaris IgG to induce acantholysis through signaling occurring downstream of autoantibody binding. Thus, the p38 inhibitors prevented pemphigus vulgaris IgG induced blistering *in vivo* by blocking mechanistic events within the target keratinocytes that contribute to loss of cell-cell adhesion. Following studies showed that p38 and HSP27 are also activated in pemphigus foliaceus and that p38 inhibitors similarly block blistering in the pemphigus foliaceus passive transfer mouse model [338]. Importantly, pemphigus vulgaris and pemphigus foliaceus skin biopsies also show increased phosphorylation of p38 and HSP27 compared to normal controls, pointing out the activation of these signaling molecules first observed in pemphigus tissue culture and animal models also occurs in the human disease [337]. Activation of p38 in pemphigus has afterwards been remarked by other investigators [51, 385-8]. Several events have been shown to be downstream of p38 activity in the cascade of steps that contribute to loss of cell-cell adhesion; i.e., pemphigus vulgaris autoantibody binding to cell surface desmoglein 3 results in depletion of desmoglein 3 from the keratinocyte cell membrane [352], Delva et al., [389], and Calkins [390], have explained that desmoglein 3 is endocytosed, exiting from the cell membrane in a clathrin- and dynamin independent process. Detailed cell biologic experiments by this group have showed co-localization of internalized desmoglein 3 into early endosomes. Restraint of p38 blocks pemphigus vulgaris IgG-induced desmoglein 3 endocytosis suggesting that pemphigus vulgaris IgG-induced depletion of desmoglein 3 is also mediated downstream of p38 [391]. Similarly, pemphigus vulgaris IgG induces structural alterations to both the keratin intermediate filament and actin cytoskeletons, and these are also blocked by p38 inhibition [342]. In part, this may be mediated by HSP27; however, Waschke et al. [388] have provided more evidence involving RhoA control of actin in pemphigus vulgaris IgG-mediated loss of adhesion and that RhoA activity is also downstream of p38. Another second messenger that regulates events downstream of pemphigus vulgaris IgG binding to keratinocytes is cyclic adenosine monophosphate or cAMP [392]. Intracellular cAMP levels are increased by treatment of keratinocytes with pemphigus vulgaris IgG; this increment appears to be in part mediated via protein kinase A activity as a protective compensatory mechanism directed to partially attenuates the acantholytic effects of pemphigus vulgaris IgG. Pharmacologic elevation of cAMP by the β-receptor agonist isoproterenol, blocked loss of intercellular adhesion, depletion of cellular desmoglein 3, and pemphigus IgG induced cytoskeletal changes in cultured keratinocytes. cAMP may be working through p38 since elevating cAMP levels blocked pemphigus vulgaris IgG increased p38 activity in both *in vitro* and *in vivo* models.

These observations provided the mechanistic rationale to explore the use of p38 inhibitors for treating patients and led to the design and implementation of a multicenter open-label clinical trial of an oral p38 inhibitor for treating pemphigus vulgaris [393]. This non-placebo-controlled trial was successful in enrolling 15 patients with pemphigus vulgaris. Various assessment tools were utilized to measure disease activity [394-5]. Outcome measures included decreased disease activity as well as the ability to taper systemic corticosteroids during the 12-week course of the trial. Unfortunately, systemic toxicities and off-target effects of the investigational drug used in this trial limited its dosing, and the trial was terminated before completion. Targeting p38 for pemphigus vulgaris will require developing a new generation of inhibitors with better efficacy and safety profiles.

The presence or absence of adhesion requires a major shift in the biology of a cell; i. e. proliferating cells contact and form adhesive junctions with one another; they typically will stop proliferating. This is called *contact inhibition* and is a regulatory feature typically lost during malignant transformation. Analogously, the loss of cell adhesion may result in cells undergoing apoptosis, alternatively, in the context of development or wound healing, loss of adhesion could trigger migration and proliferation. Therefore, it is possible to find a complex interaction between structures that regulate and mediate cell adhesion with cellular systems that regulate such basic processes as cell growth, migration, and apoptosis.

Consistent with this, another keratinocyte signaling proteins have been identified in pemphigus. For example, plakoglobin, a component of both adherens junctions and desmosomes, have an essential role in pemphigus acantholysis. Muller et al., [396] has shown that cells lacking plakoglobin are resistant to the acantholytic effects of pemphigus vulgaris IgG.

Also, they have suggested a role for c-myc. Other signaling proteins that have been suggested to contribute to the mechanism of acantholysis include: Src kinase [397], EGFR [398], Protein kinase C [399-400], Protein kinase A (PKA) [392], Akt and mTOR [401], Cholinergic receptors [402], C-myc [11], Phospholipase C [403], Calmodulin [400]. In the following lines, we discuss the rol of apoptosis in pemphigus development.

4.2. Apoptosis

Apoptosis is a cell death characterized at the morphological level by chromatin condensation, nuclear fragmentation, and plasma membrane blebbing. The apoptotic machinery centers on the activity of various members of the caspase family. The intrinsic apoptotic pathway is mostly triggered by UV radiation and is mediated in mitochondria via the release of cytochrome C that complexes with apoptotic protease activating factor-1 that recruits and activates the initiator caspase-9, which in turn, activates caspases 3 and 7 leading to DNA fragmentation.

The extrinsic apoptotic pathway is triggered by death ligand binding to death receptors. Fas ligand or FasL recruits the initiator caspase-8, with resulting activation of the effector caspases 3 and 7 followed by DNA fragmentation [404]. Several lines of evidence indicate that apoptosis is involved in the pathomechanisms of pemphigus [405]. The first observations of apoptotic mechanisms operating in pemphigus were reported about 10 years ago and mostly overlooked [347]. In a genome-wide study using single-nucleotide polymorphism in a subpopulation of pemphigus patients has revealed a significant association of a genomic segment on chromosome 8q11.23 that spans the ST18 gene, with pemphigus [406].

Pemphigus is more common in certain groups, such as Ashkenazi Jews and those of Mediterranean origin. In particular, it is between 3-fold and 45-fold more prevalent in patients of Jewish descent, compared with other populations [407]. Sarig et al., [406] have nicely shown a significant association of ST18 gene in a Jewish and an Egyptian cohort of pemphigus patients, but not in a German group, suggesting that ST18 gene may predispose to pemphigus in a population-specific manner. Interestingly, the ST18 gene regulates apoptosis

[408] and is overexpressed in non-lesional epidermis of patients with pemphigus. This pattern of expression correlates with previous observations demonstrating TUNEL-positive cells in perilesional pemphigus skin [345], which has been interpreted as pointing out that keratinocyte apoptosis occurs before cell-to-cell detachment (acantholysis). The presence of TUNEL-positive cells both in the floor and in the roof of the blisters [409], reinforce previous statements. Interestingly, TUNEL reactivity that co-localized with nuclear fragmentation was detected in close vicinity to intraepidermal blisters by Schmidt et al., [341, 349] who consider apoptosis in pemphigus as a secondary phenomenon.

Nevertheless, more specific apoptotic markers are detected in lesional pemphigus skin before acantholysis [410] and pemphigus vulgaris IgG induces keratinocyte apoptosis *in vitro* [411] and cell detachment by enrichment in caspase 8 and activation of caspase 3 [412]. Also, caspase inhibitors prevent pemphigus vulgaris IgG-induced acantholysis *in vitro* [413]. The critical role of caspases in the pathogenesis of pemphigus is further confirmed by the use of caspase 3 and 7 as well as by pan-caspase inhibitors that protect mice from developing blisters induced in the passive transfer pemphigus mouse model by pemphigus foliaceus IgG [344]. Pacheco-Tovar et al., [414] showed that pemphigus vulgaris IgG induces apoptosis in perilesional keratinocytes before acantholysis, while the pan-caspase inhibitor prevents blister formation. Besides autoantibodies, pemphigus serum contains non-IgG substances that can cause a sharp reduction of keratinocyte viability and weaken intercellular adhesion strength [415].

The serum factors involved in pemphigus pathomechanisms include TNFα [416], nitric oxide [417], kallikreins [418], and anti-mitochondrial antibodies [51]. The latter factors are pathogenic and induce the release of cytochrome C, suggesting to involve the intrinsic apoptotic pathway in pemphigus. This is related to the observation that intravenous immunoglobulin, an effective treatment in pemphigus, upregulates serum level of the "inhibitor of apoptosis" proteins or IAPs, that in turn block the caspase 9/mitochondrial pathway [419]. Recent evidence points to the Fas/FasL system as key pathway for pemphigus pathogenesis [58]. Indeed, FasL and Fas are significantly increased in sera from pemphigus patients [420]. Original immunohistochemical studies revealed Fas receptor on keratinocyte membranes of pemphigus lesional epidermis [421] FasL contained in pemphigus sera induces apoptosis in normal human keratinocytes, via caspase-8 activation [347]. In addition, pemphigus vulgaris IgG treatment induces an mRNA upregulation of proapoptotic molecules in keratinocytes, including FasL [422], and the secretion from cells of soluble FasL. This is an important fact since pemphigus vulgaris IgG treatment induces a co-aggregation of FasL and Fas receptor with caspase-8 [413]. FasL acts synergistically with pemphigus vulgaris IgG and TNFα in inducting acantholysis in an organ culture model of pemphigus [423].

Neutralization of FasL prevents caspase-8 activation and decreases the number of apoptotic cells after treatment of keratinocytes with pemphigus sera [347]. Anti-FasL neutralizing antibody protects desmogleins from caspase-induced cleavage, thus preventing pemphigus vulgaris IgG-induced acantholysis. Also, anti-FasL inhibits the pemphigus vulgaris IgG-induced activation of caspase 8 [405].

These observations defined a role for apoptosis in the pathogenesis of blistering in pemphigus, time course studies in both *in vitro* and *in vivo* pemphigus models suggest that apoptosis may not be a primary event, but a secondary one that may contribute to blistering by sensitizing cells to the acantholytic effects of pemphigus IgG [342]. In pemphigus tissue culture and mouse models, two peaks of p38 activation have been reported, (1) an early peak that occurs within minutes of exposure to pemphigus vulgaris IgG and is activated by binding of pemphigus vulgaris IgG to desmoglein; and (2) a second late peak occurring hours after exposure to pemphigus vulgaris IgG that represents stress response signaling secondary to pemphigus vulgaris IgG-induced adhesive changes. Giving p38 inhibitors before pemphigus IgG injection blocked both peaks of p38 phosphorylation and blister formation; however, administration of the inhibitor after the first peak, but before the second peak of p38 activity, blocked only the later peak of p38 activation and failed to block blistering. Examination of the temporary relationship of p38 phosphorylation and apoptosis showed that apoptosis occurs at or after the second peak of p38 activation. The time course of p38 activation and apoptotic markers as well as the ability of inhibitors of p38 to block activation of the proapoptotic proteinase caspase-3 suggest that activation of apoptosis is downstream to, and a result of p38 activation in pemphigus acantholysis. Further, we may assume the earlier peak of p38 activation is an important part of the mechanism leading to acantholysis; whereas, the later peak of p38 and apoptosis may not be essential for acantholysis and thus, the blistering process. The observation the activation of proapoptotic pathways is a late event and may not be essential for blistering in pemphigus does not exclude the possibility that activation of components of apoptotic signaling, including caspase family member proteinases, could augment the blistering response as downstream effects of p38 activation. This is supported by the observations that in staphylococcal scalded skin syndrome, direct proteolysis of the desmoglein 1 ectodomain induces loss of cell-cell adhesion [424]. Also, caspase inhibitors block pemphigus IgG-induced acantholysis in the passive transfer mouse model [344]. Parts of the desmosome including desmoglein 3, 1, plakoglobin, and desmoplakin, as well as intermediate filaments [344, 424], have all been shown to undergo caspase-dependent cleavage suggesting that caspase-dependent proteolysis may disrupt these structures, weakening cell adhesion and augmenting the pathogenic response in pemphigus. Although induction of apoptosis may be a secondary response in the mechanism of acantholysis, blocking caspase-dependent desmoglein degradation may augment cell-cell adhesion and decrease keratinocyte sensitivity to the acantholytic effects of pathogenic pemphigus IgG.

Finally, several theories have tried to explain the mechanism by which pemphigus IgG induced loss of adhesion, including steric hindrance, activation of proteolysis, and signaling. These are not mutually exclusive, but complimentary for acantholysis. Pemphigus vulgaris IgG likely acts as competitive inhibitor for endogenous homophilic and/or heterophilic desmoglein binding at the EC1/EC2 extracellular domains. Disrupting endogenous desmoglein molecular interactions (steric hindrance) activates a variety of intracellular signaling events, including p38 and HSP27 phosphorylation that lead to desmoglein endocytosis and reorganization of the keratin intermediate filament and actin cytoskeletons (signaling). Because of changes in the cellular adhesive structures, some keratinocytes undergo apoptosis, activating and releasing proteolytic enzymes (proteolysis) including caspases and metalloproteinases that have the potential to digest desmoglein and other components of the desmosome adhesion complex on alongside cells, further weakening and/or disrupting cell-cell adhesion.

Targeting many of these components can antagonize the acantholytic effects of pemphigus vulgaris IgG providing multiple potential targets for blocking blistering in this life-threatening autoimmune disease.

4.3. APOPTOLYSIS

The term "apoptolysis" links the basal cell shrinkage to suprabasal acantholysis and cell death, and highlights that apoptotic enzymes contribute to acantholysis in molecular events. (Figure 6) It postulates that cell detachment and death in pemphigus vulgaris develop through the following five major steps: (1) binding of pathogenic antibodies to keratinocytes by a receptor-ligand sends an array of the agonist- and antagonist-like signals; (2) activation of signaling elements (Src, EGFRK, p38 MAPK, mTOR) downstream of ligated pemphigus vulgaris antigens and elevation of intracellular Ca^{2+}, altogether, initiate cell death enzymatic cascades; (3) suprabasal acantholysis starts when basal cells shrink due to reorganization of cortical actin filaments, collapse and retraction of the tonofilaments cleaved by executioner caspases, as well as dissociation and internalization of intercellular adhesion complexes caused by phosphorylation of adhesion molecules and their cleavage by caspases; (4) acantholysis advances due to continued degradation and massive collapse of structural proteins by the same cell death enzymes, leading to separation and rending of preexisting desmosomes from the cell membrane by shear forces, thus separating the collapsing cells and stimulating production of secondary (scavenging) antibodies; (5) rounding up and death of acantholytic cells in the lower epidermal compartment follows irreversible damage of mitochondrial and nuclear proteins [49].

The mechanism of apoptolysis in pemphigus vulgaris encompasses several tiers of events triggered through distinct antigen-antibody systems. Because apoptolysis develops in a stepwise fashion, late morphologic features of apoptosis, such as rounding up, nuclear fragmentation, and plasma membrane blebbing, do not become clear until the keratinocyte death in the last step. Signaling mechanisms may vary from patient to patient because a unique composition of the pool of autoantibodies determines the principal pathway. The desmoglein 3-dependent late peak of p38 MAPK activity and activation of JNK represent the pathways mediating processing and use of internalized desmoglein 3, rather than a primary downstream signaling emanating from the cell membrane. The theory has several important implications: (1) it links several seemingly unrelated, and previously held contradictory, observations on the events surrounding acantholysis; (2) it opens new avenues of investigation into the pathomechanism of pemphigus; and (3) it creates new approaches to treat pemphigus based on interfering with or blocking the signaling pathways and enzymatic processes that lead to blistering [49].

Chapter 5

GENETIC AND ENVIRONMENTAL RISK FACTORS OF PEMPHIGUS

5.1. GENETIC SUSCEPTIBILITY

Many studies provide support for the importance of genetic factors in pemphigus vulgaris [425-6]. As for many autoimmune conditions, several lines of evidence make a compelling argument for a complex, polygenic basis for disease involving multiple, but an unknown number of genetic loci, as well as non-genetic factors. The strong linkage disequilibrium within the HLA genetic region on chromosome 6 has placed barriers to the clear description of disease-associated alleles. Genetic and non-genetic/environmental elements are believed to contribute to the dysregulation of normal immune tolerance that lastly leads to develop autoimmunity in the skin. The full complement of susceptibility loci remains unidentified, and it is not possible to identify individuals at risk. The overall prevalence and incidence of pemphigus is low, but it varies significantly in various ethnic populations (Table 1).

Table 1. MHC genes identified in pemphigus vulgaris and foliaceous

Population	Alleles Pemphigus vulgaris	Alleles Pemphigus foliaceous
Ashkenazi jews	DR4, DQw8	
French	DRB1*0402, 1401; DQB1*0302; 0503	DRB1*0404; DRB1*0102
Indians	DRB1*1404; DRB1*0202; DQA1*0101; DQB1*0503	
Italians	DRB1*0402, DRB1*1401; DQB1*0503	DRB1*04; DRB1*1404; DQB1*0503
Sardinians	DRB1*0402; DQA1*0301; DQB1*0302	
Pakistani	DRB1*1404; DQA1*0101; DQB1*0503	
Spanish	DRB1*0402, 1401; DQB1*0503, 0302	
US	DR4	
Japanese	DRB1*0403, 0406; DRB1*1401, 1405, 1406	DRB1*04; DRB1*0403, *0406; DRB1*14; DRB1*1401, *1405, *1406
Brazilians		DRB1*0102, *0404, *0406; DRB1*1406, *1602
Tunisians		DR4

Molecular sequencing and genotyping methods have provided the strongest evidence for DRB1*0402 and DQB1*0503 as pemphigus vulgaris risk alleles [155, 427-9], over 95% of non-Asian pemphigus vulgaris patients type as such. A meta-analysis identified 18 studies on the association of pemphigus vulgaris with alleles of the HLA-DRB1 gene. The frequencies of three genotypes, DRB1*04 (odds ratio 3.6), DRB1*08 (odds ratio 2.3) and DRB1*14 (odds ratio 6.5), were significantly increased in pemphigus vulgaris. Three other alleles, DRB1*03 (odds ratio 0.28), DRB1*07(odds ratio 0.45) and DRB1*15 (odds ratio 0.35), were significantly decreased [430]. Most recently, HLA-E*0103, a non-classical class IB allele, has been linked to pemphigus vulgaris susceptibility [431]. It remains to be determined the extent to which the HLA genotype affects the specificity of the autoimmune response within individual patients and in turn affects clinical phenotype and therapeutic response to given medications.

A north-south gradient has previously been observed in type 1 diabetes mellitus and multiple sclerosis and has been suggested to be related to the relative dominance of Th1-type versus Th2-type pathogens in particular geographic locations. It remains to be determined how specific genetic and environmental factors influence developing pemphigus vulgaris across the globe. Similarly, the literature and our own studies point out a female predominance in pemphigus vulgaris, as is often reported in autoimmune conditions. The female/male ratio ranges from 1.1:1 to 2.25:1 [425]. This female bias can be interpreted as evidence for the role of genetics in disease.

Nongenetic mechanisms may be involved, influencing the expression of pemphigus vulgaris in women rather than men. For several autoimmune conditions, twin and adoption studies have been able to provide strong evidence for genetic susceptibility [425]. Future work aimed at more precisely linking HLA genetic profiles to a patient's clinical profile will be important to advance towards the path of personalized medicine.

An association of pemphigus vulgaris with a non-HLA marker, encoding for the pro-apoptotic molecule ST18, has also been recently identified [406]. Taking advantage of the relatively high prevalence of the disease among Jewish populations; Sarig et al., [406] conducted the first genome-wide association study in pemphigus vulgaris. Besides the major histocompatibility complex locus, a genomic segmenton 8q11.23 that spans the *ST18* gene was also found to be significantly associated with pemphigus vulgaris. This association was confirmed in an independent Jewish group of patients as well as in an Egyptian replication set but not in a German patient sample, suggesting that *ST18* -associated variants may predispose to pemphigus vulgaris in a population-specific manner and, thereby, contribute to population specific differences in pemphigus vulgaris prevalence. ST18 regulates apoptosis and inflammation, two processes of direct relevance to the pathogenesis of pemphigus vulgaris [408]. Further supporting the relevance of ST18 to pemphigus vulgaris, this gene was found to be overexpressed in the skin of pemphigus vulgaris patients as compared with healthy individuals [406]. Non-endemic pemphigus foliaceus is predominantly associated with HLA-DRB1*04 and DRB1*14. Carriers of the TNFα polymorphic are found more frequently in pemphigus foliaceus (odds ratio 8.1) [432]. In France, paraneoplastic pemphigus was strongly associated with the DRB1*03 allele [433]. In Chinese patients, the disease seems associated with HLA-Cw*14 irrespective of the underlying tumour [434].

The comparison of concordance rates among monozygotic versus dizygotic individuals allows a focus on the relative contribution of genetic risk to disease. However, because largescale population-based assessments are required and the prevalence of pemphigus vulgaris is low, twin and/or adoption studies are not available [425]. Additional support for the genetic basis of disease comes from the increased incidence of autoimmunity in blood relatives of autoimmune patients [435-7]. In one survey of 171 patients with pemphigus, it was found that 48% reported having one or more relatives with autoimmune disease. Type 1 diabetes was reported most commonly, followed by autoimmune thyroid disease. Pemphigus itself was reported less commonly, occurring in the relatives of 2.9% of patients. Although family cases of pemphigus vulgaris have been cited in the literature [438-41], this seems to be rare. Multiple pemphigus vulgaris cases within families are most likely to occur in first-degree relatives. There is a significantly higher incidence of all autoimmune diseases in first degree relatives of patients with pemphigus vulgaris compared to second-degree and third-degree relatives. These findings, in which autoimmunity correlates more strongly with an increased genetic commonality (first > second > third degree), strongly support the genetic basis of the disease. However, the influence of environmental factors cannot be ruled out.

Genetic-based tools are likely to provide a scientific rationale behind future clinical decision making by physicians and facilitate the implementation of individually tailored therapy.

5.2. Environmental Risk Factors

Various environmental and pharmacologic risk factors have been reported in pemphigus. These factors include medications, pesticides, malignancy, ultraviolet radiation, and stress [442-9]. Foods containing an allium, phenol, thiol, or urushiol group have also been reported to trigger pemphigus [450-1]. Non-thiol drugs such as cephalosporins are also among the drugs which may induce or worsen pemphigus vulgaris.

Drug-induced pemphigus is a well-recognized complication (Table 2). While in the past most cases of drug-induced pemphigus were associated with penicillamine, various other drugs have been implicated in recent decades. Some of these drugs are thought to induce pemphigus via the same immunological mechanisms that are found in primary pemphigus.

Other drugs are postulated to cause acantholysis directly, through biochemical processes. A combination of both mechanisms may be involved in many cases of drug-induced pemphigus. Pemphigus-inducing drugs can be broadly divided in two categories: thiol and non-thiol drugs.

Thiol drugs contain a sulfhydryl group (-SH) in their chemical structure and are the commonest cause of drug-induced pemphigus. Penicillamine and the angiotensin-converting enzyme inhibitor captopril, both drugs that contain a thiol group, are the most often reported culprits [445, 452-3]. About 7% of patients treated with penicillamine for at least 6 months develop pemphigus. The sulfhydryl groups have been speculated to interact with desmogleins, increasing their antigenicity and leading to autoantibody production. Thiol drugs have also been shown to induce acantholysis *in vitro* without antibody formation. The potential mechanisms for thiol-induced direct acantholysis include restraint of enzymes of keratinocyte aggregation, disruption of cell adhesion by thiol–cysteine bonds and activation of proteolytic enzymes such as plasminogen activators.

Table 2. Drugs implicated in pemphigus

Thiol (SH) drugs	Non-thiol drugs		
D-penicillamine	Phenol drugs	Pyrazolone derivatives	Other
Bucillamine	Rifampicin	Oxyphenbutazone	Penicillins
Captopril	Cephalosporin	Aminopyrine	Quinolones
Gold sodium thiomalate	Aspirin	Azapropazone	ACE inhibitors
Thiopronine	Levodopa	Phenylbutazone	Angiotensin II receptor blockers
Piroxicam	Progesterone	Aminophenazone	Phenytoin
Carbimazole	Heroin		Carbamazepin
Methimazole	Phenobarbital		NSAIDS
5-thiophyridoxine	Pentachlorophenol		Chloroquine/ hydroxychloroquine
Pyritinol			Montelukast
Mercaptopropionylglycine			Interferon a, b
			Nifedipine
			Propranolol
			Glibenclamide
			Isotretinoin
			Imiquimod

Non-thiol drugs associated with pemphigus include penicillins, cephalosporins and angiotensin-converting enzyme inhibitors other than captopril. Additional drugs have been recently reported to induce pemphigus, for instance, angiotensin II receptor blockers, anticonvulsants and glibenclamide. Some non-thiol drugs, such as penicillins and piroxicam, have sulphur in their chemical structure, which may be metabolized *in vivo* to form thiols. These are termed masked thiols, and their mechanism of acantholysis may be similar to thiol drugs [445]. Other non-thiol drugs contain phenol groups, for example, levodopa and rifampicin. Phenol drugs have been postulated to induce acantholysis by causing release of cytokines (TNF-α, IL-1) from keratinocytes, which participate in the regulation and synthesis of complement and proteases. An active amide group is also found in the structure of many non-thiol drugs, and its role in the pathogenesis of drug-induced pemphigus has not been elucidated. Non-thiol drugs are more likely to induce pemphigus via immunological mechanisms. Studies have shown the presence of antibodies to pemphigus antigens, desmoglein 3 and desmoglein 1, in most cases of thiol and non-thiol-induced pemphigus; however, 4–5% of rheumatoid arthritis patients treated with thiol compounds produce antibodies to non-conformational epitopes of desmoglein 1 or 3 without developing pemphigus, suggesting that such antibodies alone are not enough to induce acantholysis [454].

Whereas in patients who had received thiol compounds pemphigus foliaceus predominates and the pemphigus disease remitted spontaneously in up to 50%, only 15% of cases induced by other drugs showed spontaneous recovery, most of them were pemphigus vulgaris [453]. Recently, a reversible relapse in a patient with pemphigus foliaceus was observed in an area treated with topical imiquimod for superficial basal cell carcinoma [455].

This case points to a role of local inflammatory mediators such as various cytokines in the development of pemphigus lesions.

Patients with drug-induced pemphigus have been found to carry the same susceptibility alleles HLA-DR4 that are thought to predispose to primary pemphigus vulgaris, thus, drugs are capable of triggering pemphigus in genetically susceptible individuals. Drug-induced pemphigus usually begins a few weeks to several months after initiation of an offending agent, although the onset of pemphigus after 6 years of anticonvulsant therapy has been described [456]. The latency period may be much shorter on repeat exposure to the culprit drug.

Two controlled studies identified exposure to pesticides and metal vapour [444] and history of smoking as risk factor for pemphigus [457]. A case report and two retrospective studies suggest that smoking affects pemphigus development and healing of lesions. Smokers respond faster to treatment when compared with nonsmokers. Furthermore, the percentage of smokers and ex-smokers (15%) among pemphigus patients is lower when compared to the general population (47%) [458-60]. The impact of nicotine, a cholinergic agonist, in pemphigus may be explained by the observation that cholinergic agonists are able to reduce pemphigus vulgaris IgG autoantibody-induced acantholysis *in vitro* [461]. Interestingly, while smoking increases the exacerbation risk in most autoimmune conditions, current smokers have a reduced risk for Behcet's disease and aphthous stomatitis [462]. Furthermore, stressful life events were common in pemphigus patients [463]. In a multicenter case-control study in Tunisia, traditional cosmetics, Turkish baths, cutting raw poultry, contact with ruminants and wasp, bee and spider stings were found to be associated with an increased risk for pemphigus [464]. Finally, pemphigus has been anecdotally described after exposure to ultraviolet light, ionizing radiation, burns and surgery [465]. A role for dietary factors has also been claimed [466]

On the other hand, Brazilian pemphigus, also called pemphigus brasiliensis and *fogo selvagem*, occurs in some subtropical areas of Brazil, as well as in northern Colombia. Data have been extensively collected in the Limao Verde Amerindian reservation in the state of *Mato Grosso do Sul*. Most patients affected by *fogo selvagem* are young adults and children, live in forest areas near rivers and streams and are outdoor workers (farmers or their family members). Most patients live in poor hygiene and housing conditions. The decreased prevalence of *fogo selvagem* in Sao Paulo and Parana was linked to improved living conditions [467-8]. A strong association has been proven between the occurrence of *fogo selvagem* and the infestation of the similar areas with some insects including *Simuliids* (also called black fly) with the greatest number of new cases at the end of the rainy season [285]. The same ecological system found in the pemphigus area overlaps with that for vector-borne diseases such as Chagas disease, leishmaniasis and onchocerciasis.

Anti-desmoglein 1 antibodies are often detectable in normal subjects living in these endemic areas, in which a significant proportion of patients also had onchocerciasis and leishmaniasis.

This temporary and geographic clustering suggests there is an environmental triggering antigen(s) showing molecular mimicry with desmoglein 1 [469]. There is some evidence suggesting the anti-desmoglein 1 response in *fogo selvagem* patients living in endemic regions of Brazil is antigen selected [281]. In individuals with the known HLA susceptibility allele and living in endemic areas, the development of *fogo selvagem* is associated with a subclass switch of the IgG antibody response (from the IgG 1, 2 and 3 subclasses to the IgG4 subclass) as well as with a change of the antibody reactivity (epitope spreading with development of a reactivity from the EC5 domains of desmoglein 1 to the EC1 and EC2 domains) [282, 312, 470]. A strong association of *fogo selvagem* with HLA-DRB1*1402 and DRB1*04040 was identified [471].

Tunisian pemphigus, an endemic type of pemphigus foliaceus is also associated with poor economic conditions [472]. Some familial cases have been described [473]. Similar to pemphigus brasiliensis, a high prevalence of anti-desmoglein 1 antibodies has been reported in people living in endemic areas, as well as among people genetically related or unrelated to the patient [474-5]. Interestingly, the highest prevalence of antidesmoglein1 antibodies in the healthy relatives (up to 22%) was observed in the rural localities. As observed in Brazil, a high prevalence of antidesmoglein1 antibodies in sera from patients with hydatidosis and leishmaniasis (but not-affected by pemphigus) has been described [476-7]. Antibodies against *P. papatasi*, the main vector of *Leishmania major* leading to cutaneous leishmaniasis, have also been found in 25% of pemphigus foliaceus patients but only in 6 and 3% of healthy controls and patients with bullous pemphigoid [477].

A significant case–control study investigating potential environmental factors contributing to pemphigus was a multicentre study conducted in Bulgaria, Brazil, India, Israel, Italy, Spain and the United States [444]. Involving 126 pemphigus patients and 173 controls from the dermatology outpatient clinics of participating hospitals; the study showed a lower rate of current or past smokers among pemphigus patients; supporting a previous clinical report which suggested that smoking was beneficial for lowering the risk of developing pemphigus [459]. Although there were some variations in environmental factors between countries, overall, exposure to gardening materials, pesticides, metal vapour, chronic wounds, drug reactions and pregnancies were significantly greater in the pemphigus group. However, despite having a greater variability in subjects due to the multicentre design, the study had a relatively poor ratio of approximately 1.37 controls *per case*. Furthermore, the controls chosen were consecutive dermatology outpatients of the participating hospitals, where attendances depend on the nature of the patient pool; and thus increasing selection bias. Additionally, due to the multicentre approach, a single interviewer could not survey all subjects, adding to observer bias. The inverse relationship between the prevalence of smoking and pemphigus was also noted in an Iranian study. The study involving 210 pemphigus patients and 205 controls of Razi Hospital revealed a higher proportion of smokers in the control group (17.1% of cases vs. 27.3% of controls). Total duration of smoking and the mean number of cigarettes smoked *per day* were also significantly lower in controls. Furthermore, oral contraceptive use was significantly higher in women with pemphigus (43.8%) than matched controls (30.5%) with an odds ratio of 1.78, while pesticide exposure was significantly greater in pemphigus cases (14.8%) than controls (5.4%) with an odds ratio of 3.06 [457]. Although this study had many patients, there were not enough controls to match them, with a control-to-case ratio of around 0.98: 1. The controls themselves had dermatological problems other than bullous disorders, and were only age and gender matched to the cases. *Fogo selvagem*, the endemic form of pemphigus foliaceous in Brazil, was found to be associated with black fly bites in a hospital-based study of 52 *fogo selvagem* patients and 52 controls (odds ratio 4.7) [478]. A more recent and larger population-based study of 30 *fogo selvagem* cases, 108 community controls and 90 family controls supported this association; and further added kissing bug and bed bug bites as potential risk factors for *fogo selvagem*. The study also found that rustic houses with thatched roofs, adobe walls and poorly fitted doors were significantly more common among pemphigus patients [479].

As for endemic Tunisian pemphigus, a multicentre study found that Turkish baths, traditional Tunisian cosmetics, cutting raw poultry, contact with ruminants and insect stings were possible risk factors [464]. This study involved all dermatological departments of Tunisia and had a relatively high control-to-case ratio of 2.37: 1.

Further environmental and occupational factors found to be associated with pemphigus in other case-control studies include high UV exposure, high consumption of spices, low vitamin D levels and low serum zinc and copper [480-1]. The results of these studies, however, are statistically powerless and inconclusive due to their small sample sizes.

The human herpesvirus type 8 or HHV-8 has been found to be positively associated with pemphigus in an Iranian case-control study of 41 pemphigus patients (37 with pemphigus vulgaris, 4 with pemphigus foliaceous) and 21 age- and sex-matched cosmetic surgery patients (HHV-8 was present in 36.6% of pemphigus vulgaris cases and 50% of pemphigus foliaceous cases vs. 0% of controls) [482]. Another Iranian study of 24 pemphigus vulgaris cases and 24 healthy controls matched by age and sex showed a positive correlation between elevated serum prolactin levels and pemphigus vulgaris (mean serum prolactin level of 21.66 ng/mL in cases compared to 11.38 ng/mL in controls) [483]. However, both of these studies were statistically weak due to small sample sizes and poor control-to-case ratios.

An Israeli study of 255 pemphigus patients and 509 controls (age and sex matched) over 20 years-old, revealed a diagnosis of dyslipidaemia in 65.5% of patients versus 47.8% among the controls [484] However, the observed dyslipidaemia was predominantly caused by the corticosteroid treatment, not solely pemphigus itself [485]. Other factors that were investigated by case–control studies but showed no significant associations with pemphigus include autoimmune thyroid disease, Coxsackie virus infection and raised or decreased serum leptin level [486-8].

The skin, nervous system, and immune system are interconnected, and functionally represent a unique system, which can well account for a pathogenic link between an intensive emotional stress and the onset (or the worsening) of an autoimmune skin disorder. Several cases of pemphigus vulgaris triggered by emotional stress have been reported [444, 448]. The stressing events more often associated were environmental disasters, partner's or near relative's death, separation from partner, sexual aggression or sex-related disturbance [444]. In each case, these events had been lived in an emotional way.

The role of psychological stress in triggering pemphigus vulgaris is still underestimated and, in most cases of seemingly spontaneous pemphigus vulgaris, both patient and doctor overlook the intervention of an emotional precipitating factor. A recent study has shown that stress can play a triggering part in pemphigus apart from any underlying personality disorders [463]. Therefore, these events can be pathogenically interconnected: emotional stress and outbreak or worsening of pemphigus vulgaris.

The possible intervention of the environment in the outbreak of pemphigus is far more perceived by clinicians. In fact, there are some reports of induced or triggered pemphigus claiming more than one environmental factor as causal or precipitating agent (eg, penicillamine and captopril acting simultaneously) [445], two viral infections (common cold and herpes simplex labialis) treated with a combination drug composed of paracetamol, caffeine, chlorpheniramine maleate and phenylephrine HCl [445], surgical trauma and sunbathing occurring in different times, concurring action of sun-bathing [449], aspirin, other

NSAIDs, and progesterone, combined effect of contact dermatitis and sun exposure [446]. It is also of note that several drugs that are able to induce pemphigus share an active amide group in their molecule [453], which might lead to considering further pathomechanisms of induction.

Probably, in the future, the more patients' clinical history and laboratory investigations (aimed at the search for possible environmental-inducing factors) are meticulous and exhaustive, the fewer cases of spontaneous pemphigus will be found. Even today, the assumption that genetic factors alone are not enough to provoke the outbreak of pemphigus; inevitably raises a provocative question: Does spontaneous pemphigus exist or is the outbreak of the disease always a result of an interaction between an individual pemphigus-prone genetic background and environmental-inducing agents, often hidden or seemingly harmless such as diet ingredients or emotional stress?

We think that a thorough investigation on induced or triggered pemphigus aimed at detecting environmental provoking or precipitating factors and relative pathogenic mechanisms, is of the utmost importance for both speculative and practical purposes.

No case-control studies were found studying the potential link between pemphigus and drugs. Therefore, a case-control study with a powerful design addressing this issue would contribute to our understanding of what begins pemphigus vulgaris.

PART 3. EPIDEMIOLOGY

Chapter 6

EPIDEMIOLOGY OF PEMPHIGUS

Autoimmune bullous diseases comprise a large group of potential devastating diseases, which also differ in their epidemiological characteristics. Recent high-quality epidemiological studies have provided valuable new knowledge in this broad area.

The incidence of various autoimmune conditions, e.g., type I diabetes mellitus, multiple sclerosis, and systemic lupus erythematosus, varies considerably between different geographical regions. The latter observation cannot be explained by simple ethnic and genetic differences alone [489]. In this context, the emerging field of preclinical epidemiology addresses the result of autoantibody-bearing individuals without clinical disease, by providing new relevant information about the interplay of genetic and environmental predisposing factors. For example, the relevance of preclinical epidemiology studies has been shown in systemic lupus erythematosus [490], as well as in other autoimmune diseases, such as endemic pemphigus foliaceus [62, 282, 312, 491].

6.1. PEMPHIGUS VULGARIS

Pemphigus vulgaris and pemphigus foliaceus are the two major types of pemphigus. The first one is associated with mucocutaneous lesions with an immune response directed against desmoglein 3 and eventually desmoglein 1, while in pemphigus foliaceus, involvement is restricted to the skin and circulating autoantibodies are directed against desmoglein 1 [492]. The relative incidence of pemphigus vulgaris and foliaceus within a population varies in different countries with the relative frequency of pemphigus vulgaris ranging between 92% (in India) and 13% (in Mali) [493-508]. The high incidence of pemphigus foliaceus in well-defined areas of South America and North Africa (such as Tunisia and neighboring countries) is reflected by the endemic variants of pemphigus foliaceous that are discussed further.

6.1.1. Incidence

Pemphigus is a rare disease and the incidence differs between different populations. Pemphigus vulgaris occurs with a worldwide incidence of 0.1–0.5 *per* 100,000 populations and is higher in Middle Eastern populations and their descendants [509]. It ranges from 0.6 to

0.76 per million *per year* in Switzerland and Finland to 8.0 and 10.0 in Greece and Iran [510-2]. The highest incidences, 16.1 and 32/million/year, were found in the Jewish population [513-24]. The variability is most likely explained by different genetic backgrounds and trigger factors. In addition, data quality of most epidemiological studies is hampered by their retrospective design and the inability to define the study populations, i.e., to ensure that all patients within a certain area are included. The latter shortcoming does not apply for three recent studies from Switzerland, the UK, and Taiwan that reported incidences of 0.6, 6.8, and 4.7/million/year, respectively [511, 522-3]. Limitations of the latter studies, however, include the relatively low number of pemphigus patients in the Swiss study and the use of a general practitioner-based registry that may have included inadequately diagnosed patients in the UK population [525].

In India, Malaysia, China, and the Middle East (particularly Iran), pemphigus vulgaris accounts for 70% of all pemphigus cases and may be the most common autoimmune blistering disease [495, 516, 526]. While the prevalence of pemphigus vulgaris in men and women is thought to be roughly equal [527-8], some data show that pemphigus vulgaris may affect women more than men [506, 529]. The average age at the onset is between the fourth and sixth decades but can also arise in children and older people [523, 529-30].

6.1.2. Mortality

Mortality of pemphigus vulgaris and foliaceus has been dramatically reduced with corticosteroids in the early 1950s from 75 to 30% [531]. The adjuvant use of immunosuppressants in the 1980s probably contributed to the further decrease in mortality to below 5% of the study populations and 0.021 *per* 100,000 inhabitants of the USA [531-3]. In two recent studies from the UK and Taiwan, the risk of death was calculated to be two- to three-fold higher compared to the control population [532-3]. Infections, in particular pneumonia and septicemia, were the most frequent causes of death in different study populations [533-4]. Cardiovascular diseases and peptic ulcer disease were also significant reasons for death compared to the control population [533].

6.1.3. Associated Diseases

In two controlled studies an increased association of pemphigus was found with autoimmune thyroid disease and rheumatoid arthritis [535]. A case-control study revealed a higher incidence of autoimmune diseases in first-degree family members of pemphigus vulgaris patients [535]. A dramatically higher percentage of osteoporosis was diagnosed in pemphigus patients (40%) compared to controls (6.5%) [536], highlighting the importance of surveying affected patients. This notion was confirmed in a controlled study in patients with immunobullous disorders, including pemphigus [537].

6.2. Endemic Pemphigus (Brazilian Pemphigus)

Brazilian pemphigus, also called pemphigus braziliensis and *fogo selvagem*, occurs in some subtropical areas of Brazil, as well as in Northern Colombia [538]. Data have been extensively collected in the Limao Verde Amerindian reservation in the state of Mato Grosso do Sul. Most patients affected by *fogo selvagem* are young adults and children, live in forest areas near rivers and streams, and are outdoor workers (farmers or their family members). The prevalence of the disease in this population is between 3 and 5% [539]. There is no sex or racial tendency. Most patients live in poor hygiene and housing conditions. The decreased prevalence of *fogo selvagem* in Sao Paulo and Parana was linked to improved living conditions [468, 539].

The existence of other foci of endemic pemphigus foliaceus has been reported in the El Bagre area in Northern Columbia [540]. Patients affected with the disease also lived in rural areas. However, most of endemic pemphigus foliaceus patients are men (95%). Similar to the braziliensis type, most patients with the called Columbian pemphigus are illiterate and poor and perform outdoor activities. The prevalence of the disease among the rural population is close to 5% [540]. The significance of the presence of autoantibodies against the neural and cardiac antigens in El Bagre in pemphigus foliaceus patients remains unclear [541-2].

Endemic Tunisian pemphigus mainly occurs in the southern area of Tunisia, in Algeria, Morocco, as well as in some sub-Saharan countries, such as Mali [499]. Overall, the incidence of Tunisian pemphigus is six to seven cases *per million* inhabitants *per year*. However, this incidence increases up to 20 cases *per million* inhabitants *per year* in some areas of South Tunisia, in particular in young adult women. Indeed, a predominance of cases among women aged 25–34 years has been described [517].

6.3. Paraneoplastic Pemphigus

Paraneoplastic pemphigus is a rare syndrome [543-4], invariably associated with a neoplasm [290]. While in Chinese patients, Castleman's disease is the predominate underlying neoplasm, in Europe, Japan, and the USA, non-Hodgkin's lymphoma and chronic lymphocytic leukemia account for about two third of the neoplasms followed by Castleman's disease, thymoma, and other diseases [545-6].

In general, the prognosis of paraneoplastic pemphigus is poor with a mortality rate approaching 90%. The prognosis is better when the disease is associated with benign tumors and may even remit when tumors such as thymoma and Castleman disease are excised. The outcome of paraneoplastic pemphigus, however, does not simply parallel the course of the underlying malignancy. Complications resulting from paraneoplastic pemphigus and its treatment contribute significantly to morbidity and mortality. Death usually results from complications of the disease or treatment, such as sepsis, multi-organ failure, gastrointestinal haemorrhage and respiratory failure (from bronchiolitis obliterans) [544]. The occurrence of bronchiolitis obliterans heralds a poor prognosis. Pulmonary involvement occurs in 30 to 92.8% of patients and it is estimated that one-third of the deaths in paraneoplastic pemphigus are due to pulmonary insufficiency. It is known that constrictive bronchiolitis can continue to worsen despite improvement in mucocutaneous manifestations after immunosuppressive therapy and resection of tumour [544].

PART 4. CLINICAL PRESENTATION OF PEMPHIGUS

Chapter 7

CLINICAL PRESENTATION OF PEMPHIGUS VULGARIS

Pemphigus, the term derived from the Greek word *pemphix,* meaning bubble or blister, is a rare, chronic, life-threatening autoimmune blistering disease characterized by intraepithelial blister formation [181, 359, 547]. Damage to intercellular adhesion structures, desmogleins, is the target of circulating IgG (and occasionally, IgA) autoantibodies resulting in the hallmark of this condition, acantholysis [256, 548]. Pemphigus can be divided into four major types: vulgaris, foliaceus, paraneoplastic, and IgA pemphigus (Table 3); pemphigus vulgaris is the commonest type of pemphigus [41-2]. In pemphigus vulgaris, the blister occurs above the basal layer in the deep part of the epidermis [62].

Table 3. Clinical classification of pemphigus

Main type	Subtype	Autoantigen
Pemphigus vulgaris		Dsg 3, 1 (Dsg 4), acetylcholine receptor. Dsc 1-3.
Pemphigus vegetans	Type Neumann	Dsg 3, 1, Dsc 3.
	Type Hallopeau	Dsg 3, 1, Dsc 3
Pemphigus herpetiformis		Dsg 1 (Dsg 3)
Pemphigus foliaceous	Pemphigus seborrheicus	Dsg 1 (Dsg 4), plakoglobin
	Endemic form (Fogo selvagem)	Dsg 1
	Pemphigus erythematosus (Senear Usher)	Dsg 1 and lupus-type antigens
Paraneoplastic pemphigus		Dsg 3, 1, desmoplakin 1, 2, envoplakin, periplakin, A2ML1 (170kDa protein), plektin, Dsc 1-3, BP230.
Drug-induced pemphigus		Dsg 1 (Dsg 3)
IgA pemphigus	Subcorneal pustular dermatosis type	Dsg 3, 1, Dsc 1 (IgA)
	Intraepidermal neutrophilic dermatosis type	Dsg 3, 1, Dsc 1 (IgA)

7.1. CLINICAL PRESENTATION

Pemphigus vulgaris has two clinical subtypes: mucosal dominant type and mucocutaneous type; the cutaneous type will not be described in this review. Patients with the mucosal dominant type show mucosal erosions mainly in the oral cavity with minimal or limited skin involvement. Patients with the mucocutaneous type show extensive flaccid blisters and erosions on the skin as well as the mucosal erosions. (Figure 7) Mucosal erosions usually precede the cutaneous manifestations of the disease and often result in a protracted course of misdiagnosis with other conditions such as aphthous ulceration [549-50]. The mucous membranes most often affected are those of the oral cavity, which is involved in up to 80% patients with pemphigus vulgaris. In some cases, oral ulceration may be the only manifestation of the disease. (Figure 8) Any stratified squamous epithelia where desmoglein 1 or 3 are expressed can be involved in pemphigus vulgaris. Mucous membrane lesions are usually seen as painful erosions. Intact blisters are rare, probably because they are fragile and break easily. Scattered and often extensive erosions may be seen on any part of the oral cavity. Extensive erosions and painful lesions in the mouth may result in decreased food and drink intake. Involvement of throat may produce hoarseness and difficulty in swallowing. The erosions may spread to involve the pharynx and larynx, producing hoarseness and difficulty in swallowing. Esophageal involvement is a rare but serious occurrence producing dysphagia or odynophagia [551]. Ocular involvement is rarely seen in pemphigus vulgaris and is frequently associated with a more severe course of disease. The most common ophthalmologic involvement is conjunctival but without progressive scarring such as occurs in ocular cicatricial pemphigoid [552]. Conjunctival involvement may occur in a one-sided or two-way fashion: the presentation may range from mild hyperemia to conjunctivitis, resulting in symptoms of irritation and excessive watering of the eyes as well as the sensation of having a foreign body in the eye [553]. Genital involvement is less common than oral involvement and may be overlooked on superficial clinical examination [554-9].

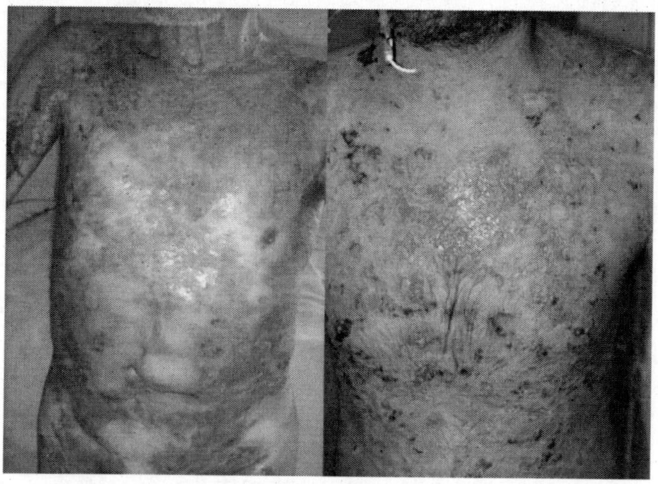

Figure 7. Extensive flaccid blisters and difficult to heal and painful erosions cover the skin of the patients as well as mucous membranes.

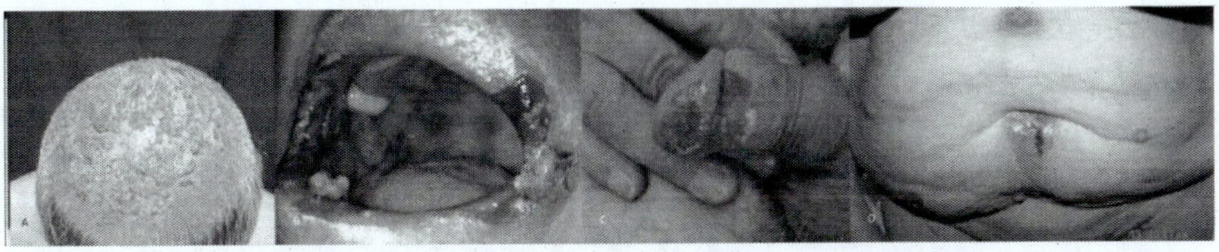

Figure 8. There are several sites where the disease arise; mucous membranes like the oral cavity, are the most commonly affected, and often, oral ulceration may be the only manifestation of the disease.

Cutaneous involvement may be localized or generalized. Skin lesions can appear anywhere on the skin surface and arise on either normal- appearing skin or erythematous bases, but they have a preference for the trunk, groin, (Figure 9) axillae, scalp, (Figure 10) face, and pressure points [560]. Flaccid blisters develop on these sites and may coalesce. The fluid within the bullae is at first clear but may become hemorrhagic or turbid (Figure 11) and decantate by gravity resulting in a pear shape. (Figure 12) These blisters eventually rupture and result in erosions. Erosions have a tendency to spread at their margin.

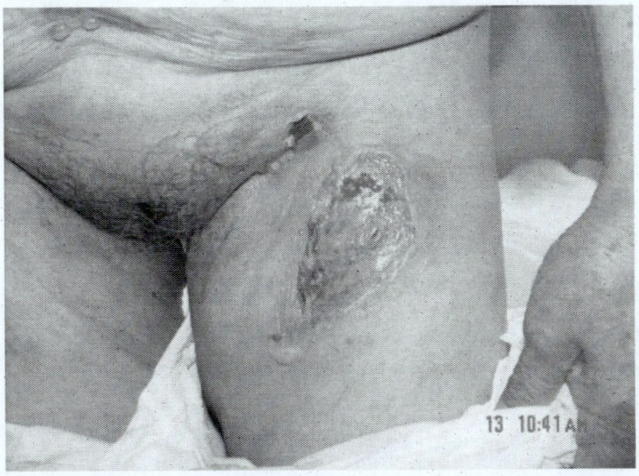

Figure 9. Case of pemphigus vulgaris affecting the groin.

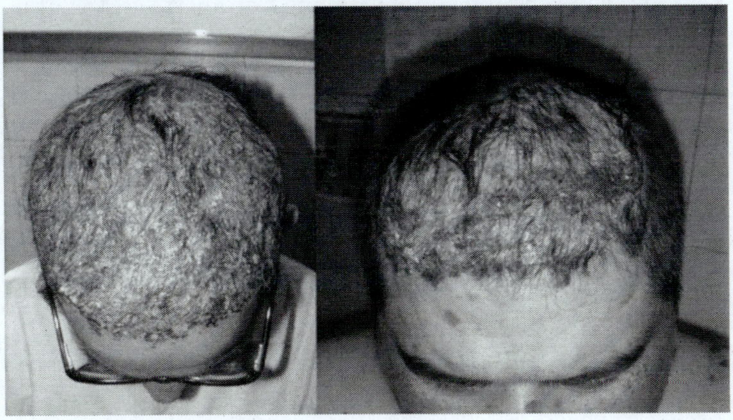

Figure 10. Cases of pemphigus vulgaris affecting the scalp.

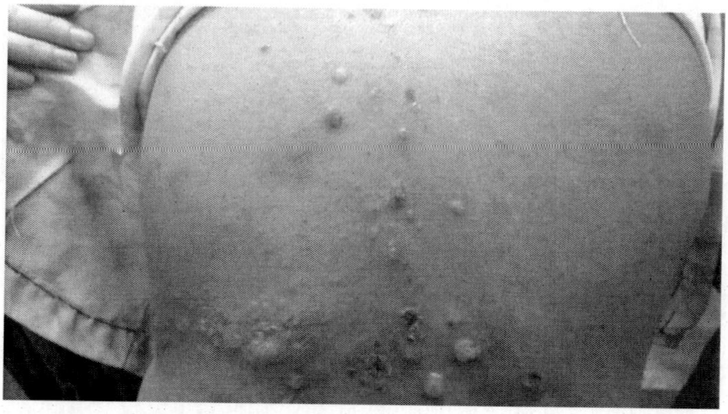

Figure 11. Case of pemphigus vulgaris with several bullae, some of them with turbid fluid. This fluid is aseptical and usually antibiotics are not required.

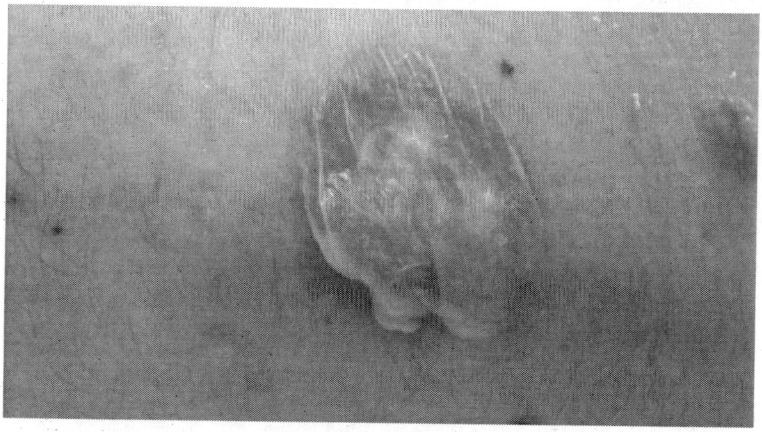

Figure 12. Old blister that become flaccid and acquire a pear-like shape due to weight of the exudates, resembling a rubber sack filled with fluid in a patient with pemphigus vulgaris.

Erosions are more obvious at the margin of the lesion; the center is usually covered by a remnant of the skin, probably the roof of the blistered or unaffected skin; this resembles an island surrounded by water. (Figure 13)

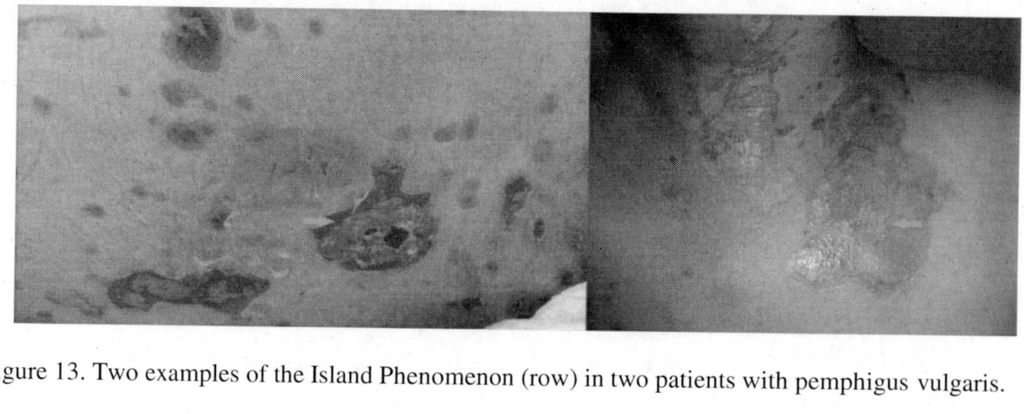

Figure 13. Two examples of the Island Phenomenon (row) in two patients with pemphigus vulgaris.

The diagnosis of pemphigus vulgaris tends to be delayed in patients presenting with only oral involvement, as compared to patients with skin lesions. The primary skin lesions of pemphigus vulgaris are flaccid, thin-walled, easily ruptured blisters that appear anywhere on the skin surface (Table 4). The blisters arise on normal-appearing skin or erythematous bases. The blisters are fragile and soon rupture to form painful erosions that ooze and bleed easily. (Figure 14) The erosions soon become partially covered with crusts that have little or no tendency to heal. Without appropriate treatment, pemphigus vulgaris can be fatal because a large area of the skin loses epidermal barrier function, leading to loss of body fluids or secondary bacterial infection. Because of the absence of cohesion in the epidermis, the upper layers are easily made to slip laterally by slight pressure or rubbing in active patients with pemphigus (Nikolsky sign). Nikolsky's sign has been divided in two forms, the form I (normal or direct Nikolsky's sign), is defined as the ability to split the epidermis on skin areas distant from the lesions of normal appearing skin by a lateral pressure with a finger, whereas the type II (marginal or indirect Nikolsky's sign), is defined as the ability to split the epidermis of the skin far beyond the preexisting erosion, extending to a great distance on the normal appearing skin, by pulling the remnant of a ruptured blister or rubbing at the margin of existing lesions. These signs are not always 100% reliable for the diagnosis of pemphigus vulgaris, but they are suggestive if present [532, 561]. The experts also subdivide Nikolsky in wet (exudative, seen in deep pemphigus) and dry (seen in superficial pemphigus) types.

The Asboe-Hansen's or Lutz' sign (blister spread or marginal spread) is the ability to enlarge a blister in direction of the margin by applying mechanical pressure on the roof of intact blister.

Sheklakov's sign (perifocal subepidermal separation), also called the false Nikolsky sign, is the ability to extend to a limited distance a lesion in direction of the margin by pulling the remnant of a ruptured blister, producing erosions that are limited in size, do not have a tendency to resulting spontaneous extension, heal fast, and may show a drop of blood. Examples are seen in subepidermal blistering diseases.

The Pseudo-Nikolsky's sign also called epidermal peeling is the ability to peel off the entire epidermis by a lateral pressure (rubbing) only on the erythematous skin areas. This sign is frequently seen in toxic epidermal necrolysis or Lyell syndrome, Stevens Johnson syndrome, burns and bullous ichthyosiform erythroderma

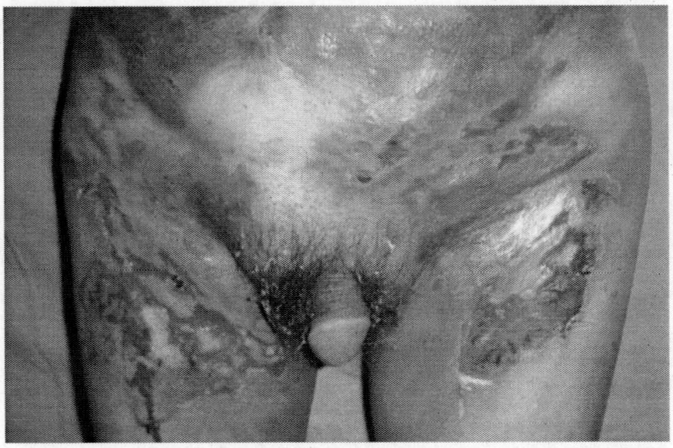

Figure 14. When blisters rupture to form painful erosions, we may observe that ooze and bleed easily.

Table 4. Pemphigus vulgaris diagnostic criteria

Criteria	Description
Clinical diagnosis parameters.	Multiple faccid, easily ruptured bullae on the skin.
	Progressive refractory erosions secondary to blisters, or scaly or crusted lesions.
	Non-infectious blisters or erosions on the visible mucosal areas, including the oral mucosa.
	Positive Nikolsky sign.
Histopathological diagnostic parameter	Detection of intraepidermal blister formation due to loss cell-cell adhesion of keratinocytes (acantholysis).
Immunological diagnostic parameters	Demonstration of *in vivo* IgG (sometimes complement) deposition on keratinocyte cell surfaces of the skin and mucosa, either in lesions or in apparently healthy skin by direct immunofluorescence.
	Detection of circulating IgG autoantibodies against keratinocyte membranes or intercellular spaces of the epidermis or anti-desmoglein IgG autoantibodies by indirect immunofluorescence or enzyme-linked immunoassay.
Assessment and diagnosis	Those cases that satisfy at least one of the diagnostic parameters of each category are diagnosed as pemphigus.
	Those cases that satisfy at least two of the clinical parameters and also satisfy both immunological parameters are diagnosed as pemphigus.

As we previously mention, pear sign refers as old blisters that become flaccid and get a pear-like shape because of weight of the exudates, resembling a rubber sack filled with fluid, we have seen this sign in IgA pemphigus, Sneddon and Wilkinson disease and even pemphigus vulgaris.

The presence of Koebner phenomenon is frequently seen, mainly as a surgical sequelae. (Figure 15) The erosions soon become partially covered with crusts that have little tendency to heal. Those lesions that do heal often leave hyper, hypopigmentation or milia, (Figure 16) rarely with scarring alopecia. (Figure 17) Acanthomas may occur at sites of previous blisters [562]. Cases of cutaneous only pemphigus vulgaris are increasingly recognized [563]. In these cases, the antibody reactivity is still against desmoglein 3 and why the oral and other mucosae are spared is not yet understood. Involvement of the nails in pemphigus vulgaris is rare and is usually seen when the disease is severe [564]. The most common clinical manifestations include nail dystrophy, paronychia, and subungual hematomas [564-5]. Fingernails are more often involved than toenails. Pemphigus vegetans is a clinically distinct variant of pemphigus vulgaris which mainly affects large skinfolds such as the groins and axillae, eventually lesions may arise in other sites. (Figure 18) Clinically, vegetating painful erosions are the major hallmark of this clinical variant. Pemphigus herpetiformis is also considered as a clinical variant of deep or superficial pemphigus which is characterized by vesicles, blisters and erosions (Figure 19) which are grouped in a herpetiform pattern (Table 5). Oral involvement is rare. Recent evidence suggests that pemphigus vegetans and pemphigus herpetiformis are associated with a particular autoantibody profile, i.e., the presence of IgG autoantibodies against desmocollin 3 [308]. The pathological role of these autoantibodies is not yet fully elucidated.

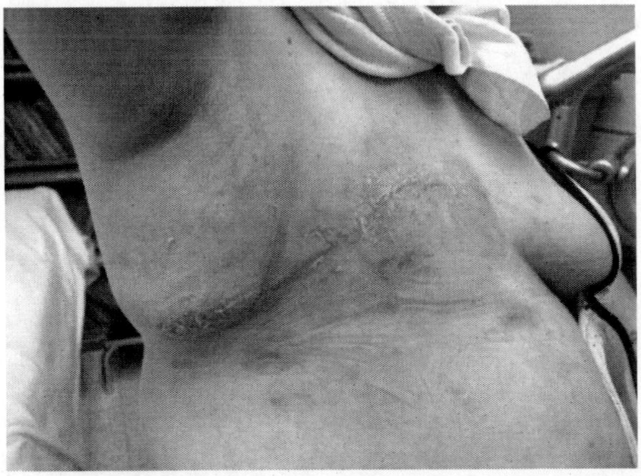

Figure 15. Koebner or isomorphic phenomenon in a patient previously treated for pemphigus vulgaris, with mastectomy related to a breast tumor.

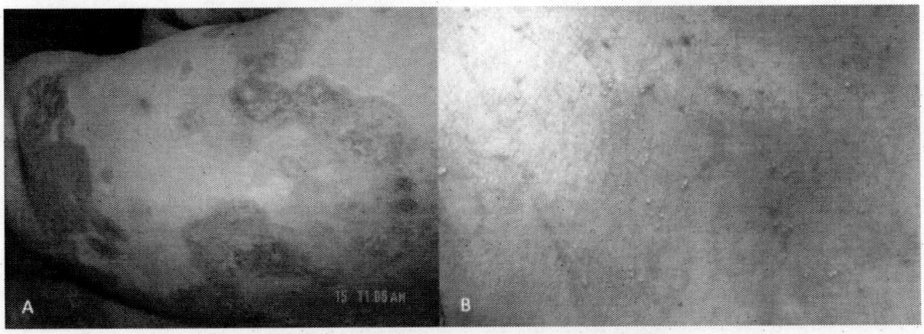

Figure 16. Sequelae in patients with pemphigus vulgaris. (A) hyperpigmentation and (B) milia cysts.

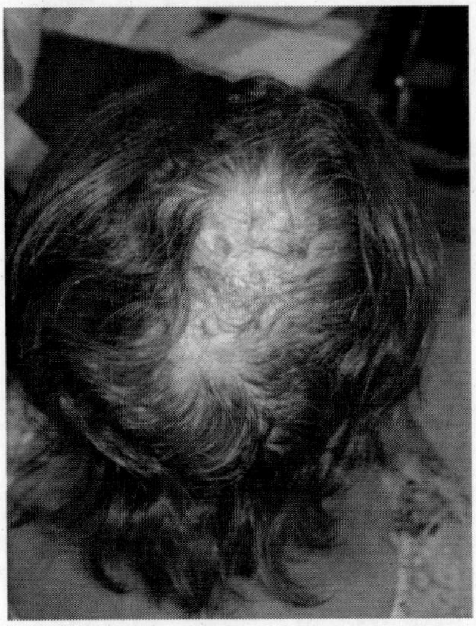

Figure 17. Patient previously treated for pemphigus vulgaris, that developed scarring alopecia.

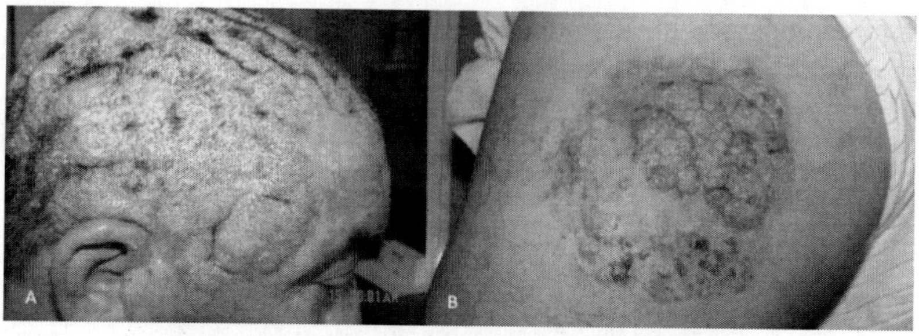

Figure 18. Two cases of pemphigus vegetans arising in less commonly seen sites.

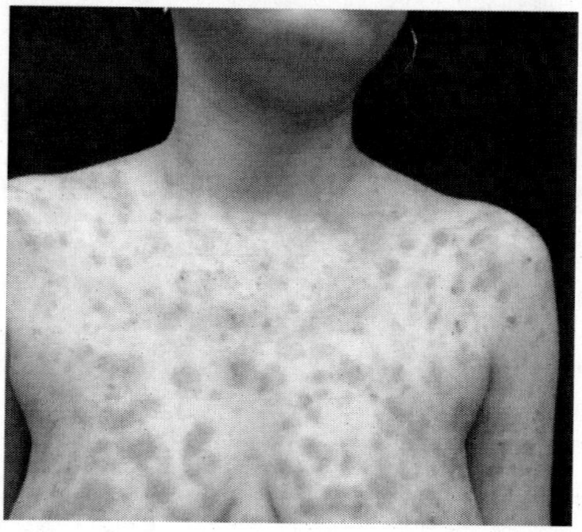

Figure 19. A case of pemphigus herpetiformis that resemble a superficial pemphigus.

Table 5. Diagnostic criteria for pemphigus herpetiformis

Characteristic	Mandatory
Grouped (herpetiform) distribution of itching erythematous vesicular/bullous/popular lesions, often in an annular-shaped pattern.	Yes
Eosinophilic/neutrophilic spongiosis/intraepidermal pustules with or without acantholysis	No
Skin-bound epithelial cell surface IgG and/or C3	Yes
Circulating epithelial cell surface IgG	No
Detection of circulating IgG autoantibodies against desmoglein 1 and/or 3 and desmocollin 1 and/or 3.	No

At least one of the two criteria (positive IIF or detection of specific autoantibodies) should be fulfilled if DIF is not available.

There is a variety of blistering conditions that should be considered when seeing patients with pemphigus vulgaris including those of autoimmune, infectious, or inflammatory etiologies. The differential diagnosis for mucosal lesions includes stomatitis secondary to herpes simplex virus, aphthous ulcers, lichen planus, paraneoplastic pemphigus, lupus erythematosus, Behcet's disease, or dermatitis herpetiformis. The differential diagnosis for cutaneous involvement includes pemphigus foliaceus, pemphigus vegetans, IgA pemphigus, paraneoplastic pemphigus, bullous pemphigoid, linear IgA disease, erythema multiforme, candidosis, Crohn's disease, Grover's disease, and Hailey-Hailey disease (Table 6).

Table 6. Clinical and histopathologic differential diagnosis for pemphigus vulgaris

Characteristic of pemphigus	Differential diagnosis
Mucosal involvement	Acute herpetic stomatitis
	Aphthous stomatitis
	Erythema multiforme
	Stevens-Johnson syndrome
	Lichen planus
	Systemic lupus erythematosus
	Mucous membrane pemphigoid
	Paraneoplastic pemphigus
Cutaneous involvement	Pemphigus foliaceous
	Linear IgA bullous dermatitis
	Hailey-Hailey disease
	Grover´s disease
Histological	Paraneoplastic pemphigus and other types of pemphigus.
	Hailey-Hailey disease
	Darier´s disease
	Grover´s disease

7.2. Disease Activity Categorization

An international consensus statement on Disease Endpoint and Therapeutic Response for Pemphigus [394] divides pemphigus disease activity into the following stages of clinical evolution: early endpoints; baseline; control of disease activity; end of consolidation phase; late endpoints; complete remission off therapy; complete remission on therapy; minimal therapy; minimal adjuvant therapy; partial remission off therapy; partial remission on minimal therapy; relapse/flare; treatment failure.

Early endpoints provide a useful clinical sign for clinicians about the beginning to defer treatment regimes. The *baseline* is classified as the day the treating practitioner starts treatment. *Control of disease activity* is defined as the time at which there is cessation of new lesions with the healing of preexisting lesions. Usually, the expected time period in this stage is weeks. The *end of the consolidation phase* is the time period in which no new lesions have developed over a minimum period of 2 weeks. This phase is also characterized by the healing of most lesions, and most dermatologists would consider the weaning of steroids during this time period. (Figure 20) Late endpoints of disease activity may be achieved with or without therapy. *Complete remission off therapy* is characterized by the absence of new lesions over a 2-month period after cessation of therapy. *Minimal therapy* constitutes treatment with less than or equal to 10 mg/day of prednisone or the equivalent or the use of minimal adjuvant therapy for a duration of at least 2 months. *Minimal adjuvant therapy* comprises of half the dose needed to be defined as treatment failure. *Partial remission off therapy* is classified as development of lesions after cessation of treatment that heals within 1 week without treatment. Patients must be off systemic therapy for 2 months to be classified in this category. Patients may suffer a partial remission on minimal therapy when they develop new lesions that heal within 1 week while receiving minimal therapy. Topical steroids also constitute minimal therapy.

A *relapse/flare* is defined by developing three or more new lesions that persist without healing for greater than 1 week or by the extension of preexisting established lesions. Treatment failure results when there is no change in disease activity despite treatment on therapeutic doses of systemic steroids and other agents whose doses and durations were agreed by international consensus [394].

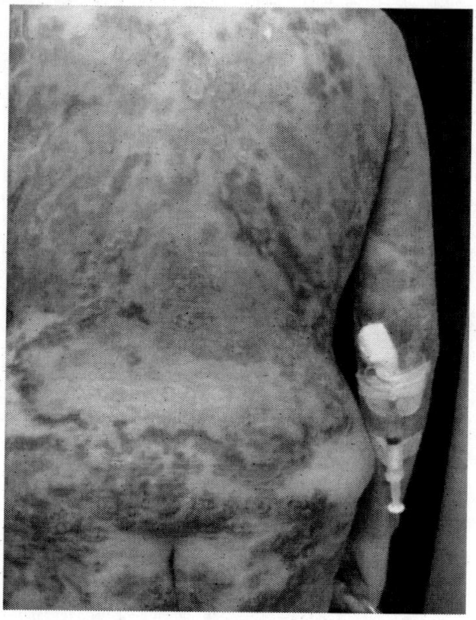

Figure 20. Pemphigus vulgaris patient in a consolidation phase.

Chapter 8

Clinical Presentation of Pemphigus Foliaceus

Pemphigus foliaceus can be separated into two general subtypes: non-endemic and endemic. Endemic pemphigus foliaceus is also known as *fogo selvagem* and is linked to several distinct geographical areas. Other variants of pemphigus foliaceus include pemphigus erythematosus (Senear-Usher syndrome), drug-induced pemphigus foliaceus, and pemphigus herpetiformis [566-7].

8.1. Disease Presentation

Both non-endemic and endemic pemphigus foliaceus begin with forming blisters on the skin. These blisters are superficial, making them fragile and prone to rupture. Therefore, it is not uncommon for some patients to be unaware of blisters and report only a history of shallow sores or areas of crusting. Lesions most commonly occur in seborrheic areas, including the trunk, neck, face, and/or scalp. Pain and/or a burning sensation localized to the areas of the lesions may be noted. Unlike pemphigus vulgaris, there is usually no history of oral or other mucosal lesions. The skin lesions may be worsened by sun exposure, remain localized, or become widespread and progress in weeks or months. Patients with the mildest form of pemphigus foliaceus may only report a history of a small, solitary, recurrent, scaly, and crusty lesion of the face [568]. Patients with untreated localized pemphigus foliaceus may achieve spontaneous remission, remain stable, or progress to more extensive skin disease. Severe pemphigus foliaceus may result in the rapid formation of many blisters and sores all over the body and subsequently requiring hospitalization. (Figure 21) In some cases, generalized pemphigus foliaceus can be fatal [569]. In cases of pemphigus erythematosus, patients report the development of lesions in sun-exposed areas of the face, scalp, and upper chest and back, similar to the distribution of lesions seen in lupus erythematosus. (Figure 22)

Non-endemic pemphigus foliaceus and *fogo selvagem* differ in their geographical distribution, average age of onset, and the high family incidence of *fogo selvagem* [285, 538, 570]. *Fogo selvagem* has a unique geographic and temporal clustering of cases. There are foci of *fogo selvagem* found in Brazil, Colombia, Peru, and Tunisia [281, 517, 539-40, 571]. In contrast to non-endemic pemphigus foliaceus symptom onset typically occurring in patients between 40 and 60 years old, *fogo selvagem* affects a larger number of children and young adults as symptoms usually begin during the second or third decade of life [571]. Non-endemic pemphigus foliaceus and *fogo selvagem* are typically seen equally in men and women and affect those of all races and ethnicities. However, there are populations of *fogo selvagem* that may deviate from the average. For example, epidemiological studies in Tunisia found the female-to-male ratio of incidence rate to be approximately 4 to 1 [472]. Various medications have been associated with developing pemphigus foliaceus. Drug-induced pemphigus foliaceus may either clear after the inciting medication is withdrawn or persist. Medications that contain or are metabolized to yield thiol groups have been most commonly involved although there have been cases associated with non-thiol drugs [445]. These include penicillamine, angiotensin-converting enzyme inhibitors, rifampicin, and topical imiquimod treatment [572-5]. Exposure to ultraviolet and ionizing radiation may also result in pemphigus foliaceus [576-7]. Several autoimmune diseases have been associated with pemphigus foliaceus, including bullous pemphigoid, myasthenia gravis, systemic lupus erythematosus, lichen planus, and psoriasis [578-82]. Pemphigus foliaceus has also been associated with certain neoplastic conditions including B- and T-cell lymphomas, prostate cancer, and cutaneous squamous cell carcinoma [583-6]. Some patients with pemphigus vulgaris have been reported to have a clinical, histopathological, and serological disease transformation to pemphigus foliaceus [587-8]. Conversely and even more rarely, pemphigus foliaceus may progress to other forms of pemphigus or even to other autoimmune blistering diseases [589-90].

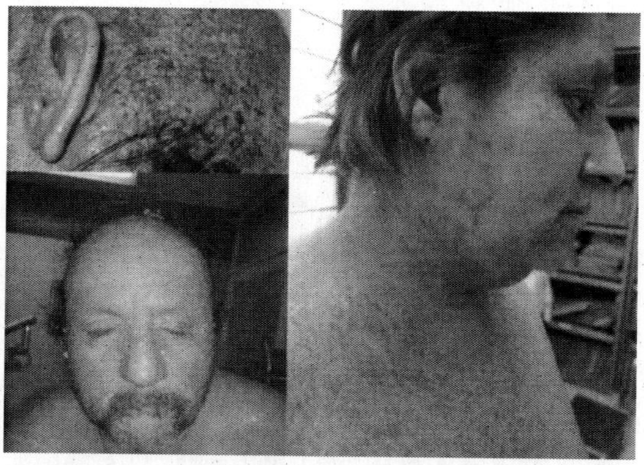

Figure 21. Severe cases of pemphigus foliaceus that required inpatient treatment.

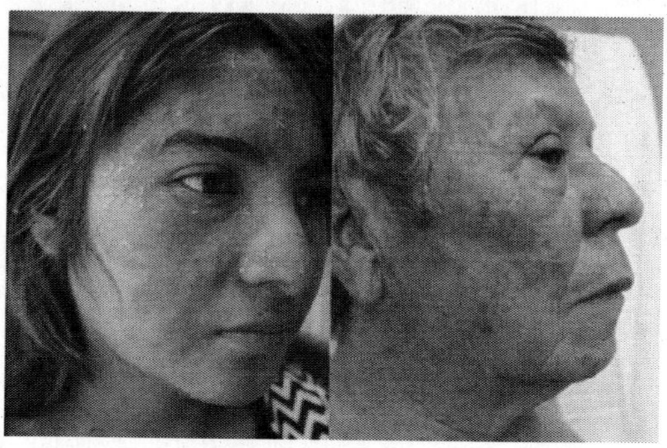

Figure 22. Two cases of pemphigus erythematosus with lesions in sun-exposed areas of the face.

8.2. PHYSICAL FINDINGS

Clinical findings of non-endemic and endemic pemphigus foliaceus are nearly identical [467]. Patients with pemphigus foliaceus develop scaly, crusted erosions, often on an erythematous base in the skin; mucosal membranes are rarely, if ever, affected, even with widespread disease. The absence of oral involvement may be a clue to clinically differentiate pemphigus foliaceus from pemphigus vulgaris. The onset of disease is often subtle, with a few scattered crusted lesions that come and go, and are frequently mistaken for impetigo. These lesions are usually well demarcated and scattered in a seborrheic distribution, including face, scalp, and upper trunk. (Figure 23) Because the vesicle is so superficial and fragile, often only the crust and scale that result from ruptured vesicles are seen. Disease may stay localized for years or may rapidly progress, in some cases, to generalized involvement resulting in an erythrodermic exfoliative dermatitis. Nikolsky sign is present. Detachment of the stratum corneum from the underlying stratum granulosum (the location of intraepidermal acantholysis) leads to scaling. Crusting, representing dried serous exudate from erosive lesion(s), is also commonly present.

On physical exam, the clinician can usually elicit a positive Nikolsky's sign, which is performed by applying a tangential force (i.e., rubbing) to the margin of an existing primary or secondary lesion. If positive, the force will result in the separation of the upper layer of epidermal skin from the underlying lower layers. Nikolsky's sign has been shown to be moderately sensitive but highly specific in diagnosing pemphigus [532]. The extent of skin involvement in pemphigus foliaceus can range from mild to severe. In mild, localized pemphigus foliaceus, the lesions tend to be smaller and/or solitary and are localized to a specific seborrheic area, such as the face or neck. Localized pemphigus foliaceus is known as an incomplete form or *forme fruste*. Severe, generalized pemphigus foliaceus can either result in exfoliative erythroderma characterized by diffuse erythema, scaling, and crusting of the cutaneous surface or in a bullous invasive form [479]. If the scalp is involved, alopecia may be present [288]. Circinate, erythematous plaques on the trunk resembling *tinea imbricate* may also be present. Pemphigus erythematosus is a distinct variant of pemphigus foliaceus that has clinical features similar to those of both pemphigus foliaceus and lupus erythematosus. Flaccid vesicles and/or erosions are present on seborrheic areas of the skin. Like lupus erythematosus, lesions are photodistributed on areas of the upper chest and back and in a malar pattern on the face. Lesions, especially those on the face and scalp, are often hyperkeratotic with thick, greasy scales and yellow crusts [591].

Pemphigus foliaceus may occasionally present with atypical skin findings. Several cases have described pemphigus foliaceous presenting as an acute eruption of many hyperpigmented and hyperkeratotic verrucous papules and plaques that closely resemble the appearance of seborrheic keratoses [592-3]. Children with pemphigus foliaceous may present with flaccid vesicles and bullae and/or erosions in an arcuate, circinate, and/or polycyclic pattern [594]. Pemphigus foliaceus presenting as an isolated erythematous plaque on the cheek with a "peau d'orange" appearance has also been reported [595].

The clinical features of drug-induced pemphigus are similar to the primary disease although pruritus is more common. Pemphigus foliaceus is the most common pattern of drug-induced pemphigus, observed in up to 70% of thiol-induced cases. It is characterized by multiple, superficial, fragile blisters over the seborrhoeic areas of the body, which easily rupture, evolving into erythematous, crusted and scaly erosions and plaques. The scalp, face and upper trunk are the common sites of involvement. Skin lesions may coalesce to cover large areas of the body and occasionally progress to an exfoliative erythroderma. The cutaneous lesions are often associated with itching and burning. The mucous membranes are typically spared. Drug-induced pemphigus may also present as pemphigus erythematosus, which is a variant of pemphigus foliaceus localized to the malar region of the face and sometimes associated with the laboratory features of systemic lupus erythematosus.

Pemphigus induced by non-thiol drugs tends to manifest as pemphigus vulgaris. Most patients develop mucosal lesions, with painful erosions of the oral cavity being the commonest presenting feature. Other mucous membranes can be affected, in particular the conjunctiva, esophagus and genitalia. Cutaneous involvement manifests with flaccid blisters, which soon rupture, producing painful erosions that tend to ooze and bleed. The Nikolsky sign can usually be elicited. The prognosis seems to be more favorable in drug-induced pemphigus caused by thiol drugs. Withdrawal of the drug results in remission in up to 50% of thiol-induced cases of pemphigus compared with only 15% of patients with pemphigus induced by non-thiols.

This observation led some authors to term thiol and non-thiol-related disease "drug-induced" and "drug-triggered" pemphigus, respectively. In patients who do not remit on drug withdrawal, the course and prognosis of drug-induced pemphigus is similar to that of primary pemphigus. The first and crucial step in the treatment of drug-induced pemphigus is to identify and stop the offending drug. If the patient is taking any implicated drug, consider stopping it even if there has been a delay between drug initiation and disease onset. This may result in remission in many, but not all, patients and reduced disease severity in others. A rapid decline in circulating anti-desmoglein antibodies, associated with clinical improvement, has been observed after withdrawal of the offending drug [596].

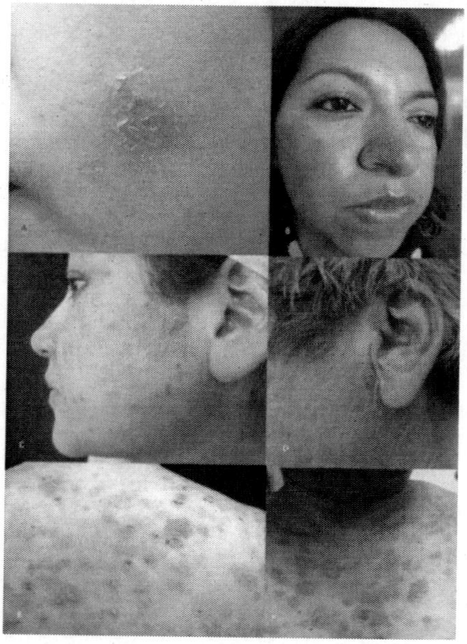

Figure 23. Cases of seborrheic pemphigus with well demarcated lesions and scattered in a seborrheic distribution.

Patients in whom the disease persists after cessation of the associated agent, require therapy with systemic corticosteroids and/or immunosuppressants as for primary pemphigus. Proper skin care is also an important part of management.

8.3. PROGNOSIS

Death occurs in 5–10% of *fogo selvagem*/pemphigus foliaceus patients and usually results from complications of prolonged systemic immunosuppressive therapy or secondary infections. Eczema herpeticum (herpes simplex), spread *Strongyloides stercoralis,* or bacterial sepsis may be fatal [479]. Generally patients with pemphigus foliaceus are not severely ill.

Chapter 9

PARANEOPLASTIC PEMPHIGUS

Paraneoplastic pemphigus was first described in 1990 by Anhalt et al., [290] as an autoimmune mucocutaneous eruption that occurs in association with benign or malignant neoplasms. It is unique and distinct from the classic forms of pemphigus vulgaris and foliaceus by clinical, histologic, and immunopathologic criteria. The associated neoplasms are non-Hodgkin's lymphoma (42%), chronic lymphocytic leukemia (29%), Castleman's tumor (10%), malignant and benign thymoma (6%), spindle cell neoplasms (reticulum cell sarcoma) (6%), and Waldenström's macroglobulinemia (6%). Combining non-Hodgkin's lymphoma and chronic lymphocytic leukemia represents almost two thirds of cases. Castleman's disease, which is a very rare lymphoproliferative lesion, is the third most commonly associated neoplasm. The absence of common tumors (adenocarcinoma of breast or bowel and squamous cell carcinomas), is notable [286, 597].

The most constant and distinctive feature of paraneoplastic pemphigus is the presence of severe, intractable stomatitis, a polymorphous cutaneous eruption, (Figure 24) humoral immunity against plakin proteins, and progressive respiratory failure. The severe stomatitis is usually the earliest presenting sign, and after treatment it is the one that persists and is resistant to therapy. This stomatitis consists of erosions and ulcerations that affect all surfaces of the oropharynx and characteristically extend onto the vermillion of the lip. Most patients also have a severe pseudomembranous conjunctivitis with scarring. Esophageal, nasopharyngeal, vaginal, labial, and penile mucosal lesions may also be affected. The cutaneous lesions are polymorphic and may appear as erythematous macules, flaccid blisters and erosions resembling pemphigus vulgaris, tense blisters resembling bullous pemphigoid, erythema multiforme-like lesions, and lichenoid eruptions. Extensive cases show clinical resemblance with toxic epidermal necrolysis. The occurrence of blisters and erythema multiforme–like lesions on the palms and soles can be used to clinically differentiate paraneoplastic pemphigus from pemphigus vulgaris. Cutaneous lichenoid eruptions are very common associated with severe stomatitis. In the chronic form of the disease lichenoid eruption may predominate over blistering lesions (Table 7).

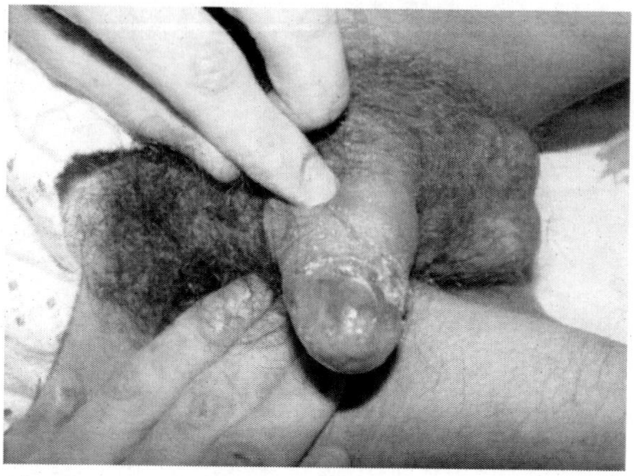

Figure 24. A case of paraneoplastic pemphigus showing the antibody mediated manifestation (stomatitis) and the cell mediated cytotoxicity (lichenoid lesions).

Table 7. Diagnostic criteria of paraneoplastic pemphigus

Criteria	Description
Clinical *	Painful mucosal erosions with a polymorphous skin eruption culminating in vesicles and/or bullae in the context of an occult or evident neoplasm.
Histology	Intraepidermal acantholysis, vacuolar interface changes, and keratinocyte necrosis
Direct Immunofluorescence	Deposition of complement and IgG in intercellular epidermal spaces and in the basement membrane zone in linear granular fashion.
Autoantibodies *	Detection in serum a similar pattern than in pemphigus vulgaris (desmogleins 1 and 3) and other autoantibodies (envoplakin, periplakin, bullous pemphigoid antigen 1, desmoplakin 1 and 2, plectic). Characteristic complex of four proteins immunoprecipitated from keratinocytes with serum autoantibodies. Indirect immunofluorescence staining with rat bladder epithelium.

* Major criteria.

The term paraneoplastic "pemphigus" is too restrictive to adequately describe the multiorgan syndrome under consideration. The term paraneoplastic autoimmune multiorgan syndrome properly encompasses the diverse group of signs and symptoms associated with this distinct and challenging paraneoplastic process (Table 8) [598]. There have been over 400 cases of paraneoplastic autoimmune multiorgan syndrome reported in the literature. There is a slight male predominance with most cases occurring between 45 and 70 years old. Interestingly, there is a significant association between patients with paraneoplastic autoimmune multiorgan syndrome and HLA-class II DRB1*03 and HLA-Cw*14 [433-4]. This differs from HLA associations in pemphigus vulgaris and foliaceous which are strongly associated with HLA-class IIDRB1+4 and DRB1*14. Most cases of paraneoplastic autoimmune multiorgan syndrome occur in association with a lymphoproliferative disorder. In a study of 163 cases, non-Hodgkin's lymphoma (38.6%), chronic lymphocytic leukemia

(18.4%), Castleman's disease (18.4%), and thymoma (5.5%) are the most commonly reported concurrent neoplasms [599]. Castleman's disease appears to be reported in much higher frequency in children [600-1] and in Chinese paraneoplastic autoimmune multiorgan syndrome (77%) [602]. Of several cases reported to occur in association with thymoma and Castleman's disease, further pathologic examination revealed concurrent follicular dendritic cell sarcoma [603-4]. Follicular dendritic cells are non-phagocytic and non-lymphoid accessory cells of the immune system which are essential for antigen presentation and regulation of the immune responses in the lymph node germinal centers [605-6]. Terminal deoxynucleotidyl transferase (TdT)-positive T cells have been identified in follicular dendritic cell sarcoma that may serve to amplify $CD8^+$ cytotoxic T-lymphocyte (CTL) responses and potentially autoimmunity, including autoreactive T cells directed against lung and other epithelial antigens [607-9]. This provides a potential novel understanding applicable to mechanisms underlying autoimmunity. (Figure 25) Additionally, Wang et al., [610] have shown auto reactive B-cell clones produce autoantibodies against plakin proteins in follicular dendritic cell sarcoma, Castleman's disease, as well as thymomas. These results suggest the presence of B-lymphocyte clones may be a common mechanism in paraneoplastic autoimmune multiorgan syndrome associated with various tumors.

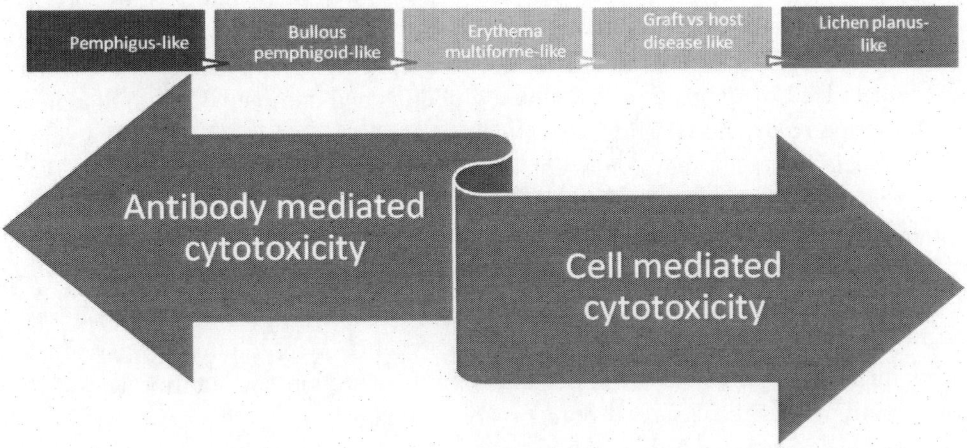

Figure 25. Clinical manifestations of paraneoplastic pemphigus according to predominance of antibody-mediated versus cell-mediated cytotoxicity.

Table 8. Curth's criteria for the diagnosis of cutaneous paraneoplastic syndromes

Criteria
Both conditions began simultaneously (neoplasia and paraneoplasia).
Development of a parallel course (treatment of the neoplasia results in regression of the skin lesion; recurrence of the neoplasia implies recurrence of the skin lesion).
The skin lesion is not associated with a genetic syndrome.
There is a specific type of neoplasia that occurs with paraneoplasia.
The dermatosis is rare in the general population.
There is a high frequency of association between both conditions.

9.1. Clinical Features

Paraneoplastic autoimmune multiorgan syndrome presents with a polymorphous cutaneous eruption that has been reported on a spectrum ranging from blisters, erosions, patches, papules, and plaques. Several subsets have been described: (1) bullous pemphigoid-like [611-3], (2) pemphigus-like [614], (3) pemphigus vegetans-like [615-6], (4) erythema multiforme-like [617], (5) graft-versus-host disease-like [618], and (6) lichen planus-like [619-20]. Severe, more recalcitrant oral mucosal lesions are the hallmark of the disease and usually are the first manifestation [621]. Pemphigus vulgaris fundamentally differs clinically from paraneoplastic autoimmune multiorgan syndrome in several ways. Paraneoplastic autoimmune multiorgan syndrome may affect any cutaneous surface including the palms and the soles, and lesions tend to be polymorphous and not limited to flaccid bullae and erosions as seen in pemphigus vulgaris. While both have oral mucosal disease, in pemphigus vulgaris oral mucosal lesions are discrete and more demarcated with areas of sparing. In paraneoplastic autoimmune multiorgan syndrome, the oral involvement is more diffuse, resulting in a generalized erosive stomatitis. As well as conjunctival and esophageal mucosa, paraneoplastic autoimmune multiorgan syndrome may also affect gastric, duodenal, respiratory, colonic, and urogenital epithelia that are spared in pemphigus vulgaris [622-3]. Affected respiratory mucous membranes in paraneoplastic autoimmune multiorgan syndrome lead to bronchiolitis obliterans, resulting in rapidly progressive and often fatal respiratory failure characterized by deposition of immunoglobulins and complement in pulmonary tissue [624]. Furthermore, paraneoplastic autoimmune multiorgan syndrome has been reported to occur in association with glomerulonephritis and a paraneoplastic neurologic syndrome, further expanding the multiorgan involvement of this disease [625]. Paraneoplastic autoimmune multiorgan syndromes has an overall mortality of 90% despite therapy, as opposed to that of pemphigus vulgaris, which is now about 5–7% with therapy. Most cases of paraneoplastic autoimmune multiorgan syndrome occur in association with a lymphoproliferative disorder, but at the time of presentation, nearly a third of patients have no known or identified malignancy [611]. Paraneoplastic autoimmune multiorgan syndrome is not infrequently misdiagnosed as chronic, erosive stomatitis or atypical erythema multiforme and, in more severe cases, as Stevens-Johnson syndrome (Table 9). Severe, more generalized cases may be referred to burn centers or intensive care units before the correct diagnosis is established [626]. It is important to perform an exhaustive medical examination to uncover potential underlying neoplastic or malignant conditions. Skin biopsy for routine histology and immunopathology as well as serologic screening should be included in the laboratory evaluation of suspected patients with paraneoplastic autoimmune multiorgan syndrome to avoid overlooking the correct diagnosis, pursuing indicated imaging studies, and instituting appropriate therapies. Respiratory failure is one of the most common causes of death in paraneoplastic autoimmune multiorgan syndrome. Patients develop a constrictive and obstructive pattern of respiratory failure with features of bronchiolitis obliterans and a functional pattern of obstructive or restrictive bronchiolitis similar to that observed in allogenic lung transplantation [627]. In a study of pulmonary involvement [628], two thirds of patients with constrictive bronchiolitis expired during the follow-up period, in contrast to only one third of those without this type of pulmonary disease. Resection of the neoplasm or induction of a complete response in cases of malignancy, despite resolution of other mucocutaneous features of paraneoplastic autoimmune multiorgan syndrome, often does not change the rapid and fatal course of the progressive respiratory failure.

9.2. PATHOPHYSIOLOGY

Paraneoplastic pemphigus is the only form of pemphigus that has involvement of non-stratified squamous epithelia. Around, 30% to 40% of patients develop pulmonary symptom. The earliest symptoms are progressive dyspnea, and pulmonary function studies show airflow obstacle, involving large and small airways, as seen in bronchiolitis obliterans, which can be fatal through respiratory failure.

Both humoral and cytotoxic immunities are involved in the development of paraneoplastic autoimmune multiorgan syndrome. Passive transfer of immunoglobulins isolated from patients with paraneoplastic autoimmune multiorgan syndrome produced mucocutaneous supra-basilar acantholysis in mice providing evidence that these antibodies are pathogenic [290]. Exposure of epithelial cells to autoantibodies against the linker subdomain of plakin proteins envoplakin and periplakin from paraneoplastic autoimmune multiorgan syndrome sera, leads to internalizations of these antibodies and retraction of keratin filaments [348]. Both these observations point to the pathogenesis of autoantibodies in developing paraneoplastic autoimmune multiorgan syndrome. In fact, cell cultures from resected Castleman's disease, thymoma, and follicular dendritic cell sarcoma have all been shown to produce autoantibodies to desmosomal and hemidesmosomal proteins [610, 629]. Deposition of polyclonal IgG autoantibodies and complement is found in multiple organ systems including mucocutaneous, conjunctival, bronchial, muscle, urinary bladder, and renal glomeruli [598]. Immunoglobulins produce three distinct or overlapping staining patterns: (1) fishnet-like intercellular staining of the epithelium (pemphigus-like), (2) linear staining at the basement membrane zone (pemphigoid-like), or (3) homogenous within the cells (apoptosis-like). Serum antibodies have been detected by indirect immunofluorescence technique using a variety of epithelial and non-epithelial tissue substrates including monkey esophagus (86% sensitivity), murine tongue (100% sensitivity), and mouse bladder (75% sensitivity) [630]. Immunoprecipitation has detected circulating autoantibodies that recognize keratinocyte proteins of various molecular weights: 40, 60, 70, 80, 95, 105, 130, 150, 170, 190, 210 (doublet), 230, and 250 kDa [290, 598]. Most sera recognize members of the plakin family including desmoplakin I, desmoplakin II, BPag 1, envoplakin, periplakin, and plectin. Antibodies against envoplakin and periplakin are consistently recognized and believed to be the most sensitive and specific indicators of disease [631]. Occasionally, decline of envoplakin and desmoglein 3 antibodies have been associated with improved clinical response in benign tumors, such as thymoma, treated with prednisone [632]. However, developing anti-keratinocyte autoantibodies has been reported as delayed in onset, limited, or absent in several cases [619, 633-4]. The 170 kD antigen target has been identified as a protease inhibitor, α-2 macroglobulin-like (A2ML1) protein, though its pathogenic role in disease development and tissue injury remains unknown [289]. The role of desmoglein antibodies in the pathogenesis of paraneoplastic autoimmune multiorgan syndrome is controversial. An increasing number of reports point out that these antibodies are present in only a minority of cases and, when present, are not consistently pathogenic [545-6, 635-6].

Indirect immunofluorescence studies on COS-7 cells transiently transfected with desmocollin 1–3 cDNA showed the presence of serum IgG and IgA antibodies to desmocollin 3, as well as IgG antibodies to desmocollin 2 [620]. Therefore, humoral immunity in paraneoplastic autoimmune multiorgan syndrome, unlike other autoimmune blistering diseases, is more varied, inconsistently positive, and not completely understood.

Cytotoxic cell-mediated immunity and antibody-dependent cellular cytotoxicity are involved in the pathogenesis of paraneoplastic autoimmune multiorgan syndrome. Cytotoxic T lymphocytes, NK cells, and monocytes and macrophages localize to the epidermal-dermal junction [598]. Immunohistochemical staining shows mostly $CD8^+$ cytotoxic T lymphocytes within the basal and suprabasal epidermis, alongside to apoptotic keratinocytes. Also, $CD68^+$ monocytes and macrophages (effectors of natural cytotoxicity) surround the subepidermal clefts. The infiltrate is similar to other inflammatory, autodestructive dermatoses characterized by keratinocyte apoptosis, erythema multiforme, GVHD, and lichen planus. Interferon γ and tumor necrosis factor appear to be central to the development of the graft-versus-host disease-like form of paraneoplastic autoimmune multiorgan syndrome [637]. Infiltrating $CD68^+$ monocytes and macrophages stain for inducible nitric oxide synthase in paraneoplastic autoimmune multiorgan syndrome pointing out they are activated and involved in its pathogenesis [598]. Nitric oxide may increase Fas-induced apoptosis in basal keratinocytes, explaining one possible mechanism for the loss of adhesion within the tegumental epithelium [638]. Epitope spreading, the development of autoimmunity following exposure to previously hidden self-antigens is also suggested by several observations. At the time of first presentation, immunofluorescence studies may be negative, reflecting a lack of humoral immunity. In one study, indirect immunofluorescence identified autoantibodies which reacted with rat bladder epithelium consistent with paraneoplastic autoimmune multiorgan syndrome [639]. These antibodies, however, were not detectable until 1 year following the initial clinical presentation. The heterogeneous clinicopathological presentation is likely a direct reflection of the diverse immunologic mechanisms of autoimmunity involving diverse effectors of humoral and cellular cytotoxicity. Bullous eruptions of paraneoplastic autoimmune multiorgan syndrome have a strongest humoral response as originally reported by Anhalt et al., [290] where passive transfer of paraneoplastic autoimmune multiorgan syndrome sera led to suprabasal acantholysis in mice. Lichenoid eruptions have been exclusively linked to cytotoxic infiltrates without detectable antibodies [619]. The spectrum of paraneoplastic autoimmune multiorgan syndrome likely includes patients with disease predominantly or exclusively mediated by cytotoxic T lymphocytes and others mainly by autoantibodies.

9.3. HISTOPATHOLOGY

The histopathologic hallmark is an interface reaction pattern, characterized by basal cell vacuolar degeneration and dyskeratotic and necrotic keratinocytes with lymphocytic inflammation and lymphocytic exocytosis. The reaction pattern may include either scattered lymphocytes at the basement membrane zone (interface vacuolar reaction pattern) or a band-like infiltrate in the upper dermis (interface lichenoid reaction pattern). Intraepidermal blisters and subepidermal blisters with acantholysis may be present and are less prominent features than in pemphigus vulgaris or bullous pemphigoid [640]. Postmortem pulmonary specimens in paraneoplastic autoimmune multiorgan syndrome show individual cells and clusters of epithelial cells in the tracheal, bronchial, and small-airway lumen with complete plugging of the alveoli [598].

9.4. MANAGEMENT

In patients without a known malignancy, a complete blood count; serum protein electrophoresis; computerized tomography of the chest, abdomen, and pelvis; and diagnostic biopsies (i.e., bone marrow, lymph nodes, or solid tumor), as indicated, should be obtained. According to Yong et al., [641] treating paraneoplastic pemphigus can be categorized into three steps, not necessarily in that order: (1) management of the underlying tumor; (2) management of autoimmune phenomena; and (3) management of associated complications. In step 1, treatment is difficult and the best outcomes have been reported in cases of resectable tumors [288, 642]. Complete resection of 20 cases of neoplasia associated with paraneoplastic autoimmune multiorgan syndrome led to sustained mucocutaneous improvement in 15 patients; however, respiratory symptoms and compromised pulmonary function persisted in most of these cases [642].

In step 2, these patients are often resistant to all conventional therapies. A combination of prednisone (0.5 – 1 mg/kg) and cyclosporine (5 mg/kg) ± cyclophosphamide (2 mg/kg) may be the most suitable pharmacotherapy [643]. In addition there have been many case reports showing promise with another agents including immunoablative high-dose cyclophosphamide without stem cell rescue, immunoapheresis, intravenous immunoglobulin, rituximab, alemtuzumab, as well as pyridostigmine bromide [644-9].

Table 9. Clinical and histopathologic differential diagnosis for paraneoplastic pemphigus

Characteristic of pemphigus	Differential diagnosis
Clinical	Pemphigus vulgaris
	Cicatricial pemphigoid
	Erythema multiforme
	Stevens-Johnson syndrome
	Lichen planus
	Graft-versus-host disease
	Persistent herpetic stomatitis
	Stomatitis due to chemotherapy
Histological	Pemphigus vulgaris and other types of pemphigus.
	Drug eruption
	Lichen planus
	Erythema multiforme
	Graft-versus-host disease

In step 3, pulmonary involvement is often progressive and irreversible despite tumor resection and treatment of mucocutaneous disease. However, it appears that some cases of constrictive bronchiolitis exhibit a more protracted and less aggressive course. In the cases when the neoplasm was resected early and immunosuppressive treatment, including parenteral corticosteroids, cyclosporine, cyclophosphamide, and methotrexate, was timely initiated, the respiratory disease was substantially slowed and residual pulmonary function stabilized. Nonetheless, destruction of the lung airways and development of fibrosis and obstruction are usually non-reversible and result in chronic supplemental oxygen requirement. In these cases, lung transplantation may be the only choice for intervention. In unresectable disease, treatment of the underlying malignancy is often not associated with disease improvement [650].

Overall, prognosis is poor and paraneoplastic autoimmune multiorgan syndrome may have a death rate as high as 90% [651]. Most of patients succumb to sepsis, respiratory failure, or the underlying neoplasm [650]. In conclusion, paraneoplastic autoimmune multiorgan syndrome is a multiorgan autoimmune syndrome affecting both tegumental epithelium and internal organs. Patients with paraneoplastic autoimmune multiorgan syndrome differ distinctively, though at times more subtly from patients with classical pemphigus, and may have lesions that resemble not only pemphigus but also pemphigoid, erythema multiforme, lichen planus, lichen planus pemphigoides, and graft-versus-host disease. Mucocutaneous lesions in these patients occur as a result of both humoral and cell-mediated immune mechanisms. Cell-mediated cytotoxicity in paraneoplastic autoimmune multiorgan syndrome involves both autoreactive lymphocytes and circulating autoreactive IgGs that recruit peripheral blood mononuclear cells into antibody-dependent cellular cytotoxicity against self-epithelium. Detachment of bronchial epithelial cells can contribute to occlusion of the small airways that provides a likely pathologic mechanism for the respiratory failure that frames a terminal event in many of these patients [598]. Treatment is difficult, and these patients often do not respond to therapies directed toward the underlying malignancy.

Based on these more recent and clinically better defined understandings of the disease, new therapeutic approaches with more potent pharmaceutical agents targeting the immune system should be developed to improve the often fatal course in patients with paraneoplastic autoimmune multiorgan syndrome.

Chapter 10

IGA PEMPHIGUS

Pemphigus is a life-threatening autoimmune blistering disorder characterized clinically by flaccid bullae or erosions on the skin/oral mucosa and histopathologically by intraepidermal acantholytic blisters [303]. Pemphigus is caused by circulating autoantibodies, mainly IgG antibodies. IgA pemphigus is a rare autoimmune vesiculopustular skin disease with exclusive IgA antibodies to keratinocyte cell surfaces. IgA pemphigus is subdivided into two types: subcorneal pustular IgA pemphigus and intraepidermal neutrophilic IgA pemphigus [652-4]. The autoantigen of the former is desmocollin-1, one of the constituents of desmosomes, but that of the latter is still unknown. IgA pemphigus was previously called as different names, including intraepidermal neutrophilic IgA dermatosis, intercellular IgA dermatosis, intercellular IgA vesiculopustular dermatosis, intraepidermal IgA pustulosis, IgA pemphigus foliaceus, and IgA herpetiform pemphigus [655-7].

10.1. EPIDEMIOLOGY

More than 60 cases with IgA anti-cell surface autoantibodies have been reported thus far. The incidence and racial distribution of IgA pemphigus are currently unknown. A male-to-female ratio of IgA pemphigus was reported to be 1:1.33. The age distribution is from 1 month to 85 years old (average 53 years old). No patients have been reported to have died because of IgA pemphigus.

10.2. CLINICAL MANIFESTATIONS

IgA pemphigus is a subacute vesiculopustular disease. Clinically, it usually shows translucent clear or pustular fluid-containing bullae on erythematous plaques. Subcorneal pustular IgA pemphigus shows superficial pustules, and an annular arrangement is occasionally seen [658]. Intraepidermal neutrophilic IgA pemphigus shows deeper atypical pustular lesions and sometimes shows a so-called sunflower-like configuration. (Figure 26) The major affected sites of IgA pemphigus are the trunk and proximal extremities and lower aspect of the abdomen are commonly involved. Intertriginous areas are commonly affected in Subcorneal pustular IgA pemphigus. Mucous membrane involvement is rare [659]. Pruritus is often a significant symptom. Clinically, these clinical features of IgA pemphigus cannot be distinguished from subcorneal pustular dermatosis (Sneddon-Wilkinson syndrome) or pustular psoriasis (von Zumbush type or generalized pustular psoriasis).

The patients with both types of IgA pemphigus clinically present with flaccid vesicles or pustules both on erythematous or normal skin. In the both types the pustules tend to coalesce to forman annular or circinate pattern with crusts in the central area, although a sunflower-like arrangement of pustules is a characteristic sign of the intraepidermal neutrophilic dermatosis type.

Patients with IgA pemphigus with features of pemphigus vulgaris or pemphigus foliaceus have also rarely been reported, and they were histologically identical to conventional pemphigus vulgaris or pemphigus foliaceus.

10.3. Pathophysiology

The autoantigen is desmocollin 1 in subcorneal pustular IgA pemphigus. IgA antibodies to desmoglein 1and 3 were found in rare types of IgA pemphigus foliaceus and IgA pemphigus vulgaris, respectively [660-1]. However, autoantigens for most cases of intraepidermal neutrophilic IgA pemphigus were unknown.

The pathogenesis of IgA pemphigus is unknown, but a few reports suggest some mechanisms for the beginning of skin lesions in IgA pemphigus. Activation of IL-5 and involvement of γδT cells are reported in IgA pemphigus [662]. In addition, binding of IgA antibodies to IgA-Fc receptor, CD89, is considered to cause neutrophil collection and proteolytic cleavage of the keratinocyte cell-cell junction in IgA pemphigus [663]. However, there have been no direct evidence of acantholysis caused by IgA autoantibodies in IgA pemphigus.

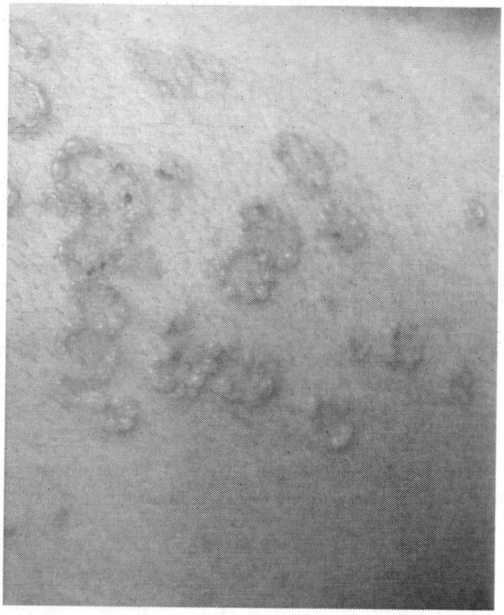

Figure 26. A case of IgA pemphigus with lesions resembling sunflower fashion.

10.4. Associated Diseases

Chronic inflammation in IgA pemphigus may increase the risk to develop several types of cancer. IgA pemphigus is reported in association with internal malignancies, mostly IgA gammopathy and lung cancer [664]. The other complications for IgA pemphigus are disease or treatment related infections. Disease-related infections occur in the blister and erosion, whereas treatment related infections occur from systemic immunosuppressions by oral steroids or other immunosuppressants.

10.5. Diagnostic Approach

10.5.1. Histopathology

Histopathologically, most IgA pemphigus skin lesions show minimal acantholysis [665]. In the subcorneal pustular IgA pemphigus, pustules are observed at the subcorneal upper epidermis, while in the intraepidermal neutrophilic IgA pemphigus, neutrophilic infiltration is observed throughout epidermis. These neutrophilic pustules are the hallmarks of IgA pemphigus.

10.5.2. Electron Microscopy

The autoantigen in IgA pemphigus was analyzed by immunoelectron microscopy. In subcorneal pustular IgA pemphigus, autoantibodies react with the extracellular space of desmosomes, which corresponds to the localization of desmocollin-1 [666]. In contrast, in intraepidermal neutrophilic IgA pemphigus, autoantibodies react with the extracellular space of interdesmosomal areas of the cell membrane [662]. Therefore, the target molecule of intraepidermal neutrophilic IgA pemphigus does not seem to be a desmosomal protein but may be adherens junction-related molecules.

10.5.3. Immunofluorescence

In direct immunofluorescence using perilesional patient skin section, IgA deposition in the cell surface of the keratinocytes was observed. IgG or C3 deposition is occasionally observed but is weaker than IgA deposition. In indirect immunofluorescence using patient sera and various substrates, including normal human skin, monkey esophagus, or other epithelia, circulating IgA anti-keratinocyte cell surface antibodies are detected in some sera. IgA antibodies in subcorneal pustular IgA pemphigus react with keratinocyte cell surface in the upper most epidermis, where desmocollin-1 exists. In contrast, IgA antibodies in intraepidermal neutrophilic IgA pemphigus react with the whole epidermis. In addition, cultured COS7 cells transfected with cDNA vectors for human desmocollin 1–3 are used as substrates for indirect immunofluorescence study to detect autoantibodies to desmocollin 1–3 [296, 300, 667-8]. By this method, IgA antibodies of subcorneal pustular type but not intraepidermal neutrophilic type, show positive signal exclusively with desmocollin-1 obtained as dotted fluorescent signals, while IgA antibodies in intraepidermal neutrophilic type do not react with any desmocollins.

10.5.4. Enzyme-Linked Immunosorbent Assay (ELISA) for Immunodiagnosis

ELISA for desmogleins and desmocollins is available for the diagnosis of IgA pemphigus. Some particular IgA pemphigus patients occasionally show IgA autoantibodies to either desmoglein 1 or desmoglein 3 in ELISA [294]. The usefulness of ELISA using baculovirus-producing recombinant proteins of desmocollins was questionable in both specificity and sensitivity [654].

10.5.5. Immunoblotting

Immunoblotting of normal human epidermal extract is not useful for the diagnosis of IgA pemphigus, in contrast of other autoimmune bullous diseases.

10.6. Treatment

IgA pemphigus is mainly treated by oral and topical corticosteroids [669]. Corticosteroids can decrease inflammation by reversing increased capillary permeability and suppressing neutrophil activity [670-1]. In addition, corticosteroids stabilize lysosomal membranes and, therefore, can suppress lymphocytes and antibody production [672]. In addition to corticosteroids, dapsone, isotretinoin, acitretin, mycophenolate mofetil, and adalimumab are also reported useful in treating IgA pemphigus [673-5].

The autoantigen for intraepidermal neutrophilic IgA pemphigus is still unknown. Possible subclass switching between classical pemphigus and IgA pemphigus should request a matter of interest for the future study. A guideline for managing IgA pemphigus as for other rare variants of pemphigus is also requested and needed.

10.7. Prognosis

Although clinical data of IgA pemphigus have not been well collected, IgA pemphigus shows a milder clinical phenotype and better prognosis than classical pemphigus. Scarring is not common in IgA pemphigus.

PART 5. DIAGNOSTIC TESTS

Chapter 11

DIAGNOSIS OF PEMPHIGUS

The diagnosis of pemphigus is generally based on combining clinical features with histological findings, as well as the results of immunofluorescence exams (direct and indirect techniques).

In general, autoimmune blistering diseases can be classified based on histological findings in two major groups: intraepidermal and subepidermal blistering diseases, in the following lines we limit the review to the first group. In addition, immunofluorescence examination will show the presence of autoantibodies attached to the skin of patients or circulating in the serum. The immunefluorescence pattern produced by these autoantibodies in each disease will further specify the diagnosis [62].

11.1. HISTOLOGY

The histological diagnosis of the different vesiculobullous diseases will depend on finding the microscopic vesicle (i.e., subcorneal, intraepidermal, or subepidermal), the presence or absence of inflammatory reaction, the type and distribution of the inflammatory reaction, and the presence or absence of epidermal dyskeratosis or necrosis. The biopsy for histology in all autoimmune blistering diseases has to be obtained from a new blister or vesicle, because obtaining a biopsy from an older lesion (of more than 24hr) may lead to an inadequate sample for histological diagnosis. For example, in old intraepidermal lesions, the blisters can erode the base and produce a false image of subepidermal blister; in old subepidermal lesions, the blisters can reepithelize from the base and produce an image of intraepidermal blister. In addition, in old lesions, bacterial superinfection (impetiginization) can result in epidermal necrosis and neutrophilic infiltrates that lead to misdiagnosis. Another important point is that when the biopsy for histology is obtained with the sample for direct immunofluorescence (i.e., generally obtained from perilesional normal skin), it is essential to avoid mixing both biopsies (send the sample for immunofluorescence for histological examination and the other way around) because this will probably lead to misleading results that will most likely require that new biopsies have to be done to the patient.

11.1.1. Pemphigus Vulgaris

The early histological finding in pemphigus vulgaris is the appearance of intercellular edema between keratinocytes that finally leads to a separation between cells and rupture of the spinous processes leading to a phenomenon called acantholysis. In pemphigus vulgaris this takes place characteristically in the suprabasal layer, producing suprabasal intraepidermal blisters, and there may be cells floating inside the vesicle, the so-called acantholytic cells. These cells are round, with a hyperchromatic nucleus and homogeneous cytoplasm. The cells of the basal layer remain attached to the basement membrane zone by their hemidesmosomal attachments and produce a characteristic image that has been compared to a *row of tombstones* [359].

In the underlying dermis there are usually mild to scarce perivascular inflammatory infiltrates of mononuclear cells and some eosinophils. Occasionally the epidermal changes are absent, and acantholysis can only be seen in the follicular epithelium selectively, without affecting the interfollicular epidermis [676]. In some patients, before blistering occurs the patients present with inflammatory plaques that show histologically spongiotic dermatitis with abundant eosinophils within the epidermis, a histological pattern that has been referred to as *eosinophilic spongiosis* [677]. Although this finding was initially described in pemphigus (both vulgaris and foliaceus), it can be seen in other autoimmune bullous diseases and in other disorders. In fact, eosinophilic spongiosis is much more often seen in the prebullous stages of bullous pemphigoid than in pemphigus.

Pemphigus vegetans is a rare vegetative variant of pemphigus vulgaris and considered to be one reactive pattern of the skin to autoimmune insult of pemphigus vulgaris. Pemphigus vegetans is characterized by flaccid blisters that become erosions and form fungoid vegetations or papillomatous proliferations, especially in the intertriginous area and in the scalp or on the face. Pustules rather than vesicles characterize early lesions but these soon progress to vegetative plaques. The findings in pemphigus vegetans show some characteristics that are different from those of pemphigus vulgaris. Although early lesions may show suprabasal acantholysis, as in pemphigus vulgaris, fully developed lesions of pemphigus vegetans will show acanthosis and papillomatosis, sometimes with prominent pseudoepitheliomatous hyperplasia, and the presence of intraepidermal abscesses of eosinophils.

Suprabasal acantholysis may be subtle and therefore may be missed occasionally [678], the differential diagnosis has to be done with conditions like pyostomatitis vegetans, Hailey-Hailey disease, or blastomycosis-like pyoderma (also known as pyoderma vegetans). Classically, pemphigus vegetans can be divided in two subtypes, the Neumann and the Hallopeau subtype, that differ clinically and histologically.

In the Neumann subtype, lesions are characterized by papillomatosis and acanthosis with intraepidermal vesiculation and suprabasal acantholysis. Intraepidermal pustules of neutrophils and eosinophils are scant or absent. In the Hallopeau subtype, lesions will also display acanthosis with occasional acantholysis, but with many and large eosinophilic abscesses, as well as areas of eosinophilic spongiosis. In late lesions the histological findings will overlap in both subtypes.

There are sporadic cases of pemphigus in association with the use of drugs, such as penicillamine and captopril. Pemphigus foliaceus is more common than pemphigus vulgaris in penicillamine-treated patients. Although most patients with drug-induced pemphigus are shown to have autoantibodies against desmoglein 1 or3, evidence suggests that some drugs may induce acantholysis without production of antibodies. Both penicillamine and captopril contain sulfhydryl groups that are speculated to interact with the sulfhydryl groups in desmoglein 1 and 3. Most, but not all, patients with drug-induced pemphigus go into remission after the offending drug is stopped.

11.1.2. Pemphigus Foliaceus and Erythematosus

The histopathological findings in endemic and non-endemic pemphigus foliaceus, pemphigus erythematosus, and drug-induced cases of pemphigus are identical. They are characterized by the presence of superficial acantholysis, just below the granular layer of the epidermis. Initial vesicles can contain abundant neutrophils or eosinophils. Occasionally, since the blisters have a thin ceiling, they break and loose the upper layer. This may give the appearance of a "normal epidermis" or even of psoriasiform dermatitis, with no clear finding of acantholysis. The clue for diagnosis in these cases is the absence of stratum corneum and parts of the stratum granulosum [679]. The main differential diagnosis here is with impetigo and staphylococcal scalded skin syndrome that are both disorders caused by the cleavage of the extracellular domain of desmoglein 1 by a toxin produced by certain strains of *Staphylococcus aureus*.

The pattern of eosinophilic spongiosis can also be seen as an early feature in pemphigus foliaceus and is also the typical histological pattern of pemphigus herpetiformis that often evolves to pemphigus foliaceus [680]. Another pattern that may be observed in early lesions of pemphigus (particularly in pemphigus foliaceus) is that of neutrophilic spongiosis [275].

11.1.3. Paraneoplastic Pemphigus

The classic pattern described in paraneoplastic pemphigus is the presence of intraepidermal blisters with suprabasal acantholysis (similar to pemphigus vulgaris), combined with lichenoid changes including interphase dermatitis, presence of necrotic keratinocytes and lichenoid inflamatory infiltrates [640]. These histological findings are not completely specific of paraneoplastic pemphigus and they have also been found in erythema multiforme, toxic epidermal necrolysis, and approximately one third of cases with other forms of pemphigus [681]. Sometimes we can observe the combination of the different patterns in different biopsies (i.e., one biopsy showing suprabasal acantholysis and another a lichenoid pattern). Eosinophilic spongiosis has also been reported in paraneoplastic pemphigus [545].

11.1.4. IgA Pemphigus

IgA pemphigus is a newly characterized group of autoimmune intraepidermal blistering diseases presenting with a vesiculopustular eruption, neutrophilic infiltration, and *in-vivo*–bound and circulating IgA autoantibodies against keratinocyte cell surfaces, but no IgG autoantibodies. IgA deposition on cell surfaces of the epidermis is present in all cases by direct immunofluorescence, and many patients have detectable circulating IgA autoantibodies by indirect immunofluorescence. There are two major clinicopathological subtypes of IgA pemphigus: (1) the subcorneal neutrophilic type and (2) the intraepidermal neutrophilic type.

In the subcorneal pustular IgA pemphigus, histological examination of the lesions shows epidermal spongiosis with exocytosis of neutrophils and some eosinophils and forming subcorneal collections of neutrophils. Acantholysis is usually not seen, and if it is present, there are usually only isolated cells. In the superficial dermis there are perivascular infiltrates of neutrophils, eosinophils, and lymphocytes. The intraepidermal neutrophilic IgA pemphigus shows epidermal acanthosis with spongiosis and exocytosis of neutrophils and eosinophils [655]. These cells tend to form microabscesses and pustules inside the stratum spinosum of the epidermis. In the dermis there is papillary edema and perivascular infiltrates with rich neutrophils, eosinophils, and lymphocytes. Acantholysis is also rare in the biopsies of these patients, although some cases have been reported where there were suprabasal blisters identical with those of pemphigus vulgaris. The exact pathogenic role of IgA autoantibodies in pustular formation in IgA pemphigus remains to be elucidated [682-3]. The differential diagnosis in this subtype of IgA pemphigus has to be done with pemphigus vegetans (Hallopeau type) and halogenodermas.

Because the subcorneal pustular IgA pemphigus is clinically and histologically indistinguishable from classical (Sneddon-Wilkinson disease), immunologic characterization is essential to distinguish the two diseases. The differential diagnosis in this subtype of IgA pemphigus must be made with subcorneal pustular dermatosis of Sneddon-Wilkinson, pustular psoriasis, acute generalized exanthematous pustulosis, or impetigo.

11.2. Immunofluorescence Studies

11.2.1. Direct Immunofluorescence Staining

Direct immunofluorescence is a technique placed between conventional histopathology and laboratory techniques. It was introduced in dermatology in the early 1960s and up to remains a useful technique for the diagnosis of different inflammatory skin diseases, and it must be considered essential for the diagnosis of autoimmune blistering diseases. Direct immunofluorescence is an immunohistological staining that allows the detection of the presence of antibodies or other proteins in skin biopsies of various skin conditions [684-5].

In general, a biopsy from patients with autoimmune blistering diseases must be taken from perilesional normal or erythematous skin (unlike other diseases like lupus erythematosus). Biopsies of vesicles or blisters should be avoided as they will often show false-negative results. Once the tissue has been obtained by punch or excision, the sample must be frozen immediately in liquid nitrogen or placed in saline solution for later freezing after a short time. In those cases where the immunofluorescence laboratory is not found near the center where the biopsy is done, the tissue has to be placed in a transport medium. The most used by dermatologists is Michel's medium, a solution that will preserve the biopsy for several days or even weeks at room temperature [686-7]. The sample can then be sent by mail to the laboratory where it will be washed in Michel's washing medium, frozen, and later processed for immunofluorescence.

It has been recently observed the best results are obtained if the biopsy is kept in saline for about 24h (instead of directly freezing the biopsy) when the sample reaches the laboratory [688]. This procedure "washes away" the tissue and decreases the background staining. Those biopsies that will arrive to the laboratory after a longer period (more than 24 h) should be sent in Michel's medium. Another concern that should be mentioned is that if a biopsy for direct immunofluorescence is accidentally immersed in formalin, this can cause both false negative and false-positive findings that make them less suitable for the diagnosis, and therefore, taking a new biopsy would be advisable [689].

In the next steps, the biopsy is frozen, and 4–6 μm section is obtained using a cryostat. Later, the sections will be incubated with polyclonal antibodies directed against human IgG, IgA, IgM, C3 fraction of complement, and fibrinogen conjugated with fluorescein isothiocyanate. Finally, after washing the biopsy several times to remove the unbound antibodies, tissue sections are examined using a fluorescence microscope. The blue light (wavelength 488 nm) emitted from the light source is capable of exciting fluorescein isothiocyanate, and this molecule will emit a wavelength of 520 nm that will be seen under the microscope with an apple green color.

11.2.1.1. Pemphigus Vulgaris

Direct immunofluorescence of perilesional biopsies obtained from the skin or mucous membranes from pemphigus vulgaris patients will show the deposition of IgG on the cell surface of epidermal keratinocytes (Figure 27) in almost all patients with active disease [690]. Although these deposits are usually found in all epidermal layers and in the adnexae (hair follicles and eccrine glands), in some patients these deposits are more intense or only found in the lower third of the epidermis. These deposits may be linear and intense and show a fishnet-like intercellular pattern, although in some patients we will observe a pattern of granular deposits on the cell surface of keratinocytes. There is also deposition of C3 in the biopsies of these patients, although, compared to IgG deposits, these deposits are always of lower intensity and found mostly in the lower layers of the epidermis. In general, most studies have shown that direct immunofluorescence is positive in more that 90% of cases of pemphigus vulgaris, being more sensitive than indirect immunofluorescence examination. Although all these findings are characteristic of pemphigus vulgaris (Table 10), they cannot be considered specific as they may also be seen in any type of pemphigus (Pemphigus foliaceus, paraneoplastic pemphigus). Besides the importance in the diagnosis of pemphigus vulgaris, direct immunofluorescence has also been suggested as a useful marker to decide whether it is advisable to suspend treatment in a patient in clinical remission, although this is still controversial. If, despite the absence of clinical lesions, direct immunofluorescence positivity persists when we perform a biopsy from normal skin, there is an increased risk of recurrence compared with patients with negative direct immunofluorescence in the same setting [691].

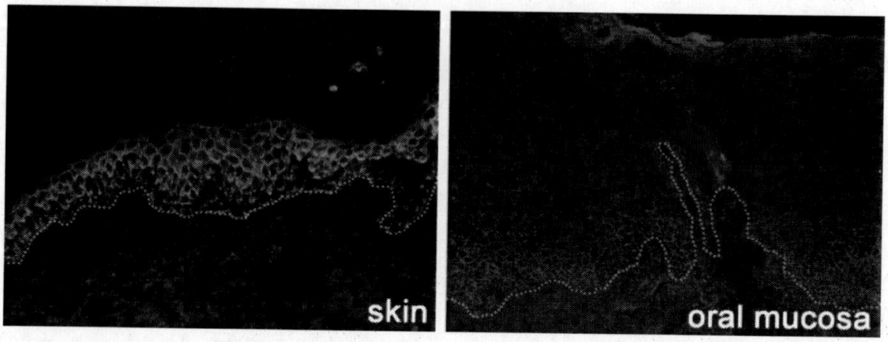

Figure 27. Direct immunofluorescence in pemphigus vulgaris. (a) Direct immunofluorescence of the cutaneous lesions revealed in vivo IgG deposition on the keratinocyte cell surface from the mid to upper epidermal layers, whereas (b) those from oral mucosa demonstrated moderate to weak IgG deposition in predominantly in the lower layers. Reproduced with permission of John Wiley and Sons from Shinkuma S, Nishie W, Shibaki A, et al. Cutaneous pemphigus vulgaris with skin features similar to the classic mucocutaneous type: a case reporte and review of the literature. Clin Exp Dermatol 2008; 33: 724-8.

Table 10. Immunofluorescence findings in pemphigus

Main type	Direct Immunofluorescence	Indirect Immunofluorescence
Pemphigus vulgaris	Intercellular IgG and C3 in the epidermis/epithelium	Intercellular IgG antibodies on monkey esophagus.
Pemphigus vegetans	Same as pemphigus vulgaris	Same as pemphigus vulgaris
Pemphigus foliaceous	Intercellular IgG and C3 in the epidermis	Intercellular IgG antibodies on monkey esophagus or guinea pig lip/tongue.
Pemphigus erythematosus	Intercellular IgG and C3 in the epidermis; lupus band (IgG and C3) at the basement membrane zone.	Intercellular IgG antibodies on monkey esophagus; ANA on monkey esophagus or Hep-2.
Endemic pemphigus	Same as pemphigus foliaceous	Intercellular IgG antibodies on monkey esophagus.
Pemphigus herpetiformis	Intercellular IgG and C3 in the epidermis	Intercellular IgG antibodies on monkey esophagus
Paraneoplastic pemphigus	Intercellular IgG and C3 in the epidermis; linear IgG and/or C3 along the dermal-epidermal junction.	Intercellular IgG antibodies on monkey esophagus and on plakin rich substrate (rat urinary bladder).
Drug-induced pemphigus	Intercellular IgG and C3 in the epidermis; sometimes linear IgG or C3.	Intercellular IgG antibodies on monkey esophagus.
IgA pemphigus	Intercellular IgA and C3 in the epidermis.	Intercellular IgA antibodies on monkey esophagus.

11.2.1.2. Pemphigus Foliaceus and Erythematosus

In pemphigus foliaceus the characteristic direct immunofluorescence findings is the presence of IgG deposits on the keratinocyte cell surface in the outermost surface of the epidermis, sometimes extending to the upper two thirds of the stratum spinosum. In many patients there are also C3 deposits with the same distribution and pattern, although they are usually less intensive.

These findings may be similar to other types of pemphigus, like pemphigus vulgaris or paraneoplastic pemphigus. Pemphigus erythematosus (also known as Senear-Usher syndrome) was described originally as an overlap between pemphigus foliaceus and lupus erythematosus. These patients can present malar rash, positive antinuclear antibodies, and granular deposition of IgG and C3 along the basement membrane zone (like a positive lupus band) besides the characteristic intercellular IgG deposits in the superficial layers of the epidermis. These findings are not specific of pemphigus erythematosus, as they may be not rarely noted in pemphigus foliaceus, as well as in paraneoplastic pemphigus, particularly the basement membrane zone deposition of C3 [692]. What is less frequent is the finding of granular IgG deposition along the basement membrane zone. It has been shown that this can occur after UV light exposure in patients with pemphigus foliaceus and that this might induce the cleavage of the desmoglein 1 ectodomain that co-localizes with IgG at the basement membrane zone [693].

11.2.1.3. Paraneoplastic Pemphigus

Direct immunofluorescence examination of perilesional skin in paraneoplastic pemphigus can usually show the presence of IgG deposits on the cell surface of keratinocytes in the epidermis and adnexa with a similar pattern to other forms of pemphigus. There are also C3 deposits in the cell surface of keratinocytes, but they are usually less intensive. Granular or linear deposits of immunoglobulins or C3 along the basement membrane zone are also a frequent finding in paraneoplastic pemphigus. They are usually of C3, but IgG may also be found, as well as IgA or IgM. This combined pattern (deposits on the surface of intercellular keratinocytes and in the basement membrane zone) despite being suggestible of paraneoplastic pemphigus is not specific for the disease since it can be observed up to 10–20% of other forms of pemphigus (primarily in pemphigus foliaceus). In addition, between 20 and 60% of paraneoplastic pemphigus patients will have only an intercellular pattern that is indistinguishable from other forms of pemphigus, like pemphigus vulgaris [545]. Another important fact in paraneoplastic pemphigus is the high proportion of false-negative findings in direct immunofluorescence that have been reported in the literature (from 14 to 28%) [693]. This false-negative rate in paraneoplastic pemphigus is much higher than in other forms of pemphigus, and therefore, if there is a high clinical suspicion, a negative direct immunofluorescence does not exclude the diagnosis.

11.2.1.4. IgA Pemphigus

The diagnosis of IgA pemphigus is mainly based on direct immunofluorescence findings. This shows the presence of intercellular IgA deposits in the epidermis. There are usually no other immunoreactants, and if they are found, the deposits are faint. The IgA deposits are usually located almost only in the upper third of the epidermis in the subcorneal pustular dermatosis subtype, while in the intraepidermal neutrophilic dermatosis subtype, the intercellular deposits of IgA can be found throughout the epidermis, but sometimes they are more intense in the lower half.

11.2.2. Indirect Immunofluorescence Examination

Indirect immunofluorescence is a widely used technique for the detection of circulating auto antibodies in the serum of patients with autoimmune blistering diseases. It is very useful for the diagnosis and characterization of these diseases, although it is far less sensitive than direct immunofluorescence (which should be positive in 100% of the patients with active disease) because circulating autoantibodies can be present at low levels and therefore are not always detectable.

For indirect immunofluorescence examination we will need to get blood from the patients, although some authors have used blister fluid or even urine for indirect immunofluorescence studies [694-5]. About 5–10 ml of blood is usually needed, and after the blood is drawn, it has to be collected in a tube without anticoagulants (like EDTA, sodium citrate, or heparin). Blood samples should be allowed to clot, and serum is then separated from the clot by centrifugation. It can then be aliquot and stored at−25°C until indirect immunofluorescence is done. Blood samples can be left in the refrigerator for 24–48 h before centrifugation or while they are waiting to be sent to the lab. It is important to note that blood samples should never be frozen if they have to be used for indirect immunofluorescence because this may cause extensive hemolysis that will alter the results. Another important issue is to avoid using tubes with anticoagulants because we would obtain plasma instead of serum and, if used, fibrinogen can lead to artifacts of non specific fluorescence.

The tissue substrate that will be used will depend on the disease that we are studying and the autoantibodies that we want to detect. The substrate slides can be obtained commercially (like monkey esophagus), alternatively the tissue can be prepared in the laboratory (like 1M sodium chloride separated a skin or rat bladder) and frozen, and 4–6 μ[mu]m tissue sections will be obtained with a cryostat. Tissue sections can then be incubated with patient serum at initial dilutions of 1:10 and 1:20 for 30 min. The slides will then be washed to remove the unbound antibodies and incubated for 30 extra minutes with polyclonal antibodies directed against humanIgG (or IgA when we are studying the presence of circulating IgA autoantibodies) conjugated with FITC. Finally, after performing several washes, the tissue sections will be mounted and examined using a fluorescence microscope.

11.2.2.1. Pemphigus Vulgaris

The presence of circulating serum antibodies against the cell surface of keratinocytes is characteristic of patients with all types of pemphigus. These antibodies bind to the intercellular spaces of stratified epithelia producing a *fishnet* pattern on indirect immunofluorescence that is indistinguishable between the different types of pemphigus. These antibodies are usually of the IgG class. Overall, it is estimated that circulating antibodies can be detected in more than 75% of the patients and in the sera of nearly all patients with active disease. When the patients have localized disease or are in clinical remission, indirect immunofluorescence will usually be negative [696].

Although the detection of these intercellular IgG autoantibodies by indirect immunofluorescence is characteristic of pemphigus (Table 10), their detection has also been observed in other entities like thermal burns, tinea, impetigo, bullous pemphigoid, mucous membrane pemphigoid, toxic epidermal necrolysis, cutaneous drug eruptions, etc. [697]

In 1964, Beutner et al. [360] showed that patients with pemphigus vulgaris had circulating antibodies against the cell surface of keratinocytes. In general, the serum titer of these autoantibodies correlates with disease extension and activity, but it is not always useful in clinical management to guide treatment or in predicting clinical relapses [698]. Different substrates can be used for IIF, yielding distinct sensitivities.

Monkey esophagus is considered the best substrate for pemphigus vulgaris, being superior to guinea pig esophagus, guinea pig lip, human skin, or other substrates [699]. Another interesting way to increase the sensitivity of indirect immunofluorescence in pemphigus is to use calcium-supplemented buffers, as the target antigen of pemphigus autoantibodies is a member of the cadherins that are calcium-dependent adhesion molecules [700].

11.2.2.2. Pemphigus Foliaceus and Erythematosus

The presence of circulating autoantibodies in the serum of patients with pemphigus foliaceus and endemic pemphigus foliaceus was also showed by the group of Beutner in the 1960s. Circulating antibody titers correlate to the extent of disease and its activity both in endemic and non-endemic forms of pemphigus foliaceus [701]. However, in some individual cases this correlation is not so clear, so it is recommended to note the patient's clinical improvement when we want to decrease treatment in each case. In pemphigus foliaceus, indirect immunofluorescence results will also vary depending on the substrate that we use. Different studies have shown the best substrates for indirect immunofluorescence testing in pemphigus foliaceus are in decreasing order of sensitivity: human skin [702], guinea pig esophagi [703], and monkey esophagus. In a similar way to pemphigus vulgaris, adding calcium to the buffers used in indirect immunofluorescence technique will increase the sensitivity of the test [700], In patients with pemphigus erythematosus (Senear-Usher syndrome), indirect immunofluorescence testing can show the presence of antinuclear antibodies, or other markers of connective tissue disease [591], concomitantly with the presence of pemphigus autoantibodies.

11.2.2.3. Paraneoplastic Pemphigus

The serum of patients with paraneoplastic pemphigus-like in other types of pemphigus contains IgG antibodies that react with the intercellular spaces of monkey esophagus epithelium or other flat stratified epithelia. The antibodies may stain the intercellular spaces, but some patients show a diffuse pattern where all the cells are stained (a diffuse cytoplasmic pattern). This is because of the presence of antibodies to intracellular proteins (like plakins). Some patients have also been described with prominent basement membrane zone staining of the esophagus, in a similar pattern to pemphigoid [704]. What is characteristic of paraneoplastic pemphigus autoantibodies is that in addition to binding to the cell surface of stratified epithelia, they also bind to other types of epithelia (simple, columnar, and transitional) and other non-epithelial substrates (thyroid, myocardium, skeletal muscle, and liver) [290]. When rat bladder epithelium is used as a substrate for indirect immunofluorescence, it is usually positive in most patients with paraneoplastic pemphigus and negative in other forms of pemphigus. At first, it was considered a specific technique (98.9%) for the diagnosis of paraneoplastic pemphigus [705]. In later studies it was observed the specificity was lower (about 83% in some series) and that circulating antibodies cannot be detected in all patients. In a series of 28 patients, 25% showed no reactivity with rat bladder epithelium, while immunoprecipitation studies confirmed the diagnosis of paraneoplastic pemphigus (sensitivity of 75%) [630]. More recent series have found sensitivities ranging between 86 and 100%, with specificities approaching 100% [545]. False positives (positive indirect immunofluorescence on rat bladder in patients without paraneoplastic pemphigus) have been reported rarely. This has been the case of patients with severe forms of erythema multiforme (which may also be confused clinically) that have circulating antibodies against desmoplakins during outbreaks [706]. Indirect immunofluorescence positivity with rat bladder and the presence of antibodies against desmoplakins (but not against other paraneoplastic pemphigus antigens) has also been reported in pemphigus vulgaris patients with significant mucosal involvement [707]. In summary, rat bladder is considered as an excellent substrate to screen sera of patients with suspected paraneoplastic pemphigus because of a combined high specificity and sensitivity.

11.2.2.4. IgA Pemphigus

IgA autoantibodies directed against the intercellular spaces can be found by indirect immunofluorescence in patients with IgA pemphigus, but the titers are substantially lower than in other forms of pemphigus. Although probably all the patients have IgA circulating autoantibodies, they are often found at low titers and can only be demonstrated in around 50% of the patients. Also, unlike other forms of pemphigus where monkey esophagus is preferred, in IgA pemphigus normal human skin appears to be the most sensitive substrate for indirect immunofluorescence, and in one study almost all patients had circulating autoantibodies using this substrate, although low titers were noted mostly [652].

Chapter 12

ELISA TEST AND IMMUNOBLOTTING

Autoimmune diseases are caused by dysregulation of the immune system, which normally works to attack and remove non-self-antigens [708]. In autoimmune disease patients, antibodies attack and damage self-antigens. The major autoimmune skin diseases are autoimmune bullous diseases [709].

Over the past two decades, the molecular pathogenesis of these diseases has been rapidly enlightened. Making use of this knowledge, molecular diagnostic methods for these diseases have also rapidly developed. Among the sophisticated methods to diagnose these diseases, enzyme linked immunosorbent test (ELISA) and immunoblotting using several different substrates are the two major tests.

12.1. MOLECULAR PATHOLOGY OF ADHESIVE STRUCTURES IN THE EPIDERMIS AS TARGET FOR PEMPHIGUS

The epidermis is composed of mainly four layers, from the upper epidermis to the deep epidermis, the cornified or corneum, granular, spinous, and basal or proliferative layers [710]. In these layers, keratinocytes tightly adhere to each other by the cell-cell adhesion apparatus, desmosomes. Desmosomes are composed of three groups of proteins, i.e., cadherins, plakins, and armadillo proteins. Major trans membrane adhesion molecules belonging to desmosomal cadherins are desmogleins 1–4 and desmocollins 1–3 [711]. The cytoplasmic tails of these proteins adhere to armadillo proteins, plakoglobin, and plakophilins 1–3 [712]. Desmoplakin tethers these armadillo proteins to keratin intermediate filaments [243]. Keratinocytes adhere to basement membrane mainly by hemidesmosomes. The core of the hemidesmosome consists of four transmembrane proteins: BP180/type XVII collagen/BPAG2, α6 and β4 integrins, and CD151 [713]. Both BP180 and α6 β4 integrin interact with laminin-332 at the extracellular space [714]. BP180 interacts with BP230/BPAG1e intracellularly, and α6 β4 integrin interacts with plectin in the cytoplasm [715-6]. Both BP230 and plectin belong to the plakin family proteins, targets for paraneoplastic pemphigus [717]. Both BP230 and plectin adhere to keratin intermediate filaments. (Figure 28) [718-9]

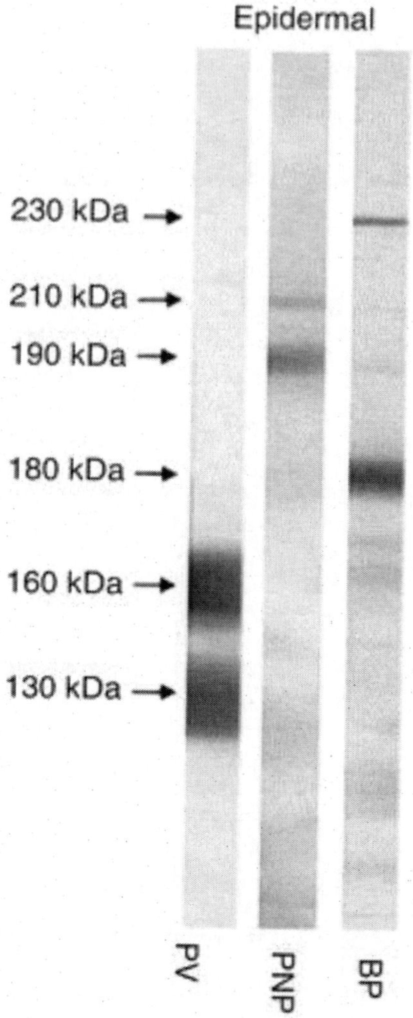

Figure 28. Characterization of antibody profiles of pemphigus vulgaris, bullous pemphigoid and paraneoplastic pemphigus sera by immunoprecipitation.

12.2. Targeting Desmosomal Proteins

Classical pemphigus is the prototype of this group. Pemphigus is an autoimmune bullous disease with autoantibodies against desmogleins. Histopathologically, pemphigus patients show intraepidermal blister and acantholysis. Classical pemphigus is divided into two major subtypes, pemphigus vulgaris and pemphigus foliaceus. The autoantigen for pemphigus vulgaris is desmoglein 3 and that for pemphigus foliaceus is desmoglein 1. Pemphigus vegetans is the variant of pemphigus vulgaris, and pemphigus erythematosus is that of pemphigus foliaceus [720-1]. Other minor subtypes of pemphigus include IgA pemphigus, pemphigus herpetiformis, and paraneoplastic pemphigus [722]. The desmoglein compensation theory can explain the phenotypic differences among the aforementioned various subtypes of pemphigus.

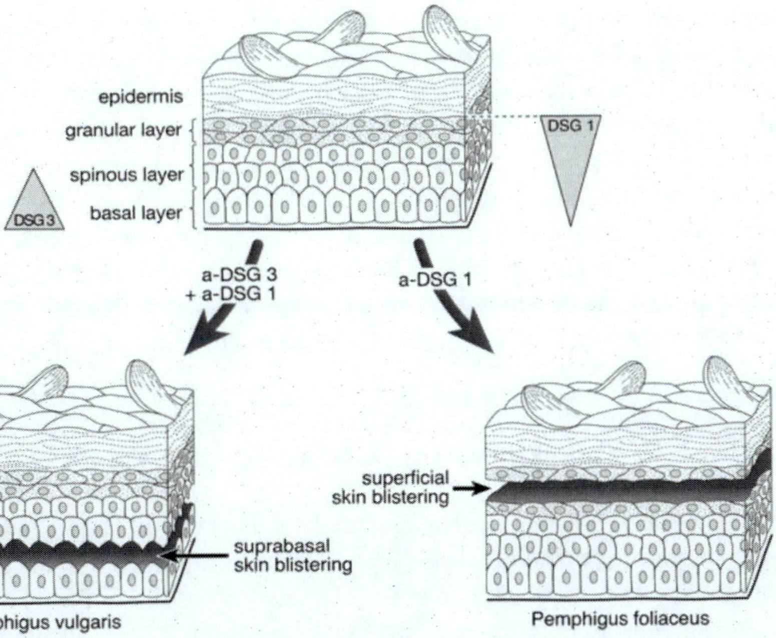

Figure 29. The desmoglein compensation hypothesis. Based on the different autoantibody profiles in pemphigus vulgaris and pemphigus foliaceous together with the findings that desmoglein 3 is present in the deep epidermis only whereas desmoglein 1 is primarily expressed in the superficial epidermis, the desmoglein compensation hypothesis has been proposed to explain the epidermal cleavage planes typical for pemphigus vulgaris and foliaceous. According to this model, blistering in pemphigus foliaceous affects the superficial epidermis because desmoglein 3 is present in the deep epidermis to compensate for the autoantibody-induced loss of desmoglein 1 binding. In pemphigus vulgaris, epidermal involvement would occur only when autoantibodies against both desmoglein 1 and 3 are present because desmoglein 1 is found in all epidermal layers and could compensate for loss of desmoglein 3 binding when antibodies to desmoglein 3 are solely present. Reproduced from Ref. 321 under the Supplemental Terms and Conditions for unrestricted reproduction in any medium with the proper cite.

12.3. Desmoglein Compensation Theory

Although disrupting desmoglein-dependent cell adhesion by autoantibodies is the basic pathophysiology underlying blister formation in pemphigus, the clinical spectrum is more complex. These complex features of pemphigus are explained by the desmoglein compensation theory: desmoglein 1 and 3 compensate for each other when they are expressed in the same cell. The intraepithelial expression pattern of desmoglein 1 and 3 is different between the skin and mucous membranes. In the skin, desmoglein 1 is expressed throughout the epidermis, but more intensely in the superficial layers, while desmoglein 3 is expressed in the lower portion of the epidermis, firstly in the basal and parabasal layers. In contrast, desmoglein 1 and 3 are expressed throughout the squamous layers of mucosa, but desmoglein 1 is expressed at a much lower level than desmoglein 3 [49].

Patients with pemphigus foliaceus have only anti-desmoglein 1 IgG autoantibodies. Patients with the mucosal dominant pemphigus vulgaris have only anti-desmoglein 3 IgG autoantibodies, whereas those with the mucocutaneous pemphigus vulgaris have both anti-desmoglein 3 and 1 IgG autoantibodies. (Figure 29) For example, when sera contain only anti-desmoglein 1 IgG, which interferes with the role of desmoglein 1, the presence of desmoglein 3 compensates for the loss of function of desmoglein 1 in the lower epidermis. In contrast, in upper epidermis, there is no compensation by desmoglein 3. Therefore, blisters only appear in the superficial epidermis of the skin because that is the only area in which desmoglein 1 is present without coexpression of Dsg3. Although the anti-desmoglein 1 IgG binds to mucosa, no blisters are formed because of the coexpression of desmoglein 3. Thus, sera containing only anti-desmoglein 1 IgG cause superficial blisters in the skin without mucosal involvement, as are seen in patients with pemphigus foliaceus [49].

12.4. Enzyme-Linked Immunosorbent Test (ELISA)

ELISA is a plate-based immunoassay which is used to detect autoantibodies in various autoimmune diseases, including autoimmune bullous diseases. In ELISA, recombinant proteins of target autoantigens are immobilized to a solid surface of the plates, which are then incubated with autoantibodies in the patient sera, followed by incubation with second antibody conjugated with horseradish peroxidase. Detection is achieved by enzyme activity of these peroxidases via incubation with chromogen [723].

ELISA test alone is not enough to diagnose autoimmune bullous diseases; the patient has to have typical clinical features, histopathology and positive direct immunofluorescence, because unaffected patients can have non-pathogenic antibodies in the sera. ELISA test is available for several autoimmune bullous diseases, including pemphigus vulgaris; pemphigus foliaceus, bullous pemphigoid, and epidermolysis bullosa acquisita, to both make diagnosis and survey the clinical course in these diseases. Historically, ELISAs are first developed for the diagnosis of pemphigus vulgaris and pemphigus foliaceus in 1997. The recombinant proteins of full-length of extracellular domains of desmoglein 3 and 1 were produced by baculovirus expression system [724]. Using ELISAs of both desmoglein 1 and 3, serological diagnosis of mucosal-dominant-type pemphigus vulgaris, mucocutaneous-type pemphigus vulgaris, and pemphigus foliaceus became possible [258]. Positive desmoglein 3 ELISA with negative desmoglein 1 ELISA means mucosal-dominant-type pemphigus vulgaris. Positive desmoglein 1 ELISA with negative desmoglein 3 ELISA means pemphigus foliaceus. Double positive by ELISAs for both desmoglein 1 and 3 means mucocutaneous-type pemphigus vulgaris. However, clinical and histopathological findings are also required to diagnose correctly these diseases. The specificity and sensitivity of desmoglein 3 ELISA for a diagnosis of pemphigus are 94 and 96%, respectively, and those of desmoglein 1 ELISA are 96 and 96% [724]. The effect of steroids and determination of steroid dose can be assessed by recording ELISA indices [725]. Also, clearance of autoantibodies before and after plasmapheresis can also be confirmed [726].

12.5. IMMUNOBLOTTING

Immunoblotting is used to identify auto antigens in various autoimmune bullous diseases. Proteins are separated by electrophoresis and then transferred onto nitrocellulose or polyvinylidene difluoride membrane [726]. The membrane is overlaid with patient sera and then with second antibodies to human IgG or IgA conjugated with horseradish peroxidase or other enzymes [727-8].

Immunoblotting is a relatively easy method to be performed in any clinical laboratories. The disadvantage of immunoblotting is low sensitivity because of degeneration of target proteins during electrophoresis procedure. By immunoblotting using normal human epidermal extract, patient IgG antibodies react with the 130 kDa desmoglein 3 in pemphigus vulgaris and pemphigus vegetans [729]; with the 160 kDa desmoglein 1 in pemphigus foliaceus, pemphigus erythematosus, and mucocutaneous-type pemphigus vulgaris [730]; with the 210 kDa envoplakin and the 190 kDa periplakin in paraneoplastic pemphigus [731].

Chapter 13

ELECTRON MICROSCOPY AND IMMUNOELECTRON MICROSCOPY

Epidermal blistering diseases affect malpighian stratified squamous epithelium lining the skin and the oral, esophageal, nasal, pharyngolaryngeal, conjunctival, genital, and anal mucous membranes; and they are secondary to binding autoantibodies on proteins of adhesion junction systems, e.g., desmosomes between keratinocytes. The electron microscopy studies allow for the analysis of these junction systems which cannot be detailed seen by light microscopy.

Two techniques of electron microscopy are available: (1) standard transmission electron microscopy and (2) immunoelectron microscopy. The standard transmission electron microscopy as the standard histology allows identifying intraepidermal and epithelial blistering diseases. Standard transmission electron microscopy also enables studying precisely the level of blister formation and the structural abnormalities of junction systems which lead to this cleavage. The direct immunoelectron microscopy as direct immunofluorescence allows the detection of *in vivo* bound IgA, IgG, IgM, and/or C3. While the direct immunofluorescence gives only general information showing immune deposits either in a net staining pattern on intercellular substance of the malpighian epithelium, direct immunoelectron microscopy shows exact *in vivo* antibody binding sites within the junction systems. The localization of the target antigens of circulating autoantibodies can be determined by indirect immunoelectron microscopy testing the serum of the patient on normal skin. Finally, standard histology and direct immunofluorescence all together allow classifying the intraepidermal autoimmune bullous group of pemphigus. Standard transmission electron microscopy and immunoelectron microscopy help in the differential diagnosis of types and subtypes of blistering diseases in each of these groups.

The minimal size of the biopsy is 3 mm for the electron microscopy and 6 mm for the immunoelectron microscopy. The sample must be immersed immediately in the acceptable medium since any delay will cause it to dry out and result in irreversible damages, rendering it partially or useless for later electron microscopy analysis.

13.1. Fixation and Specimen Processing

The basic principle of a primary and secondary fixation sequence is accepted as being the best method of fixing specimens for electron microscopy, while immunoelectron microscopy asks for a specific specimen processing. Typically the embedding and processing for standard transmission electron microscopy takes 4 days and for immunoelectron microscopy takes two extra days to perform the immunolabeling. This can be achieved with horseradish peroxidase [732-4], or colloidal gold [735-7], and before [694] after [736], or without embedding [737-8].

13.2. Results in Individual Diseases

When the patients have multiple locations of their disease, these results are the same from one location to another. The labeling by direct immunoelectron microscopy reveals auto antibodies increased in the skin or mucous membrane of the patients and is coarser than by indirect immunoelectron microscopy since the sera containing the autoantibodies are diluted before use. The techniques of immunoelectron microscopy in block before embedding can only reveal membrane or extracellular antigens. Finally, interpreting the results has to consider the ultrastructure of normal skin and mucous membranes and its variations without pathological significance [738].

13.3. Uses in the Pemphigus Group

Pemphigus is due to anti-intercellular substance autoantibodies directed, among others, against the desmosomal cadherins, desmoglein 1 and/or 3. These antibodies lead to intraepidermal and epithelial cleavage by acantholysis that is a characteristic loss of cell–cell adhesion. The two main subtypes of pemphigus are pemphigus vulgaris and pemphigus foliaceus. Immunoelectron microscopy and standard transmission electron microscopy analyses are not required to make the diagnosis of pemphigus subtypes, based on clinical examination, standard histology, direct immunofluorescence, and possibly ELISA. They have nevertheless precisely located the target antigens of autoantibodies-intercellular substance and allow to better understand the mechanisms leading to acantholysis [739]. Many studies in immunoelectron microscopy have been published with results sometimes opposed from one team to another [365, 740-1]. All authors agree that at least a fraction of anti-intercellular substance autoantibodies bind to the extracellular part of desmoglein1 and/or 3 on desmosomes. Moreover, the inversely graded desmoglein 3 and 1 densities between the basal and granular layers explain very well the difference in level of cleavage between the two subtypes of pemphigus [740]. The discussion focused on whether an interdesmosomal pool of pemphigus vulgaris target antigens exists on keratinocyte cell membranes. Recently, the identification of a pool of non-desmosomal and nonjunctional desmoglein 3 [12, 324] and target antigens other than desmosomal cadherins, such as the E-cadherin located in adherens junctions, increase the interest in these processes [283]. For some authors, the target antigens of autoantibodies in pemphigus are only the desmosomal desmoglein 3 and 1 [742-3]. These authors argue the labeling between desmosomes previously described by others [353, 744-7], was an artifact related to diffusing peroxidases they used as a marker instead of colloidal gold. Since these comments [548], also reported desmosomal and interdesmosomal pools of pemphigus vulgaris target antigen(s). They discussed possible technical problems, in particular loss of antigenicity in the post-embedding immune gold technique. More recently, such loss of antigenicity, after procedure of cryo fixation without chemical fixatives followed by cryosubstitution before immunogold labeling, has clearly been showed by Ishiko et al. [737] Finally, Shimizu et al., [365] using an active pemphigus vulgaris mouse model and immune gold immunoelectron microscopy, have showed the *in vivo* binding of Ig both at desmosomal and non-desmosomal lateral surfaces of keratinocytes in the basal layer, whereas the labeling was mainly desmosomal and a little non-desmosomal in the suprabasilar layers. Many studies using standard transmission electron microscopy have also been published, and all authors agree that acantholysis is the result of an alteration of desmosomes. However, alterations described vary from one author to another. For some, the acantholysis is the result of an extracellular split of desmosomes in half by breaking the bonds between two adjacent keratinocytes [352, 748]. Other study showed the breakdown of desmosomes is intracellular between tonofilaments and their attachment plate, leading to pseudo-half desmosomes [749]. Finally, the last ones think that keratinocytes detach due to a loss of desmosomes at cell surface, which itself would be secondary to their disintegration [750-1]. or abnormal constitution. 59 However, a widening of epidermal intercellular spaces before any change of desmosomes has been demonstrated by several authors using standard transmission electron microscopy, in patients [752-3], passive and active mouse pemphigus models [352-3], and human skin explants [754-5]. It raised many questions and discussions about the sequence of events between the fixation of antibodies on their target antigens and terminal acantholysis. For some, the acantholysis is simply and directly the result of the autoantibodies binding on the extracellular portion of desmoglein 1 and/or 3 on desmosomes, resulting in loss of their intercellular adhesive function by steric hindrance and therefore extracellular split [39]. For others, acantholysis is only the end of a much more complex process starting by binding of anti-intercellular substance autoantibodies on the interdesmosomal/non-junctional desmoglein 3 or 1 or other target antigens of the basal layer. It would be followed by endocytosis of these immune complexes with resultant depletion of desmoglein 3 and/or 1 from desmosomes and decrease of their adhesive strength [756-7]. Finally, pemphigus vulgaris IgG binding to desmogleins would also induce intracellular signaling events that lead to desmosomal dissociation, via the phosphorylation of plakoglobin in the attachment plate [39].

PART 6. GENERAL MANAGEMENT OF PEMPHIGUS

One of the main goals of treatment of pemphigus is patient education on risk factor for exacerbation and keeps the erosion without crust and aseptic. (Figure 30) Topical agents may be useful for palliative treatment of symptomatic oral lesions. Topical anesthetic rinses, such as viscous lidocaine, are often effective for temporary relief while high-potency topical corticosteroids can be prescribed in various forms (rinses, pastes, gels) and may be used as monotherapy or with systemic treatment. Topical tacrolimus has also proved some benefit in treating recalcitrant lesions. Intralesional corticosteroid injections may be used to treat oral pemphigus vulgaris lesions, but this therapy has been associated with scarring and/or mucosal atrophy.

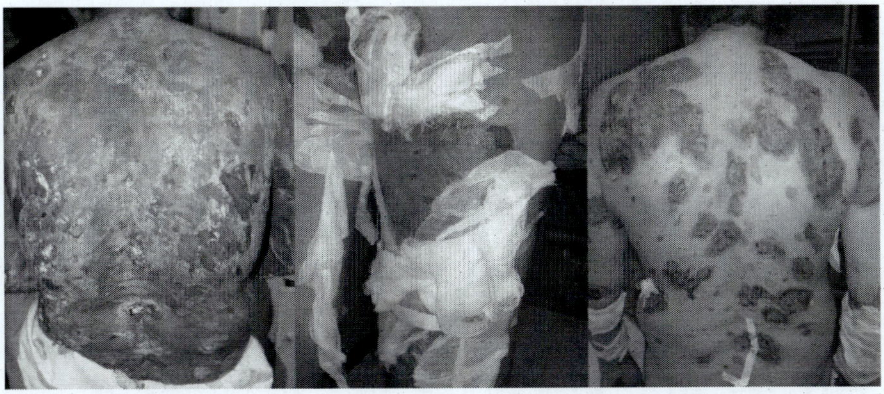

Figure 30. Negative aspects of patient auto-care. Education about the correct topical treatment as well as systemic treatment is mandatory.

Chapter 14

NON-BIOLOGICAL THERAPY

Pemphigus is a potentially life-threatening condition with chronic blistering capable of causing fluid depletion, secondary infection or sepsis, and, sometimes, death. Before the advent of corticosteroids, mortality was about 90% usually because of sepsis [758], however, currently most deaths are attributable to side effects of steroid therapy [531]. The death rate which is commonly reported in general reviews on pemphigus is around 6% [131]. However, most references cited in these general reviews referred to previous general reviews, rather than original epidemiological studies. In fact, two recent epidemiological studies performed on large series of pemphigus patients in the UK and in France have estimated the 1, 2, and 5 year survival rates at 88–90%, 75–85%, and 65–82% respectively, similar to mortality rates from 10% 1 year after the diagnosis to 18–35% 5 years after diagnosis which is much higher than the 5% mortality rate commonly reported in general reviews on pemphigus [62, 522, 759]. Thus, adjuvant therapies are commonly employed in the long-term management of pemphigus in patients who do not respond to high dose steroids, cannot tape or tolerate the steroids due to systemic complications [131]. Treatment for pemphigus can be categorized into three phases: control phase, consolidation phase, and maintenance phase [394]. The control phase is the acute phase in which high doses are required to suppress the disease. In the consolidation phase, the current dose of medications is continued until resolution of most lesions. These are about of weeks, usually. The maintenance phase consists of tapering of medications and selection of proper doses which prevent forming new lesions and is about of several months to a year. Because of their delayed onset of action, adjuvants are typically started in the maintenance phase of therapy rather than control or consolidation phases [760]. It is in this phase that complete withdrawal of all medications is attempted. A diverse group of interventions has been reported in pemphigus, (Figure 31) but there is no international consensus among experts about treatment strategy (Table 11) [761]. This is because pemphigus is an uncommon disease affecting a small fraction of the population, and therefore, producing enough numbers in clinical trials is a challenging task. About this, difference among clinical presentations, disease severity, and impact on quality of life limits the generalizability of the results gained from interventional research.

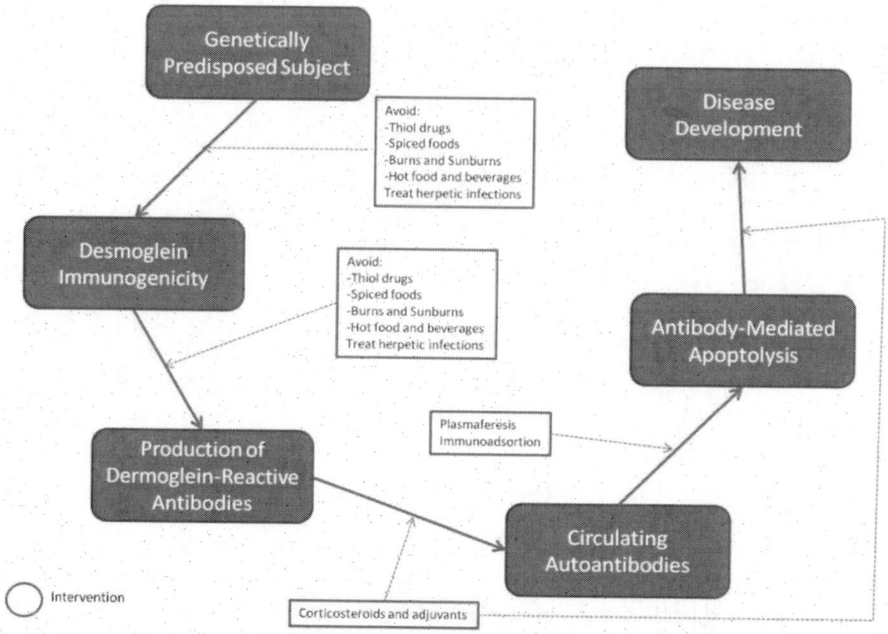

Figure 31. Interventions of pemphigus according to the steps of its pathomechanism.

Table 11. Pharmacological treatments for pemphigus vulgaris

Type of treatment	Drug
Complementary topical treatments	High-potency corticosteroids (clobetasol propionate)
	Tacrolimus ointment 0.1%
First line systemic treatments	Corticosteroids (prednisone) 1mg/kg/day (usually 60mg/day). Tapering by 25% dose reduction every 2 weeks (more extended <20 mg/day) *
	Rituximab 4 weekly infusions at 375mg/m2 of BSA (Lymphoma protocol) or 1g x 2 separated by 2 weeks (Rheumatology protocol) *
Adjuvants (mainly combined with systemic steroids)	Intravenous immunoglobulin 400mg/kg/day administered on 5 successive days (Rate of administration: maintained at 2mg/kg/min or less) *
	Azathioprine 2-4mg/kg/day (usually 100-150mg/day) +
	Mycophenolate mofetil 35-45 mg/kg/day (usually 2-3g/day) +
	Cyclophosphamide 1-3mg/kg/day (usually 50-100mg/day) *
	Methotrexate 2.5-7.5 mg/wk (maximum dose 12mg/wk, given over a 2-day period) +
	Gold
	Cyclosporine 3-5 mg/kg/day *
	Plasmapheresis (usually 2-3 times/wk, double filtration/centrifugation).
	Extracorporeal photochemotherapy
	Dapsone 50-100mg/day +
	Thalidomide 100-200 mg/day.
	TNF alpha inhibitors
	Immunoapheresis or immunoadsorption (on 3-4 consecutive days with 3-4 week intervals) *
	Pulse therapy (methylprednisolone/dexamethasone with or without cyclophosphamide)

* Efficacy on paraneoplastic pemphigus.
+ Steroid-sparing effect.

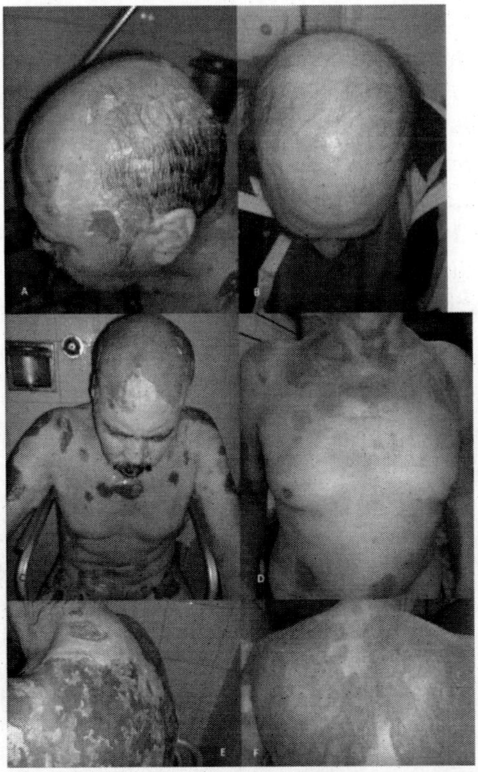

Figure 32. Therapeutic response of a patient with severe, recalcitrant pemphigus vulgaris, treated with pulse corticosteroids + cyclophosphamide pulse with excellent and sustained response.

14.1. CORTICOSTEROIDS

Systemic corticosteroids are considered the first-line treatment for pemphigus and are often used as the mainstay of treatment. Despite the benefits in reducing inflammation and inhibiting autoantibody production [762], systemic corticosteroids are associated with multiple adverse effects and may even contribute to death [534]. Because these side effects correlate with dose and duration of therapy, studies seek to find the minimum dose of corticosteroids needed to induce and uphold remission. In pemphigus higher doses are associated with greater morbidity and do not confer an advantage over lower doses [763-4]. It is therefore recommended that prednisone dosing be less than or equal to 1mg/kg/day, up to a maximum of 120 mg/day [765-6], with the use of higher doses restricted to the rapid control of acute flares. It is often stated that prednisone can be started at lower doses for pemphigus foliaceus as it is usually less resistant to treatment than pemphigus vulgaris [767]. However, some studies failed to prove any difference between pemphigus vulgaris and pemphigus foliaceus for the cumulative dose of corticosteroid [250, 768]. Clinical improvement may be observed within days of starting treatment, although ending of new blister formation may take 2 – 3 weeks [769-70], with full healing occurring on average at 6-8 weeks [771]. When improvement is noticed, prednisone can be reduced within weeks to 30mg/day and then tapered slowly over 3–4 months after that [131]. If control is not achieved with prednisolone and prednisone, it may be worth changing to an alternative corticosteroid or adding an adjuvant such as an immunosuppressant [772]. Pulse corticosteroid therapy has also been studied as a potential therapy. It is to manage high-dose steroid medications over a short time period to rapidly control disease activity. The aim of high-dose pulse steroids is to reduce the duration of therapy, cumulative dose, and iatrogenic effects of corticosteroids [760]. However, this has not been convincingly proven to be effective owing to the studies having inadequate power to exclude a beneficial effect because of the very low number of patients studied and because showing a difference with pulse steroids would need a randomized trial of patients who did not respond to normal oral steroid doses, (Figure 32) since the disorder is often responsive to normal doses of oral steroids. Attention should be paid to the treatment during pregnancy (Figure 33) or to nonclassical variants of the disease. (Figure 34)

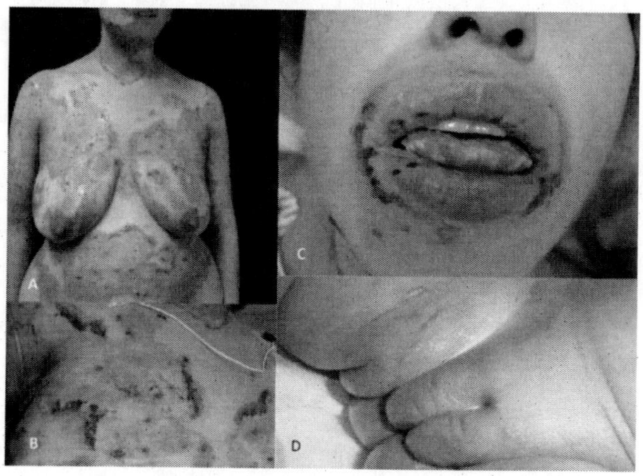

Figure 33. A case of pemphigus gestationis with transient consequences for the product.

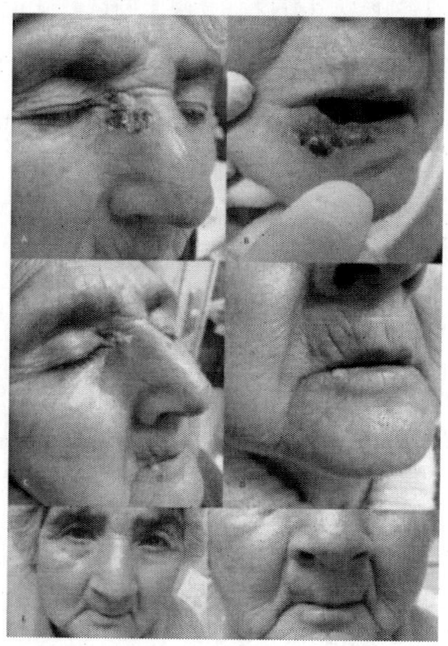

Figure 34. Rare variant of pemphigus (IgG/IgA), initially diagnosed as a malignant tumor. The patient showed an excellent response to topical corticosteroids.

The typical doses prescribed in pulse therapy are 100–200mg dexamethasone or 500–1,000 mg of methylprednisolone [773-4] Adverse effects of pulse therapy include facial flushing, mood and sleep disturbances [773].

14.2. AZATHIOPRINE

Azathioprine is one of the most often used adjuvants to treat pemphigus [767] Azathioprine has been suggested to have a steroid-sparing role in multiple case series [775-9], and it is suggested that it is therefore likely to reduce steroid-related complications [780]. However, most of the studies evaluating azathioprine have been case studies, and its use has not been evaluated in randomized controlled trials [781]. The dose of azathioprine is adjusted according to the thiopurine methyltransferase [767]. With normal thiopurine methyltransferase levels, dosage between 2.0 and 2.5 mg/kg/day is usually prescribed, whereas 1mg/kg/day is recommended for patients with reduced thiopurine methyltransferase activity [782]. Common adverse events associated with azathioprine include nausea, vomiting, myelosuppression, liver disease, arthralgia, and pancreatitis [767].

14.3. CYCLOPHOSPHAMIDE

While there are case reports of successful cyclophosphamide therapy, there are also series that suggest it has limited utility as a monotherapy [783], and the most substantive evidence for its benefit is when used in combination with corticosteroids. Cyclophosphamide appears to have a steroid-sparing effect compared with prednisolone alone based on one study with 54 participants [784]. Cyclophosphamide can be gave orally or intravenously (which is called pulse). Pulse cyclophosphamide has been tried as an alternative treatment but failed to show any benefit [778, 785]. Cyclophosphamide shows a poor safety profile, with patients at increased risk of sepsis, malignancy (especially bladder), infertility, and myocardial infarction. 786 Early use of alternate adjuvants would benefit patients with pemphigus and prevent the adverse events associated with cyclophosphamide use [131]. Refractory diseases can then be treated with cyclophosphamide.

14.4. MYCOPHENOLATE MOFETIL

Mycophenolate mofetil is effective as an adjuvant and a corticosteroid-sparing agent for treating pemphigus [131]. Mycophenolate mofetil appears to be equivalent to azathioprine in inducing disease control based on one study with 40 participants [781]. However, mycophenolate mofetil had an inferior steroid-sparing effect compared to azathioprine [131]. Mycophenolate mofetil also had an inferior steroid-sparing effect compared to cyclophosphamide based on one study with 54 participants [781]. Mycophenolate mofetil is available in 250 and 500mg capsules in an oral form to minimize gastrointestinal side effects but can also be administered in an intravenous form [787]. It is typically prescribed as 2 – 3 g/day in divided doses with reduced dosages in patients with renal impairment [788-9].

Therapy is initiated at 500mg daily and increased as tolerated by 500mg to the needed final dose. Improvement is usually noticed within 2 months of beginning [788]. Cost and availability are limiting factors in its use compared to other immunosuppressive agents [790]. Though mycophenolate mofetil is well tolerated [791], adverse effects have been reported. These are mainly gastrointestinal and include diarrhea, nausea, vomiting, and abdominal discomfort. Such gastrointestinal symptoms are dose dependent and can be reduced by change in dose, gradual dosage increments, or taking the tablet with food [790]. Other reported adverse effects include genitourinary symptoms (frequency, urgency, dysuria), hematological abnormalities (<5% of patients), and opportunistic infections secondary to immunosuppression [792]. Mycophenolate mofetil interacts with multiple medications. Accompanying use with some antibiotics, immunosuppressive agents, and antacids results in a decrease in mycophenolate levels and inadequate immunosuppressive effect. Salicylates and probenecid cause an increase in mycophenolate level and therefore a higher immunosuppressive effect. These effects need to be corrected with dosage changes of mycophenolate mofetil [788, 790]. There is no consensus or guideline for dosing or laboratory checking of mycophenolate in dermatological conditions. Complete blood count with differential liver and renal function tests should be monitored fortnightly at first, then monthly for 3 months, and then every 3 months once on a stable dose [788]. Anemia, leucopenia, neutropenia, and thrombocytopenia have been reported with mycophenolate mofetil [792-3].

14.5. Methotrexate

Methotrexate is another corticosteroid-sparing agent commonly used in pemphigus [794-7], but no controlled trials have yet been conducted researching the efficacy of methotrexate in pemphigus. Though there are concerns about the adverse effects of methotrexate, doses up to 25 mg/week for symptom control are safe. Larger doses can be associated with adverse effects. Nausea and infection, including pneumonia and activation of tuberculosis, were the most common side effects reported on the use of methotrexate in treating pemphigus [798]. There is not enough evidence to draw conclusions regarding the role of adjuvant methotrexate in pemphigus [780].

14.6. Cyclosporine

Cyclosporine has been evaluated in two studies, including comparisons with glucocorticoids alone and cyclophosphamide, but these studies have failed to prove any advantage of cyclosporine as an adjuvant therapy for pemphigus [799, 800]. Also, adverse events are more frequent in the setting of combined glucocorticoid and cyclosporine therapy [801]. It is suggested to use cyclosporine only after other agents have been tried [131],

14.7. Dapsone

Dapsone has been evaluated in one randomized controlled trial with 19 participants [802]. In this study, the authors presented some trends favoring the use of dapsone, but statistical significance was never reached. In a meta-analysis study which summarized 55 identified pemphigus patients who responded to dapsone, hemolysis was the most common adverse reaction observed [803]. In all patients, glucose-6-phosphate dehydrogenase deficiency must be excluded [767]. Dapsone appears to benefit some pemphigus patients in the maintenance phase of their disease; however, as there is little evidence to recommend the use of dapsone in pemphigus, it is difficult to evaluate its utility [780].

14.8 Tetracyclines/Nicotinamide

The evidence for the use of tetracyclines and nicotinamide in pemphigus is derived from small case-series [804-6]. However, these studies present inconsistent evidence about the use of antibiotics and nicotinamide in pemphigus. They could perhaps be considered as adjuvant treatments in mild cases, but further research including controlled trials is warranted to elicit their utility in this setting [780].

14.9. Plasmapheresis

Plasmapheresis is a procedure in which plasma is removed (and not replaced) and is therefore a less complex procedure. The role of removing plasma is to also remove the circulating antibodies from the body. The rationale behind plasmapheresis is based on the observation that there is a correlation between the levels of circulating autoantibodies and disease activity [807]. By removing plasma from the body, circulating antibodies are also removed, hence reducing the number of circulating antibodies and improving disease activity. But removal of the antibodies does not mean that production of antibodies is diminished. In fact, pathogenic B lymphocytes increase the production of antibodies in the 2 weeks following plasmapheresis to compensate for the loss of circulating antibodies. As a result, circulating levels of autoantibodies can be as high as or even higher than before the procedure. This rebound increase in antibody level can be minimized by managing immunosuppressive agents for a period of time prior to plasmapheresis [808]. Despite this rebound effect, compared to other therapies, plasmapheresis results in lower long-term pemphigus antibody levels [809]. Though small trials have proved the efficacy of plasmapheresis in getting partial or complete remission [807], a randomized controlled trial with 40 participants suggested plasma exchange with low-dose steroids is ineffective as a therapy for pemphigus [810]. Plasmapheresis may be considered for rapid control of severe or recalcitrant pemphigus as should the use of accompanying immunosuppression [780]. In clinical practice, this treatment is rarely used because of increased risk of infections and has been superseded by rituximab and intravenous immunoglobulin.

14.10. IMMUNOADSORPTION

Immunoadsorption (also known as immunoapheresis) is a more efficient form of removing pathogenic antibodies and has fewer side effects when compared to plasmapheresis [811]. By removing plasma, plasmapheresis unintentionally removes clotting factors, albumin, and hormones which need to be replaced, immunoadsorption, however, is more specific. Circulating autoantibodies and immune complexes are attracted to the adsorber and removed from the system, leading to a reduction in the number of desmoglein autoantibodies and later improvement in disease activity [812]. Immunoadsorption has been successfully used in pemphigus vulgaris, pemphigus foliaceus, and paraneoplastic pemphigus [813-5] with noticeable improvement within weeks of the procedure. However, the exact efficacy of immunoadsorption is difficult to evaluate since this treatment is most often used with concurrent immunosuppressants, intravenous immunoglobulin, or rituximab in recalcitrant cases [816].

Chapter 15

Biological Therapy

15.1. Intravenous Immunoglobulin

Intravenous immunoglobulin has been used as one part of combined therapy for severe pemphigus since 1989 [817]. Its mechanism of action is complex, targeting multiple parts of the innate and acquired immune system [818]. It suppresses the proliferation of B cells and Th1-type cells, neutralizes and inhibits autoantibodies, blocks Fc receptors, inhibits complement and cytokine production, removes pathogenic immunoglobulins, and increases sensitivity to corticosteroids [819-20]. Its complexity is a reflection of the diverse physiological role of immunoglobulins in maintaining homeostasis. In pemphigus vulgaris, intravenous immunoglobulin inhibits desmoglein 3 antibodies, decreases the number of circulating autoantibodies, and reduces blister formation in mice [821-2]. The average rate of clearance of pemphigus antibodies after 1 week ranges between 30 and 70% [823-4]. Intravenous immunoglobulin is obtained from purified human plasma from healthy donors and contains a high concentration of IgG with a small amount of IgM and IgA [818]. Intravenous immunoglobulin has a half-life of 2–3 weeks after infusion. It is supplied in two forms for intravenous use: lyophilized or liquid. The latter can be used without any modification, but the lyophilized must be reconstituted before administration [818]. Studies with differing designs and doses have led to diverse opinions about the optimal dose of intravenous immunoglobulin. Some report a single cycle of high dose intravenous immunoglobulin (200–400 mg/kg/day) is effective [817], but others claim a dose less than 2 g/kg/cycle (i.e., 667 mg/kg/day) is ineffective and will only provide partial or temporary clinical response [270]. The length of each cycle also varies among studies but is usually reported as between 3 and 5 consecutive days per month. The rate of infusion is commenced slowly and steadily increased as tolerated [818]. Before administration, routine hematological and biochemical investigations should be performed. These include a complete blood count, electrolytes, renal and liver function tests, rheumatoid factor, serum cryoglobulin, and Ig levels to exclude IgA deficiency [818].

As standardized definitions and validated outcome measures for pemphigus [395] are now available, even small randomized controlled trials in pemphigus vulgaris and pemphigus foliaceus can be compared using meta-analysis to provide useful information on the effectiveness of existing and new treatments. Until then, the approach is generally to obtain rapid disease control and then taper the steroids using steroid-sparing agents, until partial and then complete remission on minimal therapy is achieved. If the disease flared during tapering and did not respond to repeating the process with an alternative steroid-sparing agent, then IVIg or rituximab may be considered. As this is a prolonged process, minimization of steroid side effects is important. Thus far, no study has looked at whether primary treatment with rituximab randomized versus steroids would be more effective, safer, and more cost effective than dealing with the long-term after effects of steroids and other adjuvants.

15.2. Rituximab

Rituximab is a chimeric monoclonal antibody directed against the antigen CD20, which is present on the surface of pre-B cells and mature B cells. Rituximab destroys the $CD20^+$ B cells through a combination of complement, antibody, and cytotoxic activities [825]. The CD20 antigen is present on the surface of B cells but is not expressed by plasma cells, stem cells, and B-cell progenitors [826]. The selective nature of this murine-human monoclonal antibody means there is less chance of adverse effects. However, because of the close interaction between B and T cells, selective B-cell depletion indirectly results in decline of a subset of T lymphocytes [827, 262]. Autoantibody levels are expected to decrease with clinical improvement [262], but a clinical response to treatment is not always reflected by changes in autoantibody levels [261]. Some patients who have achieved remission of their mucosal lesions continue to have elevated titres of anti-desmoglein 3 antibodies. On the contrary, changes in anti-desmoglein 1 antibodies are well correlated with of the progress of skin lesions, both in pemphigus foliaceus patients and in pemphigus vulgaris patients with mucosal and skin involvement. So far, no prospective controlled clinical trial on rituximab treatment for pemphigus has been published, but Schmidt et al., [272] looked at 136 cases of pemphigus (pemphigus vulgaris 103, pemphigus foliaceus 20, paraneoplastic pemphigus 13) treated with rituximab reported in the literature. About 95% of them had at least partial remission following rituximab therapy with complete remission in 40%. Clinical remission, defined as healing of all lesions but requiring further immunosuppression, occurred in 37 and 45% of pemphigus vulgaris and pemphigus foliaceus cases, respectively. Only 12% of the total patients had a relapse, and 3% had worsening disease after treatment with rituximab. There is no accepted protocol for treating pemphigus with rituximab [767], but the typical dose of rituximab is 375 mg/m^2 weekly for 4 weeks [828]. Though some reports suggest the need for multiple cycles of rituximab [270, 829], a recent study showed remission after a single cycle [271]. Rituximab is contraindicated in patients who are pregnant or breast-feeding, hepatitis B/C, HIV, and sepsis [830]. An increased risk of infections [831] and death has been reported [832] Premedication with paracetamol and prednisone may reduce the likelihood of infusion-related adverse effects such as hypotension, coryzal symptoms, nausea, and headache. Because of the increased risk of infection, rituximab is recommended in refractory pemphigus, patients in whom it is impossible to decrease systemic corticosteroids due to relapse, and those who cannot tolerate or experience complications with immunosuppressants. The role of early treatment with rituximab about conventional therapies (e.g., immunosuppressants, intravenous immunoglobulin, or systemic corticosteroids) needs further study.

PART 7. DETAILED MANAGEMENT OF PEMPHIGUS: NON-BIOLOGICAL THERAPY

Chapter 16

COSTICOSTEROIDS

Corticosteroids have been central role to managing autoimmune blistering diseases for over 50 years. The advent of their use brought about a vast decrease in morbidity associated with these conditions [833-4]. While they can provide rapid remission and continuing control of autoimmune bullous diseases, they come with various potentially serious acute and long-term side effects. Due to the relative rarity of these conditions, large randomized controlled trials are difficult to coordinate and carry out, resulting in a lack of high-level evidence with which to evaluate the best methods of corticosteroid use in autoimmune bullous diseases. Frequent surveying of patients and simple preventative measures are effective in lessening the adverse results associated with high-dose, long-term corticosteroid use (Table 12) [62].

16.1. USE OF CORTICOSTEROIDS IN PEMPHIGUS

Measurements of equivalency for topical steroids have a much wider range than systemic steroids. This is because, dependent on the site of measurement in the skin of the active ingredient, concentrations differ [835]. Internationally agreed definitions for the various stages in therapy of autoimmune bullous diseases have only recently been published for pemphigus [394] and bullous pemphigoi [836], so many of the stages referred to in reports and studies do not conform to these definitions, further complicating to interpret the literature.

The different types of corticosteroids used in pemphigus include oral prednisone/prednisolone in remission or maintenance therapy, dexamethasone as used in oral-pulsed dosage for remission and topical application for local or mucosal disease [837-8] Intravenous therapy is used only in acute life-threatening situations. A recent systematic review and meta-analysis [837] examined a randomized controlled trial of 22 participants comparing low-dose (45–60 mg/day) to high-dose (120–180 mg/day) oral prednisolone in a cohort of newly diagnosed pemphigus vulgaris and pemphigus foliaceus patients [764]. While the low number of participants made the study underpowered, no significant difference in the time to disease control (no new lesions for 1 week and beginning of healing of existing lesions) was proved [764]. Rates of "remission" (therapy of 15 mg prednisolone per day between the high-dose and low-dose steroid group as recorded over a 5-year period) were also not statistically different [764]. On pulsed corticosteroid use, another randomized controlled trial of 20 participants [774] compared the efficacy of adjuvant pulsed oral dexamethasone

(300 mg/day for three consecutive days, monthly) versus placebo in newly diagnosed patients concurrently treated with prednisolone and azathioprine. Importantly, the rates of adverse results were significantly higher among the pulsed corticosteroid cohort when compared with the continuous dosage cohort ($P < .01$) [774]. It is important to note the patients enrolled in this study did not have severe or refractory disease and that pulsed corticosteroids may have a useful role in those particular subgroups of patient [838]. Dexamethasone was also associated with higher rates of corticosteroid-associated adverse effects [774]. This again highlights the importance of a corticosteroid regimen adapted for each patient depending on their individual disease severity, treatment response, and degree of adverse effects from therapy. Topical corticosteroid use in pemphigus vulgaris and foliaceus has been documented in a few case reports [839-40], and expert recommendations state it may be useful in localized or mild disease (Table 13) [838]. Non-controlled trials exist to formally evaluate its efficacy, but typically, highly potent corticosteroids such as clobetasol propionate ointment are used [841].

Table 12. Checklist for pemphigus treatment

Time of evaluation	Strong recommendation	Optional measures
Before the start of treatment	Confirmation of pemphigus diagnosis (based on the criteria of table).	Endoscopy (pharyngeal, laryngeal, esophageal and gastric lesions)
	Evaluation of disease severity (ABSIS or PDAI).	Tuberculin skin test and prophylactic treatment as needed.
	Urianalysis and hematology (peripheral blood, liver and kidney function, electrolytes, lipid levels. B and C hepatitis serology, diabetes mellitus protocol), C-reactive protein.	Cultures (pharynxs, skin, urine, stool)
	Chest X ray, bodyweight, blood pressure.	Diagnostic scan (ultrasound or tomography), to rule out thymoma, malignant tumor.
	Evaluation of diabetes, hypertension, gastric ulcers, tuberculosis, and other prior illness or complications, and evaluation of status.	Ocular lesion (including glaucoma and cataracts)
	Evaluation of osteoporosis (bone metabolism marker NTX in blood, bone density imaging 1-2 times/year, mostly on old, high-risk female.	IgG, IgA and IgM levels; an evaluation of CD4/CD8 could be included.
After the start of treatment	Periodic tests of peripheral blood (including blood fractions), diabetes findings (fasting plasma glucose, HbA1c), liver and kidney function, electrolytes, lipid levels, C-reactive protein.	Periodic chest X rays, depending on the severity of the case.
	Evaluation of disease activity (ABSIS or PDAI)	Antifungal preventive therapy for Candida (oral cavity)
	Periodic measurement of blood antibody titer using ELISA, if possible, every 1-2 weeks after the start of treatment and once every month after the condition has stabilized.	Cultures as needed (skin, urine, stool)

Time of evaluation	Strong recommendation	Optional measures
	From initial therapy to early-stage maintenance therapy (prednisone 0.4mg/kg/day or 20mg/day), prophylactic administration of antibiotics is recommended to prevent infection.	Antiviral agents (CMV and HSV tests)
	Careful monitoring for steroid-induced adverse drug reactions (including steroid-induced mental and neurological disorders) is required.	Patients with mucosal lesions should receive instruction from an oral care physician (oral hygiene and tooth brushing techniques).

Table 13. Grades of recommendation and levels of evidence associated to the treatments of pemphigus

Drug or treatment	Strength of recommendation	Quality of evidence
Oral corticosteroids	A	II-iii
Azathioprine	B	II-iii
Oral cyclophosphamide	B	III
Mycophenolate mofetil	B	III
Methotrexate	C	III
Chlorambucil	C	IV
Cyclosporine	C	I
Dapsone	C	IV
Pulse corticosteroids	C	IV
Pulse costicosteroids + cyclophosphamide	B	II-iii
Intravenous immunoglobulin	B	III
Gold	B/C	III
Tetracyclines and nicotinamide	C	IV
Plasmapheresis	C	I
Immunoadsorption	Unreported	Unreported

Grades of recommendation.
There is good evidence to support the use of the procedure
There is a fair evidence to support the use of the procedure
There is poor evidence to support the use of the procedure
There is fair evidence to support the rejection of the use of the procedure
There is good evidence to support the rejection of the use of the procedure.
Levels of evidence.
Evidence obtained from at least one properly designed, randomized controlled trial.
Evidence obtained from well-designed controlled trials without randomization
Evidence obtained from well-designed cohort or case-control analytic studies, preferably from more than one center or research group.
Evidence obtained from multiple time series with or without the medical intervention. Dramatic results in uncontrolled experiments also be regarded as this type of evidence.
Opinions of respected authorities based on clinical experience, descriptive studies, or reports of expert committees.
Evidence inadequate owing to problems of methodology (e.g., sample size, or length or comprehensiveness of follow-up or conflicts of evidence).

16.1.1. Adverse Effects of Corticosteroid Use

The adverse effects of corticosteroid use are both acute and chronic and involve almost all bodily systems. Some adverse effects can be life threatening if not correctly surveyed and managed during corticosteroid therapy (Table 14). Management strategies focus on prevention, continuing management, and proper treatment of adverse effects as they occur [834]. Cumulative corticosteroid dose has significant influence over the rate of adverse effects, again highlighting the need for titration of steroid use according to patient responses, both therapeutic and adverse [834].

16.1.2. Cutaneous Effects

Cutaneous effects of corticosteroid use include skin atrophy, telangiectasia, purpura, striae, and wound healing impairment with skin fragility and bleeding from mild mechanical trauma [834]. While not life-threatening, these signs and symptoms significantly affect the quality of life of individuals on long-term corticosteroid therapy [842].

Table 14. Side effects of drugs in therapy of pemphigus

Drug/Intervention	Side effects
Corticosteroids (prednisone) 1mg/kg/day (usually 60mg/day). Tapering by 25% dose reduction every 2 weeks (more extended <20 mg/day)	Hyperglicemia, osteoporosis, weight gain, Cushing´s syndrome, fluid retention, immunosuppression, glaucoma, cataract, increased blood pressure, thinning of skin, mood changes.
Rituximab 4 weekly infusions at 375mg/m2 of BSA (Lymphoma protocol) or 1g x 2 separated by 2 weeks (Rheumatology protocol)	Severe infections, deep venous thrombosis, sepsis, urticaria, arthralgia, anemia.
Intravenous immunoglobulin 400mg/kg/day administered on 5 successive days (Rate of administration: maintained at 2mg/kg/min or less)	Infusion reaction (chills, pyrexia, tachycardia), aseptic meningitis, migraine, headache, renal insufficiency.
Azathioprine 2-4mg/kg/day (usually 100-150mg/day)	Myelosuppression (mostly neutrophenia), nausea, immunosuppression, hepatotoxicity, increased risk of nonmelanoma skin cancers or lymphoma.
Mycophenolate mofetil 35-45 mg/kg/day (usually 2-3g/day)	Nausea, vomiting, reversible hematological adverse effects as leucopenia, thrombocytopenia; immunosuppression
Cyclophosphamide 1-3mg/kg/day (usually 50-100mg/day)	Hematologic, gastrointestinal, pulmonary toxicities; risk of secondary malignancies after prolonged exposure (i.e., >20g cumulative dose); gonadal toxicity and infertility after cumulative doses of >5g.
Methotrexate 2.5-7.5 mg/wk (maximum dose 12mg/wk, given over a 2-day period)	Myelosuppression, hepatic toxicity, pulmonary fibrosis.
Dapsone 50-100mg/day	Methemoglobinemia, hemolysis, agranulocytosis; very rare: hypersensitivity syndrome (dapsone syndrome) with fever, rash, eosinophilia involvement of internal organs.
Immunoapheresis or immunoadsorption (on 3-4 consecutive days with 3-4 week intervals)	Hypotension, bradycardia, sepsis (in particular with central venous line)

16.1.3. Metabolic Effects

The most common metabolic effects of corticosteroids include salt retention, increase in appetite with consequent weight gain, hyperglycaemia, hyperlipidaemia, and insulin resistance. Baseline lipids (cholesterol, triglycerides, HDL, LDL, liver function tests), weight, blood pressure, and blood glucose checking are advised before long-term glucocorticoids, with regular monitoring every 4–6 weeks, when in combination with hepatotoxic drugs such as methotrexate [834]. The patient may become cushingoid with a chubby-looking face (full moon) and "buffalo bump." These effects may take several months to reverse after tapering systemic steroids.

16.1.4. Musculoskeletal Effects

Musculoskeletal effects of systemic corticosteroids include cushingoid proximal myopathy and the unpredictable complication of avascular necrosis, commonly of the femoral head. Prevalence of avascular necrosis ranges from 5% in long-term steroid-treated systemic lupus erythematosus patients, it is thought to be less common in steroid-treated autoimmune bullous diseases patients, and disease factors are thought to contribute to the risk of developing the condition [842]. One of the most common long-term effects of corticosteroid use is steroid-induced osteoporosis. With the greatest rate of bone mineral density loss occurring in the first 12 months of corticosteroid therapy, assessment and therapy before beginning of therapy or as soon as possible after initiation of therapy is vital [843-5]. Baseline bone mineral density testing, and serum calcium, magnesium, and vitamin D levels, is necessary. The test considered most valuable for bone mineral density is dual X-ray absorption spectrometry because of a combination of its low-radiation levels and reproducibility [843-4]. Annual bone mineral density testing along with ensuring adequate calcium supplementation (recommended 1,500 mg/day) and vitamin D (recommended 800 IU/day) can help minimize osteoporosis [843-4]. Other prophylactic pharmacological therapies include bisphosphonates such as alendronate and risedronate [845-6]. Rheumatological guidelines recommend managing bisphosphonates to all individuals on long-term (>3 months) corticosteroid therapy greater to 5mg prednisone per day [844]. Non-pharmacological methods include a low-sodium diet (to help prevent calcium loss from the renal tubules) and minimizing caffeine and alcohol intake [843-4].

16.1.5. Neuropsychiatric Effects

Corticosteroids can induce both depression and hypomania at moderate doses, with psychosis and mania almost only seen at doses above 20 mg/day [847]. One retrospective study could identify individuals at risk by previous episodes of major depression before the onset of disease [847]; however, a review by Patten et al., [848] has documented that prior psychiatric illness is not a risk factor for steroid-induced affective disorder, with the risk in proportion to steroid dose (both daily and total) alone. Factor analysis in a cohort of systemic lupus erythematosus patients on systemic glucocorticoids showed that hypoalbuminaemia was a significant predisposing factor to corticosteroid-induced psychosis in that patients

[849]. Insomnia is a common complaint present at low doses, and therefore, dosing is recommended first in the morning or second dose at lunchtime if using divided doses. In elderly populations, cognitive damage may reveal [850]. Preventive measures encompass monitoring and education and proper dosing regimens, treatment for psychosis with various antipsychotic medications has been documented as effective [848-9].

16.1.6. Ophthalmological Effects

Prolonged corticosteroid use is well documented to result in ophthalmological adverse effects including posterior subcapsular cataracts. Younger patients, particularly children, are more susceptible to form cataracts, and doses equivalent to less than 10mg prednisolone per day can still cause significant increases in the rates of cataract formation when compared to matched controls [850]. Increased intraocular pressures can also occur within months of systemic corticosteroid use, mimicking open-angle glaucoma, although it is more commonly a risk with ocular use of corticosteroids [834]. Patients with preexisting glaucoma have an increased sensitivity to corticosteroids and risk of disease progression. Regular ophthalmological reviews (each 3-6 months of therapy), are necessary in surveying these patients [851].

16.1.7. Cardiovascular Effects

The risk of ischaemic cardiac events and diagnosis of cardiac failure in individuals taking long-term corticosteroids has been evaluated in a case-control study of over 50,000 individuals [852]. Results have suggested the risk of cardiovascular events is increased among individuals on long-term corticosteroid therapy greater than 7.5mg of prednisone per day (OR = 1.25, $^{95\%}$CI = 1.21–1.29) [852]. The risk was not as great for cerebrovascular disease, the results are yet to be corroborated in randomized controlled trials, and therefore general recommendations on prevention or monitoring of patients on systemic corticosteroids are inconsistent.

16.1.8. Gastrointestinal Effects

Corticosteroid use is associated with a slightly significant increased risk of peptic ulcer disease, gastritis, and gastro-oesophageal reflux disease. When used in combination with nonsteroidal anti-inflammatory drugs, a significant elevation in the risk for gastroenterological complications (above the level attributable to non-steroidal anti-inflammatory drugs alone) is detectable [850]. Experts recommend prophylaxis with proton pump inhibitors in the setting of long-term glucocorticoids [851].

16.1.9. Teratogenicity

There have been suggestions that systemic and potent topical corticosteroids may have an association with an increase in the incidence of cleft palate from 0.2 to 2% incidence (when used in the first trimester of pregnancy) and low birth weight, although a Cochrane review found no statistically significant evidence supporting such claims. Currently, no recommendations exist about limiting the use of corticosteroids in pregnancy [851-2].

16.1.10. Immunological Effects

The risk for potentially serious infection in pemphigus patients, particularly those on long-term corticosteroid therapy combined with other immunosuppressive therapies is high. Expert recommendations suggest considering prophylaxis for Candida and/or pneumocystis infections in these patients. Although no clear consensus guidelines are available concerning infectious prophylaxis in pemphigus, the topic has been reviewed recently [853] Williams et al., [834] state that trimethoprim-sulfamethoxazole and dapsone are acceptable alternatives for bacterial prophylaxis, with dapsone having another antiinflammatory properties.

Valacyclovir can be used for viral prophylaxis for herpes simplex, and chlorhexidine/miconazole mouth washes are appropriate for oral candidiasis prophylaxis [834]. Concerns over tuberculosis reactivation with individuals on immunosuppressive regimens have led rheumatological authorities to suggest baseline chest X-rays and tuberculin skin testing prior to long-term therapies. Opinions vary as to the appropriateness of these investigations in those on glucocorticoids alone, as most concern centres around the use of TNFα inhibitors such as etanercept and infliximab [834]. Drugs such as rituximab are being used as first-line treatments for pemphigus patients who have significant contraindications to high-dose corticosteroids. Cost-benefit analyses in the short-term may find that oral corticosteroids are cheaper than topical alternatives, and new biological therapies, however, in the longer-term costs of the sequelae of high-dose steroids, listed above, have yet to be properly evaluated.

Corticosteroids play a central role in the acute control and continuing long-term management of pemphigus and other autoimmune bullous and non-bullous diseases. The lack of research about their efficacy versus placebo is due to the unethical nature of such trials due to the life-threatening adverse results of steroids not being used in these conditions. Their efficacy is widely accepted, and the focus on management of these conditions is to minimize adverse effects of treatment. This is achieved by using the lowest doses of corticosteroids or alternative mode of application possible for maximum efficacy.

Chapter 17

TREATMENT AND PREVENTION OF GLUCOCORTICOID-INDUCED OSTEOPOROSIS

Systemic glucocorticoids play a central role in the treatment and long-term management of pemphigus [781]. Glucocorticoid-associated side effects, such as glucocorticoid-induced osteoporosis, are a significant source of morbidity and the primary limit to the long-term use of these medications. Effective prevention and treatment of these side effects are essential to successful therapy [62].

17.1. PATHOPHYSIOLOGY

Glucocorticoids hasten bone resorption while inhibiting bone formation. This combination leads to an early rapid decline in bone mineral density within the first 3–6 months of therapy followed by a slower yet steady rate of loss overtime with chronic use [854]. Much of this outcome is mediated by direct effects of glucocorticoids on bone cells through an array of effects on nuclear signaling and gene expression, glucocorticoids decrease the replication of osteoblast precursors, impair osteoblastic differentiation and maturation, and inhibit the function of mature cells. They also induce the apoptosis of mature osteoblasts by activating caspase-3, a common downstream effector of multiple apoptotic signaling pathways. The apoptosis of osteocytes, which play an important role in bone repair and maintenance, is induced via the same mechanism [855]. By reducing the pool of available mature and functional bone-forming and bone-repairing cells, glucocorticoids suppress the formation and maintenance of biomechanically normal bone, thereby increasing the risk of fracture and osteonecrosis [856].

At the same time, glucocorticoids favor osteoclastogenesis by increasing the expression of macrophage colony-stimulating factor, receptor activator of NF-kB ligand, and interleukin-6, all cytokines that favor the differentiation and maturation of osteoclasts [855]. In contrast to their activity on osteoblasts, glucocorticoids decrease apoptosis and prolong the survival of mature osteoclasts, thereby promoting bone resorption [857]. More effects of glucocorticoids on bone metabolism include inhibition of calcium absorption from the gastrointestinal tract [858] and calcium reabsorption in the renal tubules [859]. By opposing the actions of vitamin D, glucocorticoids create a negative calcium balance that leads to further bone resorption.

Glucocorticoids also alter the secretory dynamics of parathyroid hormone [860] and inhibit the production of insulin-like growth factor 1 [861]. Blunting of growth hormone and sex steroid secretion may contribute further to the pathogenesis of glucocorticoid- induced osteoporosis [862].

17.2. Problem Scope and Epidemiology

Fractures occur in as many as 30–50% of patients taking glucocorticoids chronically [855]. The most often involved sites are the femoral neck and the vertebrae, where fractures are often asymptomatic but highly prevalent [863]. Compared with postmenopausal osteoporosis, fractures in those taking glucocorticoids occur at higher bone mineral densities [863]. As expected, excess fracture risk correlates with increasing dose and duration of glucocorticoid therapy [864]. However, not only those on chronically high doses have an increased risk. Doses as low as 2.5–7.5mg of prednisolone daily result in decreased bone mineral density and an increased relative rate of hip (1.77) and vertebral (2.59) fracture. Further, this risk increases rapidly within the first 3–6 months of treatment, bringing harm even to those on relatively short-term glucocorticoid therapy [865]. Given these findings, it is not clear that any dose or duration of glucocorticoid therapy can be considered safe for bone health. Across the spectrum of autoimmune disease, the duration of glucocorticoid therapy needed to uphold disease control is of course highly variable and dependent on disease state and severity. The natural history of pemphigus vulgaris and other autoimmune blistering diseases is such the most of patients who need systemic corticosteroid therapy likely will require more than 3 months of it to achieve and keep disease control [866]. The significance of this reality is that patients beginning glucocorticoid therapy for treatment of autoimmune blistering disease are virtually assured of being exposed to a dose and duration of steroids which can negatively impact their bone mineral density and increase their risk of fracture. It is thus the rare patient with a blistering disease for whom the subject of prevention and treatment of glucocorticoid induced osteoporosis is not relevant.

17.3. General Preventive Measures

Early implementation of preventive measures against glucocorticoid-induced osteoporosis is recommended. All patients likely to receive therapy for three or more months should undergo risk assessment and counseling at the outset of treatment [867]. Despite this recommendation, a minority of patients receiving or starting glucocorticoid therapy undergoes bone health evaluation, and few receive recommended preventive or therapeutic medications when suggested [868-9]. Certain general preventive measures are applicable to all patients. Lifestyle adjustment, including smoking cessation (although is a contradictory measure when considering pemphigus pathogenesis), avoidance of excess alcohol, participation in weight-bearing exercise, and fall prevention should be encouraged. Increased bone loss and fracture risk are directly related to the dose and duration of corticosteroid use. Much of this excess risk appears to dissipate within about 1 year of stopping therapy [865]. Strategies aimed at limiting corticosteroid exposure therefore play a key role in osteoporosis prevention. Whenever possible, the lowest effective dose of steroid should be used, and alternative therapy should be substituted. For the initial therapy of pemphigus vulgaris, high-dose (120 mg/day) prednisolone appears to be no better than low-dose (60 mg/day) prednisolone with respect to relapse or disease-related complications [764]. “Steroid-sparing” agents may be introduced “up front” at the time of diagnosis to simplify the reduction in glucocorticoid dosage. Model therapeutic strategies for pemphigus vulgaris and pemphigus foliaceus are currently unknown [781]. Glucocorticoid dosing and tapering strategies continue to be highly variable.

17.4. Calcium and Vitamin D

Glucocorticoids decrease calcium absorption in the intestine and increase calcium excretion in the urine. To restore proper calcium levels, the American College of Rheumatology recommends all patients taking glucocorticoids at any dose and for any duration receive 1,200 mg of calcium and 800 international units of vitamin D daily through diet or supplementation [867]. A meta-analysis of 5 randomized trials involving 274 corticosteroid-treated patients showed that calcium and vitamin D supplementation prevents bone loss compared with placebo, accounting for a mean difference in lumbar and radial bone mineral density of 2.6 and 2.5%, respectively. The authors inferred that all patients starting glucocorticoids should receive prophylactic calcium and vitamin D supplementation [870]. Some epidemiologic studies have suggested a relationship between dietary calcium intake and cardiovascular disease, but results have been inconsistent, and the pooled data do not support any significant risk or benefit. Secondary analyses in existing trials suggest a neutral effect of calcium supplements (with or without vitamin D) on cardiovascular events. Though definitive data are lacking, the known benefits of calcium supplementation for bone health in those exposed to glucocorticoids outweigh possible risks [871]. Vitamin D metabolites such as calcitriol and alfa-calcidol have also shown efficacy for the prevention and treatment of glucocorticoid-induced bone loss [872]. However, there is no evidence these metabolites are superior to vitamin D for that purpose [873]. Furthermore, their use is limited by concern for hypercalcemia and hypercalciuria and because bisphosphonate therapy is more efficacious [874].

17.5. Fracture Risk Assessment

For patients at increased risk of fracture, calcium and vitamin D supplementation may be not enough. At the outset of corticosteroid therapy, patients should be screened for elevated fracture risk using a combination of bone mineral density and clinical risk factors, including advanced age, female sex, low body mass index, smoking history, excess alcohol intake, use of glucocorticoids, history of rheumatoid arthritis, personal history of fragility fracture (low-trauma fracture of the spine, hip, wrist, humerus, or pelvis), and parental history of hip fracture [875]. Bone mineral densities are expressed as a “T-score” the standard deviation difference between the patient’s score and that of a reference population of young adults. Those with T-scores < -2.5 have osteoporosis and are at greatest risk of fracture. Those with

T-scores between −1.0 and −2.5 have osteopenia and are at an increased, though somewhat lower, risk of fracture than those with osteoporosis. There are more patients with osteopenia than osteoporosis, and more fragility fractures occur in that group as a result. Overall, most fragility fractures occur in patients with T-scores greater than −2.5 [876]. For this reason, strategies for identifying patients at risk of fracture must be comprehensive and should not rely solely on measurement of bone mineral density. To help determine which patients are at risk, the World Health Organization developed a Fracture Risk Assessment Tool to predict the likelihood of hip and major osteoporotic fracture (including hip, spine, proximal humerus, and forearm) over a 10-year period for untreated patients between ages 50 and 90. To estimate this risk, the Fracture Risk Assessment Tool equation uses the aforementioned clinical risk factors and the femoral neck bone mineral density, as measured by dual-energy X-ray absorptiometry. The calculation is based on data from large prospective studies and has been validated in 11 independent cohorts. The Fracture Risk Assessment Tool is a useful screening and clinical assessment tool, but due to several limitations, it may under- or over-estimate the risk of fracture in some patients. Some of these limitations, which include failure of the Fracture Risk Assessment Tool to consider the dose and duration of glucocorticoid exposure, are listed in a position statement by the International Society for Clinical Densitometry [877]. While the Fracture Risk Assessment Tool can be used to help identify patients with an elevated risk of fracture, it provides only general guidance; treatment decisions should be made on an individual basis, incorporating the full range of unique risk factors for a specific patient.

17.6. Candidates for Pharmacologic Osteoporosis Therapy

Those at highest risk of fracture are most likely to benefit from pharmacologic therapy. Cost-effectiveness modeling has been performed in various populations to settle the 10-year fracture likelihood threshold at which treatment becomes cost-effective [878-81]. Such models consider the morbidity and cost associated with osteoporotic fracture treatment and prevention and use generally accepted cost per quality adjusted life year thresholds.

17.6.1. Proved Osteoporosis

Patients with bone mineral density T-scores <−2.5 or a history of previous fragility fracture at the time of early assessment have osteoporosis and are at high risk of repeat fracture. Such patients should be treated with bisphosphonates whether they are exposed to glucocorticoids.

17.6.2. Prevention of Osteoporosis

Postmenopausal women and men >50 years old at high risk of fracture should also receive prescription osteoporosis therapy regardless of glucocorticoid use, according to the American College of Rheumatology and the National Osteoporosis Foundation Guidelines

[867]. These high-risk patients are those with T-scores between−1.0 and −2.5 or calculated Fracture Risk Assessment Tool scores estimating the 10-year likelihood of hip or combined major osteoporotic fracture at >3% and 20%, respectively. According to US-specific cost-effectiveness analysis, a 3% 10-year risk of hip fracture, with its high morbidity and cost, is the threshold at which treatment of osteoporosis becomes cost-effective [878]. Postmenopausal women and men >50 years old who do not meet this threshold are at low or intermediate risk of fracture. They should receive pharmacologic therapy if taking >7.5mg of prednisone or its equivalent daily for three or more months. Guidelines for premenopausal women and men younger than age 50 are less well defined. The Fracture Risk Assessment Tool was not developed for use in these populations, and there is limited evidence related to glucocorticoid-induced osteoporosis and fracture risk in these groups. Clinical trials involving premenopausal women and younger men showed low fracture rates in both glucocorticoid-treated and control groups [882]. Also, the long-term safety of bisphosphonates and other medications used to treat glucocorticoid-induced osteoporosis and the effect of these medications on a developing fetus are not well-defined. For these reasons, the American College of Rheumatology recommends pharmacologic therapy only for patients with a history of fragility fracture who are clearly at high risk of more fractures and taking 7.5mg of prednisone or its equivalent for 3 months or longer [867]. Patients without a history of fragility fracture who have evidence of sped up bone loss should also be considered for therapy. Without definitive data in these groups, the decision to start pharmacologic osteoporosis therapy should be individualized and should weigh potential risks and benefits.

17.6.3. Bisphosphonates

For men and postmenopausal women, bisphosphonates are the agents of choice for the treatment and prevention of glucocorticoid-induced osteoporosis. Most data support their use, showing efficacy in randomized, controlled trials for improving bone mineral density and reducing fracture risk. A meta-analysis of 13 randomized trials with 842 patients on chronic glucocorticoid therapy showed a significant improvement in lumbar and femoral neck bone mineral density of 4.3 and 2.1%, respectively, among those taking bisphosphonates compared with placebo groups. The odds of spinal fracture were reduced by 24%, though this result was not statistically significant [OR0.76 ($^{95\%}$CI 0.37, 1.53) [883]. Clinical trials have shown bisphosphonates to be superior to calcium alone as well as to vitamin D and active vitamin D metabolites [874]. For women of childbearing potential, bisphosphonates remain an alternative in select patients despite the concerns noted above. Mechanistically, bisphosphonates are thought to promote osteoclast apoptosis and, in general, prolong osteoblast survival, opposing the effects of glucocorticoids [884-5]. However, the effects of bisphosphonates on osteoblast gene expression and survival appear to be complex, varying with the specific bisphosphonate and its concentration [886]. Of the several bisphosphonates (alendronate (Fosamax), risedronate (Actonel), zoledronic acid (Reclast), ibandronate (Boniva), pamidronate (Aredia), etidronate (Didronel), and clodronate (Bonefos)), alendronate, risedronate, and zoledronic acid are best supported by the available data and most widely used in clinical practice. Randomized trials of 5mg daily, 10mg daily, and 70mg weekly alendronate showed improvements in bone mineral density and a decrease in vertebral fractures among patients receiving glucocorticoids, benefits which were preserved for 2 years

[882]. Trials of risedronate 5mg daily or 35mg weekly similarly showed efficacy for the treatment and prevention of osteoporosis in patients taking glucocorticoids [887]. These patients upheld or increased their bone mineral density and reduced their vertebral fracture risk by 70% compared with control patients [888]. For patients who cannot take oral medications or for whom adherence is a concern, intravenous zoledronic acid at a dose of 5mg every 12 months is an alternative. It too has shown efficacy in increasing bone mineral density in patients taking glucocorticoids chronically [889]. Ibandronate, pamidronate, etidronate, and clodronate all have demonstrated efficacy for preserving bone mineral density in patients exposed to glucocorticoids. Etidronate and intravenous pamidronate are uncommonly used; in clinical practice alendronate and risedronate are favored over the former, while zoledronic acid is favored over the latter. Ibandronate is more commonly used, but there are fewer data about the use of its oral formula than its intravenous form for the prevention and treatment of glucocorticoid-induced osteoporosis.

Where available, these agents are likely to be acceptable alternatives to alendronate, risendronate, and zoledronic acid, but overall, there are fewer data to support their use in this patient population. The American College of Rheumatology has stated that it considers the amount and quality of data about ibandronate and etidronate to be insufficient to recommend their use [867]. Studies comparing bisphosphonates directly to one another have only rarely been performed, but in one trial comparing zoledronic acid to risedronate, bone mineral density improved to a greater extent among those who received zoledronic acid [889].

17.6.3.1. Bisphosphonate. Indications and Side Effects

The bioavailability of oral bisphosphonates is <1%. To aid absorption, patients should be instructed to take the medication on an empty stomach, first in the morning and at least half an hour before breakfast. If not dosed in this manner, bisphosphonates may lose some efficacy [890]. There have been rare reports of renal impairment and acute renal failure following zoledronic acid infusion, though usually this complication has occurred in the setting of multiple myeloma. As a precaution, bisphosphonates are not recommended in patients with creatinine clearance below 30 mL/min. Bisphosphonates may cause symptomatic reflux, esophagitis, or esophageal ulcers. To help prevent these symptoms, patients are advised to take bisphosphonates with a glass of water and remain upright for at least 30 min after dosing. When following these recommendations, the incidence of adverse events is very low. Clinical trials have not shown any excess risk of upper gastrointestinal symptoms in patients taking bisphosphonates compared to those taking placebo [891]. Whether bisphosphonates increase the risk of esophageal cancer is controversial. One large case-cohort study involving 46,000 bisphosphonate users found no increased incidence of esophageal or gastric cancer over 4.5 years [892] Conversely, a case-control study involving 2,954 patients with esophageal cancer showed a relative risk of 1.30 (95% CI 1.02–1.66) among those taking bisphosphonates over an average of 7.5 years of observation [191]. At present, it is not clear whether bisphosphonates increase esophageal cancer risk, but they are not recommended for use in patients with active upper gastrointestinal disease such as those with Barrett's esophagus. Osteonecrosis of the jaw, characterized by pain, exposed bone, and pathologic jaw fracture, has been described in the setting of chronic bisphosphonate therapy. The risk of osteonecrosis of the jaw is roughly 1 in 10,000 to 1 in 100,000 in those taking oral bisphosphonates for osteoporosis [893]. Factors such as multiple myeloma, high-dose intravenous bisphosphonates, long duration of bisphosphonate therapy, dental disease, dental procedures, and smoking increase that risk. Since the risk of osteonecrosis is small for most patients taking bisphosphonates for osteoporosis, there are no special recommendations for dental examination prior to starting therapy. There are also no data to support stopping bisphosphonates prior to dental surgery. However, the American Association of Oral and Maxillofacial Surgeons does recommend stopping bisphosphonates 3 months before dental surgery if the duration of therapy has been longer than 3 years. Because bisphosphonates bind to bone, however, their effects may linger for years, and it is not known whether cessation of therapy decreases the risk of complications. Individual cases of atypical femur fractures, such as subtrochanteric fractures manifest by new onset pain in the mid-thigh or groin, have been reported in patients taking bisphosphonates. Bisphosphonates prevent osteoporotic fractures in part by decreasing bone resorption. They may also prevent normal bone turnover, theoretically increasing bone fragility [894]. Population-based studies suggest the risk of atypical fractures in patients taking bisphosphonates is low and is not significantly increased with duration of therapy less than 5 years. With the use of a bisphosphonate for longer than 5 years, the risk of atypical fracture increases to 0.13–0.22% over 2 years. Conversely, the risk of typical osteoporotic fractures decreases with longer bisphosphonate use [895]. While long term bisphosphonate therapy increases the risk of atypical fractures, the absolute risk is low with uncertain clinical significance. For this reason, the recommended duration of bisphosphonate therapy is controversial. Bisphosphonates have demonstrated efficacy and safety in studies lasting as long as 10 years [896]. Pooled data on patients receiving bisphosphonates for 6 years or longer show maintenance of bone mineral density but no clear and consistent fracture prevention advantage compared to patients who switch to placebo. While these analyses are limited by statistical power and sample size, they suggest bisphosphonates may be safely discontinued in some patients without sacrificing therapeutic gains. Given the potential safety concerns associated with long-term bisphosphonate use, there is new urgency to find out which patients are more likely to benefit from bisphosphonate therapy beyond 3–5 years and which are not [897]. Stopping bisphosphonate therapy after 5 years with continued bone mineral density and risk factor monitoring may be suitable for patients at low risk of fracture, whereas those at high risk should likely continue. Ultimately, the risk of major complications associated with bisphosphonate use is low compared with their proven benefit [898].

17.6.4. Parathyroid Hormone

Parathyroid hormone (teriparatide) is another drug with proven efficacy for the treatment and prevention of glucocorticoid-induced osteoporosis [899]. Intermittent administration of parathyroidhormone produces anabolic skeletal effects and stimulates bone formation [900]. In a head-to-head randomized trial of alendronate versus teriparatide 20mcg injected subcutaneously daily, teriparatide-treated patients experienced a greater increase in bone mineral density than their counterparts taking alendronate, though both groups experienced statistically significant increases [901]. Compared to alendronate, those taking teriparatide also experienced significantly fewer vertebral fractures [902]. Despite these impressive results, teriparatide is not used as a first-line drug for most patients because of its cost, route of administration, and potential dose dependent risk of osteosarcoma, for which it has a black box warning from the Food and Drug Administration in the United States. In a meta-analysis to determine the comparative effectiveness of different pharmacologic agents in reducing fragility fractures, teriparatide was most efficacious for fracture risk reduction. However, differences between bisphosphonates, teriparatide, and denosumab were small and not statistically significant [903]. Bisphosphonates thus remain the first-line treatment option for the majority of glucocorticoid-treated patients with increased fracture risk [844]. Patients at particularly high risk of fracture, such as those who have failed bisphosphonate therapy, those who are unable to tolerate bisphosphonates, and high-risk premenopausal women, are potential candidates for therapy with teriparatide. As with the other pharmacologic option, potential benefits should outweigh potential risks.

17.6.5. Calcitonin

Subcutaneous injection or intranasal inhalation of calcitonin does not consistently prevent bone loss in patients starting glucocorticoid therapy compared with calcium and vitamin D alone [904]. Calcitonin does increase lumbar spine bone mineral density, but trials have not shown the same benefit for bone of the femoral neck, nor have they shown any reduction of fracture risk [905]. The pooled relative risk from five studies was 0.71 ($^{95\%}$CI 0.26–1.89) [906]. For this reason, calcitonin is second line for the treatment and prevention of glucocorticoid-induced osteoporosis. It may be used in patients for whom bisphosphonates and teriparatide are contraindicated or are poorly tolerated, and it may also be useful for fracture pain reduction [905-6].

17.6.6. Denosumab

Denosumab is a monoclonal antibody to the receptor activator of nuclear factor kappa B ligand. By binding this osteoclast differentiating factor, it inhibits osteoclast formation. In clinical trials, it has been shown to increase bone mineral density and reduce fracture risk [907], and there are some data to support its use in patients receiving glucocorticoids [908]. There are currently no head-to-head studies comparing denosumab to other available therapies, and its long-term safety profile is unknown. It is approved for use in postmenopausal women at high risk of fracture and inpatients who fail or cannot tolerate alternate therapies. Because denosumab is not cleared by the kidney, it may be an option for patients with renal failure who cannot take bisphosphonates. Pending further efficacy and safety data, however, it is not specifically recommended for the prevention of osteoporosis or for the treatment of osteoporosis in patients taking glucocorticoids.

17.7. Monitoring and Follow-Up

Serial bone mineral density testing by dual-energy X-ray absorptiometry scan is commonly used to monitor the response to osteoporosis therapy. There is no consensus in published guidelines with respect to the frequency of such monitoring, but annual dual-energy X-ray absorptiometry scan of the lumbar spine and hip while on glucocorticoids is likely enough. If bone loss is rapid, more frequent monitoring can be considered. If the T-score is stable or increasing (a good response to osteoporosis therapy that suggests lowered fracture risk) [909], less frequent monitoring may be appropriate [910-1]. If bone mineral density is decreasing on serial exams, the patient should be evaluated to determine whether adherence to therapy, gastrointestinal absorption, and calcium and vitamin D consumption are satisfactory. If the patient is failing therapy, switching to another regimen should be considered. If oral bisphosphonate failure, alternatives include switching to intravenous zoledronic acid or teriparatide, since these agents have some evidence of superiority to alendronate.

Chapter 18

PREVENTION AND THERAPY OF STEROID-INDUCED DIABETES

While glucocorticoids are a common cause of medication-induced diabetes, not all patients treated with glucocorticoids will develop diabetes. Risk factors include advanced age, high body mass index, increased glucocorticoid treatment, and high total glucocorticoid dose [912]. A large case-control study researching the link between oral glucocorticoid therapy with prednisone and hyperglycemia showed a relative risk of 2.23 ($^{95\%}$CI 1.92–2.59) for development of hyperglycemia in patients on glucocorticoid therapy [913]. It also showed that an increased glucocorticoid dose matched to increased risk of hyperglycemia with odds ratio of 1.77 for 1–39mg of prednisone/day, 3.02 for 40–79 mg/day, 5.82 for 80–119 mg/day, and 10.34 for 120mg/day or more [913]. Consider an average weight (83kg) adult male who receives prednisone 1 mg/kg/day for pemphigus vulgaris. This patient would have an odds ratio of 5.82, indicating a significantly high risk of hyperglycemia during treatment. In addition, glucocorticoid therapy can worsen preexisting diabetes mellitus [912]. With more than 8% of the US population affected by diabetes mellitus and more than 1.5 million new cases diagnosed each year, it is likely that practitioners treating autoimmune bullous diseases will see patients with steroid-induced or steroid-exacerbated diabetes mellitus [62].

18.1. PATHOPHYSIOLOGY

Glucocorticoids alter the body's normal response to insulin by inducing insulin resistance. In the liver, there is a decrease in insulin sensitivity and an increase in gluconeogenesis when glucocorticoids are given. In addition, muscle and fat show decreased glucose uptake, likely as a result of inhibition of the glucose transporter, GLUT4 [914]. The amount by which plasma glucose levels rise is dependent on the ability of the pancreas to oppose this insulin resistance with increased insulin secretion [912]. Eventually, if hyperglycemia continues, the pancreas cannot compensate and diabetes mellitus occurs. Autoimmune bullous diseases usually require steroid treatment duration of months to years. Studies have clearly established a link between glucocorticoid treatment of greater than 1 month and development and/or exacerbation of diabetes mellitus. The evidence for the association between diabetes and steroid therapy of less than 1 month is not as well defined.

However, even a single dose of prednisone 80mg (immunosuppressive dose) increases fasting and postprandial glucose levels [915-6], and even these temporary hyperglycemic states can be harmful. Recent studies have shown that wavering glucose levels over only 24h can lead to endothelial damage, possibly increasing the risk of diabetic cardiovascular disease [917]. As the duration of steroid therapy increases, this risk of microvascular complications increases.

18.2. Signs and Symptoms

Over 50% of patients with new-onset diabetes mellitus are asymptomatic and diagnosed only incidentally [918]. However, many patients present with symptoms such as polyuria, polydipsia, polyphagia, fatigue, and frequent infections, such as recurrent genital candidiasis. If the disease progresses, the patient may complain of extremity paresthesia (classically in a "stocking-glove" distribution), poor or delayed wound healing, visual changes (which can progress to blindness), erectile dysfunction, and even symptoms of coronary and cerebrovascular disease. These sequelae suggest the microvascular and macrovascular complications of diabetes. Uncommonly, patients will have an early presentation of non-ketotic hyperosmolar coma, a life-threatening condition because of volume depletion in patients with uncontrolled hyperglycemia.

Practitioners should use laboratory testing to confirm diagnosis. According to recommendations of the American Diabetes Association or ADA, one of the following criteria must be met to diagnose a patient with diabetes mellitus [919]: HgbA1C ≥6.5%; fasting plasma glucose ≥126 mg/dL (7.0 mmol/L); two-hour plasma glucose ≥200 mg/dL (11.1 mmol/L) following a 75 g oral glucose tolerance test; random plasma glucose ≥200 mg/dL (11.1 mmol/L) in a patient with "classic symptoms of hyperglycemia or hyperglycemic crisis." These criteria may not always be applicable when diagnosing diabetes mellitus in patients treated with glucocorticoid treatment. For example, low-dose and morning-administered glucocorticoids typically do not affect fasting plasma glucose levels [914]. Therefore, diagnosis of diabetes mellitus through fasting glucose levels may not be enough sensitive. An exception to this is twice-daily dosing or prednisone ≥40 mg/day, which can cause hyperglycemia even in the fasting state [914]. It is also important to consider that a 2-h oral glucose tolerance test may not be feasible to perform during office visits. And finally, because the A1C is a reflection of the plasma glucose concentrations over the prior 2–3 months, relying on this measure may result in delayed diagnosis of diabetes mellitus early in the treatment course. A random plasma glucose check may be the best initial test for patients receiving glucocorticoid treatment.

Testing for diabetes mellitus prior to starting glucocorticoid treatment is recommended, as initiation of therapy in some patients has been reported to cause hyperglycemic hyperosmolar syndrome and unmasking of type 1 diabetes mellitus, resulting in diabetic ketoacidosis [920-1]. If baseline testing reveals hyperglycemia, further evaluation and treatment should be performed prior to beginning glucocorticoid therapy. Once steroid therapy is initiated, patients at risk for diabetes mellitus (high body mass index, advanced age) should return in 1 week for a mid-afternoon appointment to check the random postprandial glucose level. At this time, the effects of morning-dosed steroid combined with the carbohydrate load of lunch will create maximal glucose levels [914]. Patients with glucose levels ≥200 mg/dL (11.1 mol/L) and classic diabetic symptoms should begin treatment, while patients with glucose levels <200 mg/dL (11.1 mmol/L) require further evaluation. Similar to diabetes mellitus screening after organ transplantation, maintenance screening of random glucose levels may be performed weekly for 4 weeks, then 3 and 6 months later, ending with yearly screening [922].

18.3. PREDIABETES

It is important to recognize that, while some patients may not meet the requirements for diagnosis of diabetes mellitus, and they may have levels of hyperglycemia that increase their risk for diabetes mellitus relative to the rest of the population. These individuals are said to have prediabetes, which may be diagnosed when there is one of the following [919]: Impaired fasting glucose – fasting plasma glucose of 100–125 mg/dL (5.6–6.9 mmol/L); impaired glucose tolerance with 2-h oral glucose tolerance test –plasma glucose levels of 140–199 mg/dL (7.8–11.1 mmol/L); hemoglobin A1C 5.7–6.4%. These patients are also at greater risk for developing cardiovascular disease; therefore, early screening and intervention is strongly recommended. Patients diagnosed with prediabetes should receive diabetic counseling. In addition, these patients should have a goal of losing 7% of their body weight and 150 min of moderate exercise each week [919]. Several large-scale studies have shown that lifestyle intervention alone can reduce the rate of conversion to diabetes (43% at 7 years). Lifestyle modification has been found to be more effective than metformin in some studies, but the ADA cites other studies to support the use of metformin in patients with body mass index >35 kg/m^2, those with a history of gestational diabetes, and those with severe hyperglycemia [919].

18.4. MANAGEMENT

Although it is unlikely the same practitioner carrying out glucocorticoid therapy will also introduce and manage diabetic therapy, it is important for all practitioners involved in the care of pemphigus vulgaris patients to be aware of treatment alternatives for glucocorticoid-induced diabetes. While the literature describes several different approaches to treat glucocorticoid-induced diabetes, the practitioner must eventually choose a medication regimen that is safe, effective in controlling hyperglycemia, and easy to follow. First, it is important to ensure patients are on the lowest steroid dose possible that allows proper control of their disease. Doing so will lower the incidence of diabetes as the risk of glucocorticoid-induced diabetes increases with increasing dose. Diet and exercise, while effective in treating other forms of diabetes mellitus, may be less likely in glucocorticoid-induced diabetes since diet may be hampered by the increase in appetite seen with steroid use, and patients with severe, extensive pemphigus vulgaris may be unable to take part in exercise because of the number and location of open lesions [914]. For these reasons, it is likely the patient will require medication as well as lifestyle adjustment.

18.4.1. Medical Intervention: Oral Hypoglycemics

Therapy is often initiated with oral hypoglycemic agents with selection based on the glucose levels of the patient and the side effect profile of the medication. Metformin decreases hepatic gluconeogenesis and increases peripheral insulin sensitivity [915]. It is associated with only a small risk of hypoglycemia (when used as monotherapy) and promotes modest weight loss. Gastrointestinal side effects, such as nausea, abdominal pain, and diarrhea, may be avoided by starting with a low dose and slowly increasing as tolerated [915]. There is a rare but potentially life-threatening side effect of lactic acidosis in patients with chronic kidney disease and heart failure. However, there is a lack of long-term studies to determine the safety of this medication in this population. Sulfonylureas inhibit the ATP-dependent potassium channel of β-cells, thereby increasing the release of insulin. These agents have a fast onset of action and are recommended for cases of mild hyperglycemia. Long-acting forms such as glyburide can cause hypoglycemia, especially in patients with chronic kidney disease. Glipizide may be a safer alternative. In addition, older sulfonylureas have been linked to increased mortality following myocardial infarction. Meglitinides, such as repaglinide, act in a manner similar to sulfonylureas and they too can cause hypoglycemia. Thiazolidinediones bind to PPARγ (peroxisome proliferator activator) receptors, causing transcription of genes involved in glucose metabolism. These medications require several weeks to take effect, making them a poor choice in cases of short-term steroid therapy. In addition, they have now been linked to edema, congestive heart failure, and increased cardiac events in diabetic patients with heart disease. DPP-4 inhibitors (gliptins) cause an increasein GLP-1 and GIP concentration, ultimately causing increased insulin secretion and decreased glucagon secretion. Gliptins are advantageous in that they have a low risk of hypoglycemia and a weight neutral profile. However, they produce smaller decreases in A1C than other hypoglycemic, and there have been several reports of gliptin-related pancreatitis. These inhibitors have been also associated with developing autoimmune bullous diseases (i.e., bullous pemphigoid) [923].

GLP-1 agonists, such as exenatide, bind to GLP-1 receptors in β cells and in the brain to cause increased insulin secretion, decreased glucagon secretion, increased satiety, and slowed gastric emptying. GLP-1 agonists promote weight loss to an even greater degree than metformin. However, they can also cause nausea, vomiting, and diarrhea.

Acarbose inhibits α-glucosidase in the brush border of the intestine, thereby inhibiting the digestion of carbohydrates. However, this medication can cause significant gastrointestinal distress, including diarrhea and flatulence, making it less appealing to many patients. It is however a good agent to address the postprandial glucose elevations often seen with glucocorticoid treatment.

While any of these medications may be chosen to start therapy, metformin is most commonly selected and recommended [919]. If treatment with metformin fails, a different oral hypoglycemic may be substituted or added as a second line.

18.4.2. Medical Intervention: Insulin

Insulin may be a better choice for patients with very high glucose levels or those who have failed oral hypoglycemic therapy [914], recommend starting with insulin in patients with postprandial glucose ≥300 mg/dL (16.7 mmol/L). NPH, intermediate-acting insulin, is especially useful in glucocorticoid-induced diabetes mellitus, as its action profile, including peak action and duration of effect, is similar to that of prednisone. To take advantage of this, patients should take NPH before breakfast when most glucocorticoids are administered. NPH is dosed according to the patient's weight, with recommendations varying from 0.15 to 0.4 U/kg [914]. Patients receiving large glucocorticoid doses will likely require basal doses closer to 0.4 U/kg. Patients with preexisting diabetes may add these doses to their current basal dose. Minor adjustments may then be made to postprandial glucose levels by the addition of short-acting insulin shortly before meals. While these recommendations may be sufficient for patients with elevations in only postprandial glucose levels, others, such as those on high-dose and twice-daily dosed steroids, may also have elevated fasting glucose levels. In this case, a bedtime dose of 0.1 U/kg NPH may be added, with close monitoring for early morning hypoglycemia [921]. Another simple approach can be to use premixed insulin (such as 70/30) with one half to two thirds given before breakfast and the rest at dinner [914].

18.5. Evaluating Therapy Success

Through both laboratory evaluation of glucose levels and patients' self monitoring of blood glucose, medication adjustments should be made based on the following ADA goals for diabetic therapy [919]: Hemoglobin A1C <7%; preprandial plasma glucose 70–130 mg/dL (3.9–7.2 mmol/L); postprandial (1–2 h after a meal) plasma glucose<180 mg/dL (10 mmol/L). If these goals are not met, physicians should reevaluate the therapy regimen, not forgetting to assess the patient's compliance with medication dosing and scheduling. It is important to note that therapy reducing A1C to less than 6.5% has been associated with increased mortality due to increased cardiac and hypoglycemic events and is best avoided in patients with comorbid conditions, the elderly, pregnant women, and young children [924]. When tapering glucocorticoid therapy, the need for diabetic medication will likely decrease. Since the fasting glucose levels are the first to decrease during taper, patients on evening or long-acting insulin should decrease this medication first [914]. Attention may then be turned to decreasing prandial and basal insulin. Even after patients finish glucocorticoid treatment, they remain at higher risk for development of diabetes later in life and therefore should continue to have regular diabetes screening, at least once every 3 years, preferably annually [915]. In addition, the practitioner should address any cardiovascular risk factors (such as hypertension and hyperlipidemia).

Patients with pemphigus vulgaris often require treatment of glucocorticoid-induced diabetes. The practitioner must often reevaluate the approach to the patient's care, assessing the need for continued steroid therapy and the success of diabetic therapy. Patient care should be coordinated through multiple specialists including primary care physicians, pharmacists, and diabetic specialists so the many needs of the patient may be adequately addressed, helping to ensure the patient's overall well-being.

Chapter 19

Prevention and Treatment of Infections

Autoimmune blistering diseases predispose patients to infection via several mechanisms. First, localized infection may occur due to loss of physical integrity of the skin and disruption of other antimicrobial mechanisms, such as the presence of protective normal flora and antimicrobial peptides [925]. Iatrogenic immunosuppression intended to treat the underlying autoimmune bullous disease can further compromise the body's inherent ability to fight infection by pathogenic and opportunistic organisms. Hospitalization for patients with particularly severe mucocutaneous disease exposes them to potentially more resistant nosocomial strains. Moreover, dietary modifications made by patients with oral or esophageal mucous membrane involvement may lead to nutritional deficiencies that could slow wound healing and predispose the patient to infection [926]. Finally, psychosocial stressors are known to disrupt skin barrier homeostasis [927]. The psychologic impact of having a potentially disabling disease may indirectly contribute to increased susceptibility to infection. Not only does excess microbial growth inhibit cutaneous healing, but it can also create a portal of entry for systemic infection, a serious source of morbidity and mortality [534, 853, 928-32]. Many forms of bacterial, viral, fungal, and mycobacterial infections have been reported in patients with autoimmune blistering disease, mainly pemphigus vulgaris [62, 853, 932]. For example, *Staphylococcus* sp. commonly colonizes and infects damaged skin. Serious complications, such as erysipelas, necrotizing fasciitis, and sepsis, have resulted from bacterial infection of the skin in patients with bullous pemphigoid [932].

In a published study [933], we determined the prevalence rates of the main Gram-negative bacteria in pemphigus vulgaris and their antimicrobial susceptibility patterns. Two notable findings of this study were (1) the spectrum of bacterial isolates in pemphigus vulgaris is similar in inpatients and outpatients and (2) there is increasing resistance of Gram-negative bacteria to the most frequently used antibiotics in hospitalized pemphigus vulgaris patients. Because of an impaired response to oral antibiotics, fluid and electrolytic changes and/or severe sepsis, 10% to 15% of patients with pemphigus vulgaris are admitted to our service. It is possible the increasing resistance observed in our study in inpatients is due to an increase in pathogenicity of the bacteria (community-acquired ESBL producers) and/or a decreased response to oral antibiotics (inherent resistance or acquired β-lactamase and/or ESBL related to invasive procedures, mainly catheters, prolonged hospital stay, and confinement in an inpatient unit) [933].

Data about the clinical epidemiology of Gram-negative bacteria, compared with Gram-positive bacteria, are limited. Infections and severe sepsis in pemphigus vulgaris are frequently due to Gram-positive bacteria; however, Gram-negative bacteria are emerging as important pathogens among severely ill patients, including those with pemphigus vulgaris.

The resistance observed in our study can be explained on the basis of the hospital environment, the quality of inpatient care, and the frequency of prescribing antibiotics as outpatients (which is often done on an empiric basis). Antibiotic prescriptions should be justified with microbiological studies; this will lead to the use of specific antibiotics in a given case and is more scientifically sound than empiric prescribing.

Other systemic bacterial infections, such as nocardiosis, may occur [853]. Viruses such as herpes simplex virus can infect (or aggravate) skin lesions in patients with autoimmune bullous diseases and may go unrecognized [934-5]. Patients being treated with immunosuppressive medications for pemphigus vulgaris also experience reactivation of herpes zoster virus (shingles) with greater frequency than their unaffected counterparts. A patient with pemphigus vulgaris developed Kaposi's sarcoma, a low-grade vascular malignancy associated with human herpesvirus 8, at the site of intralesional corticosteroid treatments [936]. Patients with pemphigus vulgaris may develop superficial fungal infections, such as dermatophytosis or candidiasis, or serious systemic fungal infection by organisms such as *Cryptococcus neoformans* and *Aspergillus* sp [937-8]. Patients being treated with systemic immunosuppressive medications for autoimmune bullous diseases may be at risk for potentially fatal *Pneumocystis pneumonia* [934-5]. Localized or systemic mycobacterial infections or reactivation of latent mycobacterial infection may also occur [939-40].

19.1. Prevention of Infection

Patients should try to take practical measures to reduce undue exposure to potentially pathogenic microorganisms [853]. Examples include avoidance of places with a high incidence of infection (e.g., hospitals, day-care centers, and nursing homes), environments with a high density of people or reduced air circulation (e.g., airplanes), or fomites (e.g., shared computer keyboards and telephones). Hence, if at all possible, it would be best if autoimmune bullous diseases patients being immunosuppressed could be treated as outpatients. Regular hand washing, with particular attention paid to nail hygiene, is essential. Wearing of a face mask in crowded areas or when gardening may be considered. The companionship and psychosocial benefits of a pet should be weighed against the potential for infection by zoonotic organisms, such as *Salmonella* (reptiles), group A β hemolytic streptococcus (cats and dogs), *Bartonella henselae* (cats), *Campylobacter jejuni* (dogs, cats, and birds), *Chlamydia psittaci* (birds), and dermatophytes (cats and dogs). For immunosuppressed patients who wish to keep pets at home, helpful guidelines have been developed to minimize the chance for zoonotic infection [941]. Although specific immunization recommendations have not been published for patients with autoimmune bullous diseases, those developed for immunocompromised patients in general indicate that patients should be brought up-to-date on age-appropriate immunizations where feasible [942]. Although delivery of live attenuated vaccinations, such as the herpes zoster vaccine and the live form of the influenza vaccine, is contraindicated during active immunosuppression, these immunizations can be given upto 3 weeks prior to initiation of iatrogenic immunosuppression [943]. Since immunosuppressive medications can lead to reactivation of latent infectious hepatitis or tuberculosis, high-risk patients should be screened before such medications are initiated. For patients unable to receive the recommended vaccinations, it is particularly important that close contacts and family members be up to date with their immunizations to help protect the patient via the principle of "herd immunity." An important principle in infection prevention in these patients is reduction of surface colonization and restoration of the skin barrier. This can be achieved with diligent personal hygiene practices, meticulous skin care, and implementation of localized antiseptic measures, such as distilled white vinegar wet dressings, chlorhexidine gluconate solution, potassium permanganate solution, and bleach baths [944-5]. Expert wound care consultation and home health nursing aides may be required for patients with refractory wounds or personal disability. The blister roofs should be left intact to function as a biologic barrier. The skin should not be scrubbed. The use of bland emollients can hasten healing and protect the skin. Patients using topical corticosteroid preparations in the mouth often benefit from concomitant prophylactic use of anti-candidal medications (such as clotrimazole troches). Other measures important in preventing infection include minimization of the dose and duration of immunosuppressive medications as well as smoking cessation and optimization of blood sugar levels and nutritional status. To prevent opportunistic infections, patients taking high doses or prolonged courses of immunosuppressive medications may benefit from adding *Pneumocystis* prophylaxis [946-7]. In patients who have already experienced infectious complications, such as superinfection with *Staphylococcus aureus* or herpes simplex virus, chronic suppressive antimicrobial treatments could be considered as secondary prevention.

19.2. Management of Infection

Patients with pemphigus vulgaris should be educated about the signs and symptoms of localized or systemic infection and urged to present for medical attention promptly for early evaluation and intervention. Physicians should have a low threshold to culture slow-healing skin lesions, because accurate identification of the associated organism may be essential for proper treatment. Since a common pitfall in managing pemphigus is failure to recognize superinfection with herpesviruses [934-5] or dermatophytes [144], skin swab for polymerase chain reaction or fungal culture may be helpful. Treatment for localized infections can include topical antiseptic or antibiotic preparations and other skin-directed interventions. Simple topical interventions may include distilled white vinegar wet dressings, potassium permanganate baths, chlorhexidine gluconate washes, or bleach baths. Other helpful topical antiseptic preparations include silver-containing salves or dressings or antibiotic topical preparations [925].

Patients with persistent localized infection and/or systemic infection may require oral or intravenous antimicrobial medications. Specific treatments are best selected based on the resistance profile of the particular organisms identified in patients. If these data are unavailable, medication selection can be guided by resistance patterns commonly encountered in the geographic area or patient demographic. We often use antibiotics from the tetracycline class for treatment of extensive impetiginization or localized bacterial infection because they offer the potential side benefit of anti-inflammatory activity.

The best treatment of shingles is acyclovir initiated within 24-72h of initial symptoms. Analgesics and medications to prevent and treat postherpetic neuralgia (such as gabapentin) may be required. While specific antimicrobial medications to treat serious systemic infections should be guided by the nature of the infectious organisms involved, broad-spectrum antimicrobial treatment may be started until the associated microbial agents are identified. Careful attention should be paid to patient vital signs and fluid status. Hospitalization may be necessary. Multidisciplinary care, including subspecialty infectious disease consultation, is recommended.

Chapter 20

AZATHIOPRINE

Azathioprine was developed and first used to treat leukemia and graft-versus-host disease after allogeneic tissue transplantation. Today, azathioprine is used in particular for treating autoimmune diseases, such as autoimmune blistering diseases, inflammatory bowel disease, multiple sclerosis, rheumatoid arthritis, lupus erythematosus and pemphigus. The pharmaceutical precursor of azathioprine was the antimetabolite 6-mercaptopurine. The substance was synthesized in 1951 by Elion and Hitchings. The 6-mercaptopurine was first used in 1953 in children with acute lymphatic leukemia and after renal transplantation in dogs in 1960 [948]. To change the metabolism of 6-mercaptopurine and to protect it from rapid degradation, an imidazole ring was connected via the sulphur atom at position 6 of 6-mercaptopurine. This compound had a strong immunosuppressive potential, a better therapeutic index in mice and was less toxic than 6-mercaptopurine [949]. The synthesised compound was named azathioprine and approved by the US Food and Drug Administration in 1968. The first allogenic renal transplantation using a combination of azathioprine and corticosteroids was successfully performed in 1962 [950].

20.1. MOLECULAR MECHANISM AND METABOLISM

Azathioprine is a purine analogue prodrug that requires metabolic conversion into active compounds. After oral uptake about 88% of azathioprine is ingested and 12% excreted via the gut. Nearly all of the incorporated azathioprine is metabolized, since only 2% is being excreted, unchanged, in the urine. The highest serum levels can be found approximately 2h after oral application, and the half-life is approximately 5h. The first step of azathioprine activation is the non-enzymatic removal of the imidazole ring in erythrocytes [951]. The active metabolite 6-mercaptopurine can be released from erythrocytes and taken up by other cells for further metabolization. Although most of the therapeutic effects of azathioprine are dependent on the enzymatical modification of 6-mercaptopurine, there is experimental evidence the imidazole derivatives of azathioprine might also be effective [952]. Three enzymes have been reported to compete for the cleavage of 6-mercaptopurine in the cell [951]. Thiopurine S-methyltransferase is able to catabolise 6-mercaptopurine into the non-toxic 6-methyl mercaptopurine. The enzyme is active in the duodenum, the liver and in erythrocytes. Xanthine oxidase produces the non-toxic, inactive metabolite 6-thiouric acid. A lack in one of these enzymes, xanthine oxidase and thiopurine methyltransferase, leads to an increased production of metabolites via the hypoxanthine phosphoribosyltransferase (HPRT) pathway. A lack of thiopurine methyltransferase activity is caused by genetic mutations, while xanthine oxidase might be blocked by xanthine oxidase inhibitory drugs such as allopurinol, which is one of the most commonly prescribed drugs in Europe and North America. The enzyme HPRT catalyses the addition of ribose 5-phosphate to 6-mercaptopurine and generates 6-thioinosine 5-monophosphate (6-TIMP). This product is processed by thiopurine methyltransferase to active methylated metabolites or is phosphorylated to 6-thioinosine triphosphate (6-TITP). 6-TITP is converted to 6-TIMP by inosine triphosphate pyrophosphohydrolase (ITPA). A lack of ITPA, as it is often seen in Asian populations [953], leads to an increase of the toxic 6-TITP and induces similar side effects, such as leucopenia, gastrointestinal disturbances or elevated liver function tests. 6-TIMP and its active methylated metabolites can inhibit the glutamine phosphoribosyl pyrophosphate transferase, the key enzyme of the purine *de-novo* synthesis. Thereby azathioprine contributes especially to inhibit lymphocyte proliferation, which depends on the purine synthesis for proliferation [954]. 6-TIMP is converted by the inosine monophosphate dehydrogenase (IMPD) and guanosine monophosphate synthetase (GMPS) into thioguanosine-monophosphate (TGMP). TGMP can be inactivated by thiopurine methyltransferase into methylated metabolites. TGMP escaping methylation is processed by kinases and other enzymes into the active 6-thioguanine nucleotides, which are substrates for incorporation into RNA and DNA. DNA polymerases incorporate 6-thio-GTP with similar efficacy into DNA like unmodified dGTP. 6-thio-GTP is chemically more reactive than canonical nucleotides and undergoes methylation in DNA. Targeting of modified 6-thio-GTP by DNA repair pathways can lead to apoptosis and is responsible for the cytotoxic effects of the compound [951]. In lymphocytes 6-thio-GTP is able to bind to a small GTPase Rac1, thereby modulating costimulation by CD28 in T cells into apoptosis. This seems to be a major pathway for selective T-cell inhibition [955]. In addition, inhibition of Rac1 in endothelial cells exerts an anti-inflammatory effect by modulation of cytokine secretion [956]. It has further been shown that addition of azathioprine to T-cell cultures led to an inhibition of the mRNA expression of TRAIL, TNFRSF7 and α-4 integrin [515]. TRAIL is expressed on the surface of cytotoxic T cells and NK cells and can mediate a proliferative signal for these cells [956]. TNFRSF7 is also expressed by lymphocytes and enhances activation [957]. Inhibition of this effect could contribute to the immunosuppressive potential of azathioprine. A reduced expression of α-4 integrin could inhibit T cell and monocyte migration. Azathioprine not only affects T cells but also dendritic cells by reducing their proinflammatory cytokine-producing potential and maturation [958].

20.2. Azathioprine in Pemphigus

The use of azathioprine for treating pemphigus was introduced in 1969, when Krakowski et al., [959] presented the first case report of a woman with pemphigus vulgaris treated successfully with azathioprine. At the same time, Wolff et al., [960] published a case series of four patients, describing the use of azathioprine as “steroid saving and beneficial” in pemphigus patients. In 1977, Lever et al., [794] published a retrospective analysis of 63 patients with pemphigus. Lever treated 12 patients with prednisone monotherapy and 51 patients in this cohort with a combination of azathioprine, cyclophosphamide or methotrexate and prednisone. In that report, azathioprine had a steroid-sparing effect and controlled disease. Lever's therapeutic approach is still today known as "Lever's regime." At first, patients receive a high dose of prednisone (up to 2 mg/kg body weight) in combination with azathioprine 2–2.5 mg/kg. After cessation of new blister formation and reepithelisation of erosions, the prednisone dose is reduced to 40 mg/day, while the azathioprine dose remains unchanged. Further proceedings depend individually on the clinical development. Normally, the prednisone dose is gradually reduced over several months. In most studies patients with pemphigus foliaceus were not specifically mentioned and might have been included in the pemphigus vulgaris group. There are only few prospective, randomized trials reported in pemphigus. Beissert et al., [961-2] examined patients with pemphigus vulgaris or pemphigus foliaceus and found no significant differences between treatment with azathioprine or mycophenolate mofetil (both in combination with methylprednisone) about remission of disease and corticosteroid-sparing effects. The azathioprine-treated patients received a median methylprednisolone dose of 8.916 ± 29.844 mg. In the mycophenolate mofetil-treated group, patients received a median of 9.334 ± 13.280mg methylprednisolone (P = ns). The mean duration of follow-up was 438 days in both groups. However, the time needed to achieve disease control in 50% of the patients was about 30 days in the azathioprine group compared with 75 days in the mycophenolate mofetil group. After 200 days of treatment, the patients in the mycophenolate mofetil group had a remission rate of 90%, while those patients that were treated with azathioprine had a remission rate of 75%. After 600 days, this trend persisted, because 20% of the pemphigus patients were still not achieving effective control with azathioprine compared with 10% of the patients using mycophenolate. The recurrence rate was similar in both groups.

In another study with 120 patients analyzed, Chams-Davatchi et al., [784] found no significant difference about disease remission between azathioprine and mycophenolate mofetil, but the patients treated with azathioprine showed significantly less steroid consumption. They later extended their findings by a double-blind randomized trial comparing prednisolone and azathioprine with prednisolone and placebo and found a 50% increased remission rate in the azathioprine group. Interestingly, the steroid-sparing effect was less prominent compared with previous studies [963]. Rose et al., [785] compared dexamethasone and cyclophosphamide pulse therapy with oral methylprednisolone and azathioprine therapy in pemphigus and described a tendency to methylprednisolone and azathioprine about complete remissions.

In the subtype of immunoglobulin A (IgA) pemphigus, azathioprine is not recommended for dapsone as first-line treatment [964]. For pemphigus vegetans, azathioprine appears to work in individual cases [720]. In paraneoplastic pemphigus, the therapy of the underlying malignancy is essential. Accompanying treatment with azathioprine and other immunomodulatory drugs has been reported [965]. Lam et al., [966] presented a case of a 77-year-old male with chronic conjunctivitis, acanthosis nigricans and pemphigus-like mucocutaneous lesions. Further examinations revealed an underlying bronchogenic squamous cell carcinoma. While skin lesions resolved with oral prednisone and azathioprine (100 mg/day) therapy, the conjunctivitis and mucous membrane erosions persisted. Verrini et al., [967] described another patient with paraneoplastic pemphigus who showed good response to azathioprine (100 mg/day) but died shortly after initiation of treatment. Finally, the importance of systemic corticosteroids in the treatment of pemphigus is clearly documented. Since the reports show a tendency to azathioprine concerning corticosteroid-sparing effects and no significant differences with regard to disease control, azathioprine can be suggested as first-line therapy in mild-to-moderate cases of pemphigus. Mycophenolate mofetil appears to be a valid second-line choice. In severe and rapidly progressing cases, dexamethasone/cyclophosphamide pulse therapy could be considered. Other proved treatment opportunities include immunoadsorption and rituximab [968]. Since pemphigus is a chronic disease, especially long-term follow-up studies (>3 years) are clearly needed. In a Cochrane review, the available study results showed the ideal immunomodulatory agent in treating pemphigus has not yet determined. While azathioprine and cyclophosphamide did show advantages about the steroid-sparing effect, mycophenolate mofetil showed superior disease control [781].

20.3. Azathioprine during Pregnancy

The use of immunomodulatory agents during pregnancy should always be extremely well considered. Azathioprine can cross the human placenta [969]. The fetal liver does not have the enzymes to convert azathioprine into its active metabolites, suggesting the fetus might have a certain protection against azathioprine-induced cellular toxicity [970]. Most large studies have shown that azathioprine during pregnancy is tolerated, although the rate of congenital malformations appears to be 3–9% in infants exposed antenatally [971]. Malformations including myelomeningocele, preaxial polydactyly, microcephaly, thymic atrophy, hypospadias and adrenal hypoplasia were reported. Azathioprine exposure during pregnancy of patients with lupus erythematosus was independently associated with increased needs for special education [972]. In general, azathioprine can be given during pregnancy if it is highly indicated, and pregnant women on azathioprine do not need to be switched to another treatment regimen.

20.4. Side Effects of Azathioprine

Azathioprine is generally well tolerated in most of the patients. Common side effects are leucopenia and gastrointestinal effects. In a study with 114 Japanese patients treated with 50mg azathioprine each day due to inflammatory bowel disease, 33% developed side effects over a time period of 48 months of investigation [62]. The most common side effect of azathioprine was leucopenia (WBC < or = 3,000/microL) with 18 (15.8%) affected patients. Fifteen from these patients experienced a mild leukopenia with no necessary change of dosage. Two patients (1.8%) had a severe leucopenia (less than 1,000/µl), followed by a decrease of the given azathioprine dose. While the mild forms of leukopenia occurred after an average treatment period of 13.7 months (mean, range 1–47), the severe forms of leucopenia occurred in less than 1 month. Bone marrow suppression by azathioprine is a risk for severe infection and sepsis [973] and depends largely on thiopurine methyltransferase activity, which is regulated by genetic polymorphisms in the thiopurine methyltransferase gene [974]. There are four main allele types associated with reduced activity: thiopurine methyltransferase*1 (wild-type), thiopurine methyltransferase*2 (G238C), thiopurine methyltransferase*3A

(G460A and A719G), thiopurine methyltransferase*3B (G460A) and thiopurine methyltransferase*3C (A719G) [975]. Their expression is variable among different races. While, for instance, in 4.5–3.2% of Caucasians the thiopurine methyltransferase-activity-reducing thiopurine methyltransferase*3A alleles were detected; Kumagai et al., [976] did not find this mutation in Japanese. In Japanese the allele frequency of thiopurine methyltransferase*3C was 1.6%. The same polymorphism was more common in Africans (2.4–7.6%) but rare (0.2–0.8%) in Caucasians. In Caucasians, approximately one in 300 patients has a distinct reduced thiopurine methyltransferase activity, and about 11% of Caucasian patients show a moderately reduced activity, resulting in an increased production of toxic metabolites (e.g., thioinosine monophosphates) when taking azathioprine [977]. Uchiyama et al., [953] examined the relationship between the incidence of azathioprine-associated adverse effects and either the incidence of thiopurine methyltransferase gene polymorphisms or inosine triphosphate pyrophosphohydrolase gene polymorphisms (for the metabolic mechanism of the enzyme). In five of six patients who had developed an acute bone marrow toxicity, a mutation (94C > A) of the inosine triphosphate pyrophosphohydrolase gene was detectable. 75% of the patients with agranulocytosis had the 94C>A allele. In red blood cells of patients with the homozygous 94C>A missense mutation, inosine triphosphate pyrophosphohydrolase activity was below detectable levels. The frequency of 94C>A alleles was 31 of 200 in Japanese individuals (15.5%), which is 2.6-fold higher than in Caucasians [62]. Because of the high correlation between side effects under azathioprine therapy and prevalence of the inosine triphosphate pyrophosphohydrolase polymorphism genes in Japanese, it is suggested that in Japanese patients, instead of determination of thiopurine methyltransferase gene polymorphisms or activity, a screen for inosine triphosphate pyrophosphohydrolase gene mutations or activity should be introduced. In Caucasians and Africans, it is recommended to monitor for deficiency in thiopurine methyltransferase activity before azathioprine is introduced. In a few patients, azathioprine induces hepatitis accompanied by elevated liver function tests. In most cases the increase in liver enzymes is reduced to normal after discontinuation of the treatment. The mechanism of hepatitis induction by azathioprine is not clear. A recent study showed that oxidative stress and the subsequently activated immune- and inflammation related factors are involved in azathioprine-induced liver injury [978]. Further side effects of azathioprine can be flu-like symptoms (i.e., fever, headache, rash, arthralgia, myalgia and malaise) or hair loss. The latter might improve in some patients during long-term treatment. All symptoms are usually self-limited after discontinuation of azathioprine.

On the observed side effects of azathioprine, laboratory checking including blood cell counts and serum analysis (especially liver enzymes) is recommended weekly for the first 8 weeks of treatment. After 8 weeks of treatment, the interval of laboratory monitoring can be extended to once a month. Accidental or self-intentional overdose of azathioprine with single doses from 1500mg to 7500 mg was relatively well tolerated in reported cases. The reported immediate toxic reactions in the patients were nausea, vomiting and mild abnormalities in liver functions followed by leukopenic episode in the patient receiving 7.5g [979-80]. Like all immunosuppressive drugs, long-term intake of azathioprine raises the risk of immunosuppressive- induced malignancies. In a large 20-year follow-up study, patients with rheumatoid arthritis receiving azathioprine had a ten-fold increased risk for developing immunosuppression-associated myeloproliferative disorders compared to the general population. Patients with rheumatoid arthritis without a history of azathioprine treatment had "only" a five-fold increased risk of developing myeloproliferative disorders [981]. A further population-based, nested, case-control study in the UK found the odds of diagnosing lymphoma for patients with inflammatory bowel disease treated with azathioprine were three times greater than the odds for those not treated with azathioprine. In a similar Danish patient cohort, the overall cancer risk was increased in patients treated with azathioprine (rate ratio 1.4), and the risk for lymphoid tissue cancer had a rate ratio of 2.4 [982]. The latter values were confirmed by a retrospective study by Khan et al., [983] in ulcerative colitis describing a risk ratio for lymphoid malignancies between 2 and 3.

In patients with rheumatoid arthritis treated with azathioprine, there was a significant increase of cancer development in relation to the cumulative lifetime intake of azathioprine. In 8.6% of the patients with a lifetime intake of up to 50g azathioprine, any kind of cancer developed within 20 years. And in patients with a cumulative dose of 200g azathioprine, any kind of cancer developed even in more than 20% of the cases within 20 years. In addition, the risk of developing non-melanoma skin cancers (squamous and basal cell carcinomas) was two-fold compared to the general population [981]. The increased risk for developing non-melanoma skin cancers was confirmed by a retrospective study in the Danish population where patients with myasthenia gravis and long-term azathioprine treatment had an odds ratio of 4.8 for non-melanoma skin cancers [984]. The overall cancer risk in this population after treatment with azathioprine was a ratio of 1.2 [985]. In a further cohort of rheumatic patients, azathioprine treatment increased the risk for developing squamous cell carcinoma (standardised incidence ratio 16) [986]. Taken together, long-term azathioprine treatment in different patient cohorts mainly increased the risk for non-melanoma skin cancer and lymphoproliferative malignancies. There is strong evidence for an additive carcinogenic effect of ultraviolet radiation, especially UVA (320–400 nm), in combination with azathioprine treatment concerning the development of non-melanoma skin cancers. Ramsay et al., [987] examined transplant recipients of Fitzpatrick skin types I–IV. From 361 patients, 187 (51.8%) developed histologically diagnosed non-melanoma skin cancer. The ratio of squamous cell carcinoma to basal cell carcinoma was reversed in these patients from 1:3.7 before transplantation to 2:1 after transplantation.

Non-melanoma skin cancers increased with the duration of medical immunosuppression. While 29.1% of the transplant recipients developed one or more non-melanoma skin cancers when immunosuppression did not exceed 5 years, an immunosuppression of 10–20 years led to an incidence of 72.4% of non-melanoma skin cancers in the treated patients. However, the examined patients received not only azathioprine (on average daily 100 mg), but also daily 225mg cyclosporine and 7mg prednisone (follow-up: 7.1 years). Most of the observed non-melanoma skin cancers in immunosuppressed transplant recipients developed at sun-exposed areas (80% of the squamous cell carcinoma, 71% of the basal cell carcinomas and 64% of the keratoacanthoma). One of the active metabolites of azathioprine is thioguanine nucleotide. These nucleotides are precursors for 6-thioguanine, which can be incorporated into DNA upon replication, and absorb UVA wavelengths (320–400 nm) with a maximum at 342 nm. O'Donovan et al., [988] showed that biologically relevant doses of UVA generate reactive oxygen species in cultured cells with 6-thioguanine-substituted DNA. Moreover, 6-mercaptopurine, a metabolite of azathioprine, produces reactive oxygen species when exposed to UVA [989]. In experimental cell lines (HCT116, human colorectal carcinoma cells) containing about 0.01% 6-thioguanine-substituted DNA, an irradiation with a non-toxic dose of 1 kJ/m 2 UVA led to a threefold increase in adenine phosphoribosyl transferase mutation frequencies compared to non-substituted DNA [988]. Neither 6-thioguanine nor UVA alone was detectably mutagenic. In normal DNA without substitutes, 500 kJ/m 2 of UVA irradiation was needed to induce a similar increase in adenine phosphoribosyl transferase mutation frequency. O'Donovan et al., [988] measured the amount of 6-thioguanine in DNA extracted from clinically normal skin of three azathioprine-treated patients. Around 0.02% of 6-thioguanine-substituted DNA was found. In a control group of patients who did not receive azathioprine, no substituted DNA was detectable. Studies in mice showed that incorporation of 6-thioguanine in DNA of skin is even higher compared to liver. In line with this, azathioprine-treated patients showed a reduction of the minimal erythema dose for UVA, but not for UVB. These findings suggest the mutagenic effect of UV radiation is increased under azathioprine treatment. UVA appears to play a more important role for photocarcinogenesis in these patients than UVB. In a mouse model, Reeve et al., [990] showed that azathioprine but not cyclophosphamide increased the incidence of skin tumours significantly after UV irradiation. Based on the previous results, it is recommended that patients undergoing therapy with azathioprine should use effective sunscreens and avoid unnecessary long-term exposures to the sun. Patients who require long-term treatment with azathioprine should undergo a clinical examination of the skin twice a year.

Chapter 21

MYCOPHENOLATE MOFETIL/MYCOPHENOLIC ACID

21.1. MECHANISMS OF ACTION

Mycophenolate mofetil is the 2-morpho linoethyl ester of mycophenolic acid, one of the several phenol compounds first isolated by Gosio in 1896 in cultures of *Penicillium stoloniferum*. Mycophenolic acid has been found to inhibit DNA synthesis by selectively inhibiting inosine monophosphate dehydrogenase, an enzyme that catalyzes the rate-limiting step in the *de novo* biosynthesis of guanine nucleotides [991]. Mycophenolic acid targets mainly T and B lymphocytes, which unlike other cell types are dependent almost only on the *de novo* guanine nucleotide synthesis pathway for proliferation and differentiation [992]. Mycophenolic acid is five times more potent as an inhibitor of the inosine monophosphate dehydrogenase II isoform specific to lymphocytes than of the housekeeping inosine monophosphate dehydrogenase I isoform, found in most cell types [993]. Mycophenolate mofetil inhibits T and B cell proliferation [994], induces apoptosis of T cells [995], and inhibits antibody production by B cells [996]. Besides its antiproliferative effect on lymphocytes, mycophenolate mofetil has several other mechanisms of action. Guanosine triphosphate depletion caused by mycophenolate mofetil impairs fucosylation and surface expression of adhesion molecules of lymphocytes and monocytes, preventing their attachment to endothelial cells during their recruitment to inflammation sites [992, 997]. As monocytes and macrophages are major producers of proinflammatory cytokines causing fibroblast recruitment and proliferation at the inflammation site (such as TNFα and IL-1), their depletion reduces the production of these cytokines, inhibiting fibroblast proliferation and tissue fibrosis [998]. Mycophenolic acid was shown to inhibit the surface expression of antigens responsible for maturation and efficient antigen presentation by dendritic cells, thereby suppressing immune responses [999, 1000]. GTP depletion also impairs inducible nitric oxide synthase activity, which leads to a reduction of the oxidative stress, caused by activated monocytes, macrophages, and endothelial cells [1001].

21.2. PHARMACOKINETIC PROPERTIES

Mycophenolate mofetil has 94% oral bioavailability [1002]. Following absorption, mycophenolate mofetil is converted to its active metabolite, mycophenolic acid, by plasma, liver, and kidney esterases. Mycophenolic acid is almost completely inactivated in the liver by glucuronyl transferase [1003], and a significant portion of mycophenolic acid glucuronide is secreted into the bile and recycled via enterohepatic recirculation. Mycophenolic acid glucuronide is converted back to mycophenolic acid by β-glucuronidase, found mainly in the epidermis and the gastrointestinal tract. The peak plasma level of the mycophenolic acid following orally administered mycophenolate mofetil is reached in less than 1h in healthy subjects. The mean plasma half-life time of mycophenolic acid is ~17 h, making the twice-daily mycophenolate mofetil administration reasonable. A secondary mycophenolic acid peak occurs at 8–12h and is attributed to the enterohepatic circulation [1002], Ninety-seven percent of mycophenolic acid is albumin bound. Most of the drug is excreted as mycophenolic acid glucuronide in the urine [1004].

21.3. Side Effects

The most common side effects of mycophenolate mofetil are nausea, vomiting, abdominal cramps, and diarrhea, reported in 12–36% of patients. All are dose dependent and seem to be more prevalent in transplant recipients, compared to patients with autoimmune diseases, probably owing to a higher concomitant immunosuppression of these patients [1005-7]. Enteric-coated mycophenolate sodium, in contrast to mycophenolate mofetil, allows the drug to be absorbed in the small bowel [1008] and has been designed to reduce the gastrointestinal side effects, attributed to mycophenolate mofetil. Enteric-coated mycophenolate sodium has been shown to have similar efficacy and safety to mycophenolate mofetil in transplant recipients [1009-11], and its ability to significantly reduce the rate of gastrointestinal symptoms has been debated [1012-3]. Other potentially dangerous but rare gastrointestinal side effects, such as ulceration, bleeding, and perforation, have been reported [1005]. Hematologic side effects, dose dependent and reversible upon discontinuation of the drug, include leukopenia, neutropenia, anemia, and thrombocytopenia [788]. Rare cases of pure red cell aplasia, sometimes reversible upon dose reduction and drug withdrawal, have been described in patients treated with mycophenolate mofetil [1014-5]. There are reports of genitourinary side effects of urgency, frequency, dysuria, hematuria, and sterile pyuria, which generally resolve with continued drug use [790, 1016]. Neurologic complaints (headache, tinnitus, and insomnia), skin rash, and cardiovascular effects (peripheral edema and hypertension) have also been described [788]. Mycophenolic acid/mycophenolate mofetil treatments have been associated with both bacterial and viral infections (especially herpes zoster [1017-8] and cytomegalovirus [1019-21]. Increased incidence of cytomegalovirus invasive disease but not of primary cytomegalovirus infection has been reported in renal transplant recipients given mycophenolate mofetil and concomitantly treated with other immunosuppressive agents. In stem cell transplant recipients with positive cytomegalovirus-IgG, mycophenolate mofetil use increased the risk for both cytomegalovirus infection and complicated cytomegalovirus infection, but not for cytomegalovirus disease [1019].

Polyomavirus-associated progressive multifocal leukoencephalopathy, a demyelinating disease of the central nervous system appearing in immunocompromised patients, has been reported in a few renal transplant recipients [1022-3], as well as in patients with lupus [1024] treated with mycophenolate mofetil. Therefore, a safety report was issued by FDA, informing healthcare professionals of a potential association between mycophenolate mofetil and Enteric-coated mycophenolate sodium and progressive multifocal leukoencephalopathy. The ability of mycophenolate mofetil to induce malignancy is controversial. Mycophenolate mofetil is expected to be less carcinogenic than azathioprine because it is not incorporated into the DNA and does not cause chromosomal breaks [1025]. Some studies reported a dose-dependent increase in the risk of lymphoproliferative malignancy in mycophenolate mofetil-treated organ transplant patients [1026], but this finding was not supported in a comparative study of mycophenolate mofetil based and other immunosuppressive regimens in renal transplant patients [1027]. Furthermore, mycophenolate mofetil was associated with a significantly lower risk for posttransplant malignancy, compared with azathioprine in heart transplant recipients [1028]. In dermatologic literature an early report described three cases of malignancy during mycophenolate mofetil treatment in psoriatic patients [1029]. Afterwards, Epinette et al., [1017], found no increase in the incidence of cancer in psoriatic patients treated with mycophenolate mofetil. A limited number of case reports suggested that mycophenolate mofetil exposure during pregnancy could cause serious fetal malformations, such as microtia, cleft lip, cleft palate, and atresia of the external auditory canals, as well as increase the risk for first trimester spontaneous abortion [1030-3]. Therefore, mycophenolate mofetil and Enteric-coated mycophenolate sodium is classified as pregnancy category D (there is positive evidence of human fetal risk based on adverse reaction data from investigational or marketing experience or studies in humans, but potential benefits may warrant use of the drug in pregnant women despite potential risks), and it is recommended to use two different reliable methods of birth control 4 weeks before starting and during mycophenolate mofetil therapy and continue birth control for 6 weeks after mycophenolate mofetil has been stopped. One week before mycophenolate mofetil and Enteric-coated mycophenolate sodium therapy is introduced, women of childbearing potential should have a negative serum or urine pregnancy test.

21.4. Drug Interactions

Many drugs are known to interact with mycophenolate mofetil via mechanisms of absorption inhibition (antacids containing aluminum and magnesium as well as divalent cations such as calcium and iron), disruption of enterohepatic recirculation (antibiotics, cholestyramine), albumin binding (phenytoin, salicylic acid), and prevention of kidney tubular secretion of mycophenolic acid (acyclovir, ganciclovir, probenecid) [1034]. Therefore, calcium supplementation, which is often required in patients with pemphigus concomitantly treated with steroids and mycophenolate mofetil, should not be taken at the same time of the day as mycophenolate mofetil.

21.5. Mycophenolate Mofetil in Pemphigus

Mycophenolic acid was first applied in dermatology in the1970s as an anti-inflammatory agent to treat moderate to severe psoriasis [1035-6]. However, by the end of the decade, its use was discontinued owing to the gastrointestinal side effects, increased risk of latent viral infections, and possible carcinogenicity [1029]. A decade later mycophenolate mofetil, the 2-morpholinoethyl ester of mycophenolic acid, received FDA approval as in immunosuppressive agent in renal transplant patients, with studies showing that it had better oral bioavailability than mycophenolic acid and caused fewer gastrointestinal side effects. Owing to its long-term safety and tolerability, it began to be applied in other fields, including dermatology. High-dose steroids are the traditional first-line treatment of pemphigus vulgaris, but their multiple and potentially severe side effects with prolonged use have prompted dermatologists to seek alternative/steroid-sparing agents. Today, immunosuppressive agents such as azathioprine, cyclophosphamide, and mycophenolate mofetil are widely used in treating these diseases. The early evidence of the benefit of mycophenolate mofetil for pemphigus derived from some case series, reporting the efficacy of mycophenolate mofetil as a steroid-sparing agent.

Enk et al., [1037] combined mycophenolate mofetil (2g/day) with prednisolone (2 mg/kg/day) in 12 patients with pemphigus vulgaris, who had relapsed during azathioprine and prednisolone therapy. Eleven patients responded to this therapy with no relapses during the 9–12-month follow-up period. A similar regimen was applied by Chams-Davatchi [1038], in ten patients with pemphigus vulgaris with severe resistant and recurrent disease. The lesions completely cleared in nine patients by 6–16 weeks. Five patients relapsed after mycophenolate mofetil discontinuation at a 6-month follow-up, suggesting mycophenolate mofetil should be administered for a longer period to sustain remission. Several years later, a large historical prospective trial was conducted including 31 patients with pemphigus vulgaris and 11 patients with pemphigus foliaceus, who had relapsed on prednisone therapy or had had adverse effects from previous drug therapy [1007]. Combined treatment with prednisone and mycophenolate mofetil (35–45 mg/kg) led to complete remission in 71% of the pemphigus vulgaris group and 45% of the pemphigus foliaceus group. The meantime to remission was 9 months, and the remission was maintained throughout the 22 months of follow-up.

Powell et al., [786] reported treating 16 refractory pemphigus vulgaris and pemphigus foliaceus patients with mycophenolate mofetil (starting at 500 mg/day and increasing as tolerated up to 3.5 g/day) and prednisone. Clinically inactive disease was achieved in seven patients. The much lower doses of prednisone at the time of mycophenolate mofetil initiation in this study are noteworthy and may explain the relatively low rate of clinical remission. Mycophenolate mofetil doses higher than 2 g/day were not associated with a better outcome, but increased the risk for opportunistic infections. In a retrospective study of 18 pemphigus vulgaris patients treated with 2–3 g/day mycophenolate mofetil and prednisone (ranging from 35 to 100 mg/day) and followed up for an average of 35.2 months, 86% of previously treated patients and 75% of patients with no prior therapy achieved complete disease control. In a prospective open-label study of mycophenolate mofetil as a steroid sparing agent, Esmaili et al., [1039] managed mycophenolate mofetil (2g/day) and prednisolone (2 mg/kg/day) as an initial treatment to 31 patients with active pemphigus vulgaris with a 12-month follow-up. This regimen was useful for 21 patients (67.7%), making it possible to taper prednisolone down to 7.5 mg/day in those cases. Similarly to mycophenolate mofetil, the enteric coated alternative has also been shown to be a safe and effective adjuvant to prednisone in a series of ten patients with refractory pemphigus. A prospective controlled trial was conducted by Beissert et al., [961] who randomized 96 patients with mild to moderate pemphigus vulgaris to receive mycophenolate mofetil (2–3 g/day) plus prednisolone or placebo plus prednisolone.

At the end of the 52-week follow-up, a similar treatment response rate was observed in the two groups.

The patients given mycophenolate mofetil showed faster and more durable responses, but the lack of difference in the response rate may have been attributable to the milder disease of the placebo group, which may not have needed the added immunosuppressive therapy. Similarly to the results reported by Powell et al., [786] the 2 and 3 g/day doses of mycophenolate mofetil displayed similar efficacy, but infectious adverse events were more frequent with the higher dose.

In all the before mentioned studies, the mycophenolate mofetil therapy was well tolerated. The most common side effects were gastrointestinal complaints, lymphopenia, and bacterial and viral infections. Mycophenolate mofetil and mycophenolate sodium monotherapy for pemphigus vulgaris has been reported in several small case series [1040-1]. However, owing its relatively low efficacy, this treatment regimen is not generally recommended. Many randomized open-label trials compared the efficacy of mycophenolate mofetil as a steroid sparing agent to other immunosuppressive drugs in patients with pemphigus. Beissert et al., [962] treated 40 patients with pemphigus vulgaris or pemphigus foliaceus with methylprednisolone and azathioprine or methylprednisolone and mycophenolate mofetil. There was no difference between mycophenolate mofetil and azathioprine in efficacy, steroid-sparing effect, or safety profile.

In a randomized controlled study, Chams-Davatchi et al., [784] compared four treatment regimens in 120 patients with pemphigus vulgaris: prednisolone only, prednisolone and azathioprine, prednisolone and mycophenolate mofetil, and prednisolone and intravenous cyclophosphamide pulse therapy.

There was no difference in complete remission rate between the groups (70–80% of patients). All immunosuppressive drugs had a steroid sparing effect; the most efficacious was azathioprine, followed by pulse cyclophosphamide and then mycophenolate mofetil. An intention to treat analysis of data from the study reported by Beissert et al., [962] revealed mycophenolate mofetil to be more effective in inducing disease control, as compared to azathioprine. However, combined data from the mentioned randomized open-label trials showed mycophenolate mofetil to have an inferior steroid-sparing effect compared with azathioprine [781]. A few patients with paraneoplastic pemphigus were reported to benefit from combined immunosuppressive regimens, including mycophenolate mofetil and corticosteroids [786] or mycophenolate mofetil, corticosteroids, and azathioprine [1042].

Mycophenolate mofetil is an immunosuppressive drug widely used today in multiple fields of medicine, including dermatology. Its advantages include its wide therapeutic index, mild side effects, and lack of major end-organ toxicity. Mycophenolate mofetil has been successfully applied for treating various autoimmune blistering diseases, including pemphigus, mostly as a steroid-sparing agent. According to many case series, mycophenolate mofetil could be of value in treating refractory disease. The few randomized clinical trials conducted to date of patients with pemphigus report a similar efficacy for mycophenolate mofetil to other immunosuppressants. Large-scale clinical trials are needed to further describe the value of mycophenolate mofetil in this setting.

Chapter 22

Dapsone

Dapsone is a lipid-soluble compound that penetrates well into various tissues. It is well absorbed from the gut, with an absorption half-life of about 1h [1043]. It is excreted by the kidneys with a significant enteropathic circulation. This results in an effective half-life of approximately 24–36h, allowing daily dosing [1044]. Renal impairment and high acetylator status require an adjustment in dosage; however, specific guidelines are not available. Side effects are divided into those that are pharmacologic and those that are idiosyncratic. Pharmacologic side effects include hemolytic anemia and methemoglobinemia. Patients with glucose-6-phosphate dehydrogenase deficiency are prone to dapsone-mediated hemolysis and may need to be treated with lower doses and to receive more frequent follow-up [1045]. Idiosyncratic side effects include agranulocytosis, dapsone hypersensitivity syndrome, cutaneous hypersensitivity reactions, gastrointestinal irritation, peripheral neuropathy, and psychosis. This sulfone-derived medication was first used to treat leprosy in the 1940s. Because of its antimicrobial and anti-inflammatory properties, dapsone has been used in several dermatologic conditions, particularly those with neutrophil predominance because it inhibits neutrophil activation and recruitment through several different pathways [1046]. The US Food and Drug Administration-approved indications for dapsone are leprosy and dermatitis herpetiformis. Moreover, the efficacy of dapsone has been described in neutrophilic dermatosis and vasculitis, as well as autoimmune bullous disorders. The latter group includes dermatitis herpetiformis, pemphigus, pemphigoid, cicatricial pemphigoid, bullous lupus erythematosus, epidermolysis bullosa acquisita, linear IgA bullous dermatosis, and IgA pemphigus.

22.1. Dapsone in Pemphigus Vulgaris

It is a rare group of antibody-mediated blistering diseases that affects the skin and mucous membranes. It is characterized histologically by intraepidermal blisters and immunopathologically by the finding of *in vivo*-bound and circulating IgG antibodies directed against the cell surface of keratinocytes. The two main subsets of pemphigus are vulgaris and foliaceus. Desmoglein 1 and 3 are the main targets in pemphigus vulgaris, and desmoglein 1 is the main target in pemphigus foliaceus [1047]. Immunosuppressives are the mainstay of treatment of pemphigus, and dapsone was reported as an adjunctive therapy several decades ago [1048]. There has been only one randomized, double blind, placebo-controlled trial evaluating the use of dapsone as a glucocorticoid-sparing agent in maintenance phase in pemphigus vulgaris [802]. A total of 19 subjects receiving immunosuppressive therapy were randomized to two groups treated with adding either dapsone or placebo. Success was defined by the ability to taper systemic corticosteroid to at least 7.5 mg/day within 1 year of reaching maximum dose of dapsone (200 mg/day). Of the nine patients receiving dapsone, five (56%) were successfully treated, three failed treatment, and one dropped out of the study. Of the ten patients receiving placebo, three (30%) were successfully treated and seven failed treatment.

The difference between these two groups was not statically significant ($P = 0.37$). The study was underpowered but the trend favored the dapsone-treated group. Moreover, four patients in the placebo group failed treatment and were switched to the dapsone group. Of these, three (75%) were successfully treated after introducing dapsone. Overall, 8 of 11 patients (73%) receiving dapsone versus 3 of 10 (30%) receiving placebo reached the primary outcome measure of 7.5 mg/day or less of prednisone. No adverse events requiring to discontinue dapsone were noted. In a recent retrospective review, case reports and series reporting the use of dapsone for pemphigus were summarized [803]. The authors described 26 patients who received dapsone for pemphigus vulgaris as well as the clinical trial described above, with the dosages varying between 50 and 200 mg/day. Twenty-four of the 26 (96%) patients responded to dapsone alone or in addition to other systemic immunosuppressive. In 16 of these reported cases, dapsone was added to prednisone presumably as a steroid-sparing agent; however, this was not explained in every study. In 10 of these 16 patients (63%), prednisone doses were reduced after beginning of dapsone. In 6 of 16 patients (38%), prednisone dosages could not be decreased because of either continued disease or adverse events associated with dapsone. Dapsone was discontinued in 4 of the 26 patients (15%), 3 secondary to hemolysis and 1 secondary to a hypersensitivity syndrome. About pemphigus foliaceus and the use of dapsone, 18 patients have been reported in the literature [803, 1049]. Fourteen (78%) responded to doses of dapsone of 25–300 mg/daily alone or in combination with systemic corticosteroids. Of the 18 patients, 6 had adverse events (33%) and 2 (11%) needed discontinuation of dapsone therapy because of dapsone-induced hypersensitivity and peripheral neuropathy, respectively.

22.2. Dapsone in IgA Pemphigus

IgA pemphigus is a group of immune-mediated intraepidermal blistering skin diseases. Unlike typical immunoglobulin G (IgG)–mediated pemphigus, IgA pemphigus is characterized by tissue-bound and circulating IgA autoantibodies that target the desmosomal proteins of the epidermis. IgA autoantibodies bind to desmogleins or desmocollins. However, the direct pathogenic effects of the IgA autoantibodies have not been established. Presentations of IgA pemphigus include subcorneal pustular dermatosis and intraepidermal neutrophilic IgA dermatosis [566, 1050]. In a retrospective review in early 2000, dapsone was first-line therapy in the intraepidermal neutrophilic type of IgA pemphigus in 11 cases, and systemic steroids were used as second line in seven cases [667]. Since then, sporadic case reports have described the effectiveness of dapsone alone [1051-3] or incombination with oral corticosteroids [1054-5] or acitretin [1056].

Dapsone is regularly used in treating autoimmune bullous disorders; however, only smaller studies and isolated reports point out that dapsone is effective. Larger studies are needed to determine the benefits and risks of using this medication. There are a couple of randomized and controlled trials for pemphigus vulgaris. There is an agreement that dapsone should be the first-line pharmacologic therapy for dermatitis herpetiformis. When used, the lowest effective dose should be prescribed, up to a maximum of 200 mg/day, although doses up to 300 mg/day have been reported [803]. It has been recommended the therapeutic dosage of dapsone should not exceed 1.5 mg/kg/day to minimize the risk of hemolysis. Before initiation of dapsone therapy, patients should be screened for glucose-6-phosphatase dehydrogenase deficiency, because patients with decreased activity of this enzyme show an approximately two-fold increased sensitivity toward to develop hemolysis and may need to be treated with lower doses and to receive more frequent follow-up.

Also, it has been described in small case series of patients the accompanying use of either cimetidine or vitamin E as protective agents to prevent methemoglobinemia and hemolysis. A complete blood cell count with reticulocyte count should be checked weekly during the first titration of dapsone dose, then every 2 weeks for the first 3 months after that for developing hemolytic anemia and agranulocytosis. Liver enzymes, electrolytes, and urinalysis should be also checked when using dapsone. Peripheral neuropathy, although rare, is a well-described side effect, and periodic screening for both motor and sensory neuropathy is supported.

Chapter 23

CYCLOPHOSPHAMIDE

Cyclophosphamide is an alkylating agent used widely in chemotherapy regimens and immunosuppressive regimens in several autoimmune conditions [1057]. Its role in treating autoimmune blistering diseases has been questioned in recent years due to the increased availability of medications such as azathioprine and mycophenolate mofetil with significantly increased safety profiles [962]. Cyclophosphamide's benefits include significantly lower costs and suggestions of comparable efficacy compared with other immunosuppressive medications; however these benefits are offset by its significant adverse effects and safety concerns, including haemorrhagic cystitis, bladder carcinoma and myelosuppression [1057]. However, in clinical settings in which recommended treatment regimens are prohibitively expensive or not accessible, cyclophosphamide may still be an effective alternative in managing autoimmune blistering diseases alongside proper patient safety surveying.

23.1. PHARMACOLOGY OF CYCLOPHOSPHAMIDE

Cyclophosphamide is a potent DNA alkylator and is administered in oral or intravenous forms as a pro-drug in an inactive state [962]. It is a hydrophilic compound with high plasma bioavailability (between 85 and 100%) and limited plasma protein binding (20%). It is metabolised by the hepatic cytochrome P450 enzymes including CYP3A4 and CYP2B6 to form the active metabolite 4-hydroxy-cyclophosphamide. It is highly active against lymphopoietic cells with the effect of inhibiting the production of B lymphocytes and the resultant antibodies responsible for autoimmune bullous diseases [962]. As the active hydroxylated cyclophosphamide is hydrophilic, it does not diffuse readily across the lipid bilayer into cells. It is seen to spontaneously cross the cell membrane *in vitro*, but membrane transporters are suggested to aid cell entry *in vivo* [1057]. Once intracellular, it spontaneously degrades into the cytotoxic DNA alkylator phosphoramide mustard, producing a toxic by-product, acrolein. Phosphoramide mustard produces irreversible DNA cross-links within and between DNA strands resulting in cell apoptosis. Acrolein, a highly reactive molecule, disrupts cellular functions, leading to symptoms of toxicity.

Acrolein is directly responsible for haemorrhagic cystitis and hepatic aminotransferase derangement in patients administered cyclophosphamide. In cells with high concentrations of aldehyde dehydrogenase (such as intestinal mucosa and hepatocytes), carboxy-cyclophosphamide is produced from 4-hydroxy-cyclophosphamide, with no phosphoramide mustard or acrolein being produced, therefore sparing these tissues from most of the toxic effects from cyclophosphamide [1057].

23.2. Cyclophosphamide in Pemphigus Vulgaris/Pemphigus Foliaceus

Cyclophosphamide has been examined in many randomized control trials for treating pemphigus vulgaris and pemphigus foliaceus. A study of 28 patients was conducted comparing pulsed IV dexamethasone- cyclophosphamide plus daily oral cyclophosphamide versus pulsed IV cyclophosphamide and daily oral prednisolone [1058]. This study showed earlier remission in the pulsed IV cyclophosphamide and oral prednisolone group (mean 7.3 weeks vs 3.2 weeks $P = 0.02$); however no difference was observed in overall rates of remission or relapse. When comparing cyclophosphamide against other immunosuppressive medications, no significant difference was seen in any clinical outcomes when comparing cyclophosphamide and mycophenolate [1047]. No difference in time to disease control or relapse was found when cyclophosphamide was compared with cyclosporine in a small study of 18 participants [785]. With regard to the steroid-sparing role of cyclophosphamide, Chams-Davatchi et al., [784] conducted a landmark multiarm randomized controlled trial into the steroid-sparing role of adjuvants, comparing prednisolone alone to three adjuvant agents: mycophenolate, azathioprine and pulsed cyclophosphamide. The study demonstrated a significant decrease in the total dose of glucocorticoids when prednisolone was combined with a cytotoxic agent ($P = 0.047$) using analysis of variance. The average cumulative prednisolone doses over 12 months were prednisolone alone 11,631 mg, azathioprine 7,712 mg, mycophenolate 9,798 mg and cyclophosphamide 8,286 mg. No differences were detected in clinical endpoints, including time to partial response, complete response and treatment failure. A meta-analysis conducted by Martin et al., [837] found a superior steroid-sparing role for cyclophosphamide compared with azathioprine (−564.00 mg prednisone 95% CI −1,048.54, −79.46, $P = 0.023$). However the statistical analysis conducted by the authors, which accounted for comparison of multiple groups, found no significant difference ($P = 0.971$). There was weak evidence of a benefit for azathioprine over cyclophosphamide in disease control RR (1.80, 95% CI 0.89, 3.64, $P = 0.10$); however this is based on a study with small patient numbers [785]. The evidence comparing azathioprine to cyclophosphamide is inconclusive. Martin's systematic review identified three studies which included comparisons of cyclophosphamide against glucocorticoids, azathioprine, cyclosporine and mycophenolate. There was a significant steroid-sparing effect seen when cyclophosphamide was combined with steroids (mean dose −3,355 mg; 95% CI −6,144 to −566, $P = 0.018$) [131]. The steroid-sparing effect of cyclophosphamide was found to be greater than that of mycophenolate mofetil and lesser than that of azathioprine. It must be noted however that reduction in a cumulative steroid dose is a surrogate outcome.

23.3. Cyclophosphamide in Paraneoplastic Pemphigus

Cyclophosphamide is an effective treatment modality in paraneoplastic pemphigus when used in combination with systemic steroids. Treatment modalities include both pulsed IV and oral administration with either pulsed or daily corticosteroids [1059-60]. Becker reports a case of paraneoplastic pemphigus in the setting of Waldenstrom's macroglobulinaemia treated with dexamethasone (100 mg IV at three weekly intervals) and cyclophosphamide (500 mg IV day 1–3 every 3 weeks) with complete response of desquamation and erosions as well as oral and genital lesions between 4 and 6 weeks [1060]. Herzberg et al., [1059] presents two cases of non-Hodgkin's lymphoma (one follicular NHL and one large cell NHL) who developed paraneoplastic pemphigus with buccal ulceration, haemorrhagic crusted lips, conjunctivitis and papulosquamous cutaneous eruptions with sparse bullae. Both were successfully treated with 100 mg prednisone and 150 mg oral cyclophosphamide daily. Nousari et al., [624] have also reported the effectiveness and safety of ablative intravenous cyclophosphamide (200 mg/kg daily over 4 days) in a patient with chronic lymphocytic leukaemia-associated paraneoplastic pemphigus.

23.4. Safety Profile and Adverse Effects of Cyclophosphamide

Concerns over the use of cyclophosphamide stem from its safety profile. Adverse effects of cyclophosphamide are widespread and frequent. Common adverse effects of cyclophosphamide include nausea, emesis, and alopecia, gonadal insufficiency as well as hyperpigmentation of hair, skin and nails [1061]. Haemorrhagic cystitis is a serious and common effect of therapy as well as the delayed development of bladder carcinoma [1062]. Relative contraindications include hepatic insufficiency, where commonly dosages are reduced by up to 30%, although no pharmacological or clinical evidence exists as to the benefits of such dose reductions. Use of cyclophosphamide is not recommended in the first trimester of pregnancy due to teratogenic effects on the fetus and during breast-feeding due to transmission to the infant. While many of the common adverse effects are typically reversible and dose dependent, permanent effects such as sterility can be a side effect of therapy [1061]. Haemorrhagic cystitis has a reported incidence of 12–41% of cyclophosphamide-treated individuals with rheumatological autoimmune diseases and estimated to have a similar prevalence in dermatological disease [1062]. Common complaints include suprapubic discomfort and macroscopic haematuria; however the need for blood transfusion in these patients is rare. Prophylactic pharmacotherapy to prevent haemorrhagic cystitis is recommended in the setting of IV pulsed cyclophosphamide therapy. Sodium-2-mercaptoethane sulfonate or Mesna is given intravenously with cyclophosphamide and then in an oral preparation 2 and 6h postcyclophosphamide administration [1063]. Forced IV saline diuresis is also recommended if IV cyclophosphamide is being managed, although encouraging oral hydration is acceptable prophylaxis for low-dose oral cyclophosphamide therapy. The use of cyclophosphamide also confers a significant, independent and likely dose-related increase in the risk of future bladder carcinoma. A review by Monach et al., [1062] noted that all studies examining the association between cyclophosphamide and bladder carcinoma demonstrated positive odds ratios ranging from 3.6 to 100, although a significant proportion of these populations also were current or past smokers (a strong independent risk factor for bladder carcinoma) possibly confounding the results. Monach estimates the absolute risk of bladder carcinoma in individuals given cyclophosphamide is 0.067%, compared to a population baseline incidence of 0.04% with a peak in developing bladder carcinoma 11–16 years post-cyclophosphamide administration. Haemorrhagic cystitis may also increase the risk of developing bladder carcinoma with a reported odds ratio of 7.2 ($^{95\%}$CI = 1.9–27), although these results came from studies examining the incidence of bladder carcinoma, therefore bringing into question the legitimacy of the results due to selection bias. Other rare adverse effects of cyclophosphamide and related compounds include nephrotoxicity, neurotoxicity (including encephalitis) and hepatic insufficiency, although these are much more common with ifosfamide than cyclophosphamide. No estimates of the incidence of these complications are available in the use of cyclophosphamide in autoimmune conditions as they are much more frequent during high-dose chemotherapy regimens of IV pulsed cyclophosphamide.

Cyclophosphamide is reported to be equally effective as other immunosuppressive therapies in rates of remission in pemphigus vulgaris and pemphigus foliaceus. It has a high steroid-sparing effect compared with other therapies in pemphigus vulgaris although its increased rates of adverse effects remain the largest barrier to its use. It is also used in paraneoplastic pemphigus for acute life-threatening disease. Expert opinion often recommends avoiding cyclophosphamide for safety reasons due to the increased availability of azathioprine and mycophenolate. In situations where financial or access constraints exist, cyclophosphamide's efficacy is argued to be better than no therapy or steroid therapy alone, although its adverse effect profile raises significant patient safety concerns.

Chapter 24

TETRACYCLINES

Tetracyclines are a group of bacteriostatic antibiotics known to inhibit bacterial protein synthesis by binding to its 30s ribosomal subunit, therefore inhibiting to bind tRNA to the mRNA ribosome complex. Doxycycline and minocycline are second-generation tetracyclines that have been designed to have more rapid bioavailability and better activity against *S. aureus* and community-acquired strains of methicillin-resistant *S. aureus.* This group of drugs has been indicated for treating actinomycosis, animal bites, anthrax, bacillary angiomatosis, ehrlichiosis, rhinoscleroma, rickettsial infections, syphilis, tularemia, Lyme disease, and infections with methicillin-resistant *S. aureus, M. marinum, Borrelia* sp., *Chlamydia* sp., *Nocardia* sp., *V. vulnificus,* and *Y. pestis.*

Several decades ago, tetracycline was studied and used as a modality of treatment in rosacea and acne [1064]. Currently, the tetracycline group of drugs, including its derivatives minocycline and doxycycline, is being used to treat a myriad of inflammatory dermatologic conditions that do not necessarily have a bacteriologic etiology. These inflammatory and non-bacteriologic diseases include neutrophilic disorders, such as pyoderma gangrenosum and Sweet syndrome; granulomatous diseases such as sarcoidosis, foreign body granulomas, and cheilitis granulomatosa; papulosquamous disorders such as lichen planus; ulcerative disorders such as chronic wounds; and bullous disorders including autoimmune and inherited bullous disorders [1065]. The anti-inflammatory properties of tetracycline have become well settled. The antiinflammatory activity of the tetracycline group of drugs involves the inhibition of matrix metalloproteinases, downregulation of inflammatory cytokines, inhibition of leukocyte chemotaxis and activation (including degranulation of neutrophils), and antioxidation. Recently, a drug called incyclinide has been developed that would contain the antiinflammatory properties of tetracycline and not possess its antibacterial activity [1066]. Currently, clinical studies are being conducted on incyclinide, and it has been proven by toxicology studies to be relatively safe. In one study, incyclinide, also referred to as CMT-3 or Col-3, was used in Kaposi sarcoma due to the drug's ability to downregulate matrix metalloproteinases. MMP-2 and MMP-9 have been found in increased amounts in Kaposi sarcoma [1067-8].

24.1. Tetracyclines in Pemphigus

In autoimmune bullous disorders, a pathophysiologic mechanism of this disease is that matrix metalloproteinases, particularly MMP-2, MMP-9, and MMP-13, are found in increased amounts in the lesional skin of bullous pemphigoid. Matrix metalloproteinases have been found to inactivate α1-proteinase inhibitor, which inhibits elastase from enzymatic degradation. Therefore, the tetracycline group of drugs helps prevent destructive enzyme activity in the skin by protecting α1-proteinase inhibitor from degradation by the MMPs, which are downregulated by tetracycline. Apart from their ability to inhibit matrix metalloproteinases, tetracycline, its derivatives minocycline and doxycycline, and chemically modified tetracyclines have also been postulated to be effective in the autoimmune bullous group of diseases for their ability to inhibit leukocyte activation and chemotaxis. These two mechanisms are primarily involved in the pathophysiology of autoimmune bullous disorders [1065]. Currently, evidence for the effectiveness of the tetracycline group of drugs in autoimmune bullous disorders is based mostly on case reports, case series, non-randomized clinical trials, and an open-label randomized controlled trial. Results of these studies have not been consistent, in that some have shown effectiveness of the drug while others have not [1069-70]. Further studies, particularly large randomized controlled trials, would be ideal to significantly demonstrate the use of tetracyclines in autoimmune bullous disorders and just as important, to prove the manner in which the drug is to be ideally managed. This includes dosages and mode of administration (whether it is to be given as monotherapy or in conjunction with another antiinflammatory drug, such as nicotinamide). To date, an open-label randomized controlled trial by Fivenson et al., [1070] showed that treatment using a combination of 500mg nicotinamide three times daily and 500mg tetracycline four times daily for bullous pemphigoid was not statistically significantly different from treatment with prednisone. The authors have concluded that combination treatment of nicotinamide and tetracycline for bullous pemphigoid is a sound alternative to prednisone. However, the study had low numbers of patients and was therefore underpowered to detect a true difference. Despite the need for further studies to establish the effectiveness of tetracycline in autoimmune bullous disorders, this drug has become a popular alternative treatment in patient populations where side effects from other drugs such as systemic corticosteroids or disease-modifying anti-rheumatologic drugs need to be avoided or minimized. Tetracycline therapy, particularly in autoimmune blistering conditions, has become an acceptable treatment modality among elderly individuals, particularly those with osteoporosis, diabetes mellitus, and hypertension. This drug has also been given in combination with immunosuppressive treatment for more rapid tapering of the latter.

Tetracycline has been used in the treatment of bullous pemphigoid, cicatricial pemphigoid, pemphigus vulgaris, pemphigus foliaceus, linear IgA disease, dermatitis herpetiformis, and lichen planus-pemphigoides [1071-2]. Based on studies that have been done, it has been used in combination either with systemic corticosteroids, topical corticosteroids, or with nicotinamide. For tetracycline, doses range from 500 to 2,000 mg daily, with the highest possible dose given as 500 mg four times daily. Minocycline is usually given as 100–200 mg daily, although 50 mg daily dose has also been taken. Doxycycline is usually given as 200–300 mg daily. Finally, nicotinamide, which is usually used in combination with tetracycline, is given at doses ranging from 500 to 2,000mg daily. With nicotinamide, the starting dose would be 500 mg daily; the dose is then eventually increased up to 2,000 mg daily. In a treatment modality that involves combination therapy with tetracycline and nicotinamide, either drug is gradually tapered down one at a time once blister formation has been suppressed. This is done in a course of several months to prevent flares or relapse of blisters [1073-4]. The use of the tetracycline group of drugs is not without its own share of risks and adverse effects. They should not be used in children until the second set of teeth are erupting because of staining of enamel. Tetracycline must be avoided in patients with renal impairment as it has been shown to be nephrotoxic. It has also been noted to cause gastrointestinal toxicity among patients. Meanwhile, doxycycline and minocycline must be avoided in cases of hepatic impairment. These two tetracycline derivatives are also associated with photosensitivity, vestibular problems, and hyperpigmentation. Despite improvement of the bullous conditions being treated, long-term treatment with minocycline results in hyperpigmentation of the skin, nail bed, or mucosa. Fortunately, this drug-induced hyperpigmentation is reversible once minocycline therapy is ceased, but it may take many months in elderly people with thin skin who have been on corticosteroids, compared to young people with acne [1075]. In summary, although the use of the tetracycline group of drugs in the treatment of autoimmune bullous disorders has been derived merely from case reports, case series, and non-randomized clinical trials, it has earned its popularity as an alternative treatment, either as monotherapy or as an adjunct, due to its corticosteroid-sparing antiinflammatory properties. However, it also places patients at risk for its own set of adverse effects. In the final analysis, the clinician must weigh the benefits versus the risks of administering this drug to patients with autoimmune bullous conditions.

Part 8. Specific Management of Pemphigus: Biological Therapy

Chapter 25

INTRAVENOUS IMMUNOGLOBULINS

Intravenous immunoglobulin (IVIG) is comprised of IgG fractioned from pooled human plasma. It is indicated in two main situations: as replacement therapy in diseases due to antibody deficiency or as an immunomodulator in autoimmune or inflammatory diseases [1076]. The use of intravenous immunoglobulin has dramatically increased since its introduction in an intravenous form in the 1980s, overtaking intramuscular and subcutaneous preparations. The use of intravenous immunoglobulin in autoimmune bullous diseases is often considered 'off-label' by manufacturers, and funding is not routine worldwide [1077-8]. Intravenous immunoglobulin is recommended in patients who have failed or have contraindications to conventional therapy and states that intravenous immunoglobulin should be used only for short-term therapy. However to define failing conventional therapy and what constitutes a contraindication is left to the discretion the clinicians and patients resources. The autoimmune bullous diseases are a rare group of chronic, debilitating and sometimes fatal conditions affecting the skin and mucous membranes. Included in the autoimmune bullous diseases are pemphigus, bullous pemphigoid, and mucous membrane pemphigoid and epidermolysis bullosa acquisita. Mainstay of treatment is corticosteroids, the doses of which are altered according to clinical response [62]. A significant burden of bullous diseases is due to side effects from treatment, for example, side effects from corticosteroids including immune suppression, diabetes, osteoporosis, myopathy, mood changes and peptic ulcer disease.

Immunosuppressive agents, such as azathioprine and mycophenolate, are often used for their steroid-sparing effects. However these agents in turn have their own side effects including bone marrow suppression and liver function derangement. Intravenous immunoglobulin is a third-line adjunctive therapy in treatment of autoimmune bullous diseases unresponsive to conventional therapy [270]. The action of intravenous immunoglobulin is attributed to several mechanisms [1079]: neutralization of autoantibiotics; inhibition of complement binding and activation; Fc receptor binding; enhanced clearance of pathogenic autoantibodies via saturation of the neonatal FcR salvage pathway; suppression of pathogenic cytokines; downregulation of T- or B-cell function.

There are many types of intravenous immunoglobulin solution available worldwide. Differences between products include concentration, which usually varies between 5 and 6% which in turn affects the volume of solution required. Sodium and sugar (maltose or sorbitol) content. This affects osmolality and thus has effects on water retention. Low-osmolality products are more desirable for patients with conditions such as heart failure. Plasma source. Uses volunteer remunerated and non-remunerated donors. Plasma testing. Hepatitis B, hepatitis C and HIV are generally tested for. Storage conditions: Once at room temperature, it can be kept for 3 months and for up to1-2 years.

25.1. Intravenous Immunoglobulin in Pemphigus

Pemphigus is characterised by loss of adhesion between keratinocytes, giving rise to blister formation. This loss of adhesion (acantholysis) is due to autoantibodies directed against intercellular adhesion structures which result in blisters. Disease activity matches to titres of autoantibodies, which can be measured by indirect immunofluorescence microscopy and ELISA against desmogleins 1 and 3. The location of blister formation varies. In pemphigus vulgaris, blisters are located just above the basal skin layer, whereas in pemphigus foliaceus, blisters occur within the granular layer of the epidermis. Other less common pemphigus subtypes include paraneoplastic and drug-induced pemphigus [1080-1]. Several smaller studies have shown intravenous immunoglobulin to be effective in pemphigus vulgaris and foliaceus, even more so when administered in adjunct with a cytotoxic agent such as azathioprine or cyclophosphamide. It is thought that intravenous immunoglobulin reduces serum levels of antibodies that mediate pemphigus, whilst cytotoxic agents reduce the rebound increase of the depleted antibody that can occur after administration of intravenous immunoglobulin [1082]. The first placebo-controlled study investigating the use of intravenous immunoglobulin in pemphigus vulgaris used a single patient who suffered multiple relapses of pemphigus vulgaris despite steroids and adjunctive immunosuppressant and had numerous complications related to steroid use including diabetes, osteopenia, ruptured tendons and immunosuppression. In 2004, all adjuvant therapies save azathioprine were discontinued, and he was commenced on intravenous immunoglobulin at a dose of 2 g/kg fortnightly for eight infusions. This led to dramatic improvement and allowed for prednisone to be reduced from 45 to 30 mg daily. He was then maintained on intravenous immunoglobulin at 1 g/kg monthly for 16 months. Thereafter a formal randomized double-blind placebo-controlled crossover trial was conducted. There were two phases, each consisting of six consecutive months of either IVIG 1 g/kg or placebo infusion. During the trial, azathioprine and prednisone were continued, with the patient tapering the dose of prednisone by 5 mg decrements every fortnight if the disease became quiescent. The mean subjective patient disease score decreased significantly with intravenous immunoglobulin compared to placebo (median overall scores 11.6 vs 20.6, $P < 0.0001$); pemphigus autoantibody titres improved significantly (1:80 vs 1:20, $P = 0.007$) as did desmoglein 1 and 3 antibodylevels (126 vs 94 and 126 vs 79, respectively, $P = 0.004$). Prednisone was weaned to 33.7 mgdaily on placebo versus 35.8 mg with intravenous immunoglobulin ($P < 0.0001$) [824].

There has been one multicentre randomized placebo-controlled double-blind trial by Amagai et al., [179] looking at pemphigus vulgaris unresponsive to prednisone doses over 20 mg/day. Twenty-one patients were given 2g intravenous immunoglobulin over 5 days (i.e., approximately 2.5 mg/kg for a 70 kg patient), 20 patients were given 1g intravenous immunoglobulin over 5 days, and 20 patients were given a placebo. There was a significant improvement clinically and in terms of decrease in circulating anti-desmoglein 3 IgG autoantibodies when comparing the 2g and placebo groups, but not when comparing the 1g and placebo groups. In contrast to many studies which suggest multiple treatment cycles of intravenous immunoglobulin, Amagai et al., [179] show that a single 5-day cycle has therapeutic benefits.

25.2. Limitations to Intravenous Immunoglobulin

Intravenous immunoglobulin is not only an expensive treatment, but there are costs associated with laboratory tests, infusion equipment and facility fees. Further costs to the patient include travel and time taken off work and normal activities in order to have the infusion [1083]. Given the expensive nature of intravenous immunoglobulin treatment, there are specific qualifying criteria for use of intravenous immunoglobulin in autoimmune bullous diseases in Australia, with a recommended dose of at least 2 g/kg per monthly treatment cycle. In pemphigus foliaceus, disease must involve at least 30% of body surface area. With pemphigus vulgaris, disease must be diagnosed by a dermatologist as moderate to severe. In all the autoimmune bullous diseases, there must be contraindications, unresponsiveness to or severe side effects from corticosteroid and immunosuppressive agents. Responsiveness must be demonstrated at 6 months for continuance of intravenous immunoglobulin supply. Overall, studies investigating the effects of intravenous immunoglobulin in autoimmune bullous diseases are limited by participant numbers or study design (such as absence of blinding or randomisation). There is a need for future randomized and well-controlled studies using large numbers of participants. Issues requiring more investigation include: ideal intravenous immunoglobulin doses and regimens, effect of adjuvant corticosteroid or immunosuppressive agents, criteria for intravenous immunoglobulin commencement and tapering, effectiveness in modifying the course of disease and efficacy of subcutaneous versus intravenous routes of immunoglobulin. There are also many adverse events associated with use of intravenous immunoglobulin. Most side effects, such as headache and fever, are transient and can be prevented by slowing the infusion rate or by administration of oral antihistamines prior to the infusion. There are however more serious and potentially fatal adverse events including anaphylactic reactions, acute renal failure, cardiovascular compromise from fluid overload and thromboembolic events such as pulmonary emboli. Patients who have issues with fluid balance can use higher concentration intravenous immunoglobulin which allows for smaller volume. Subcutaneous immunoglobulins are an alternative to intravenous immunoglobulin. It tends to have less systemic adverse effects compared with the IV route. Other benefits include not requiring intravenous access and the ability to self-administer. However, subcutaneous infusions require a syringe-drive pump, and there may be local tissue reactions such as swelling, induration and itching. There are also few studies researching the use of subcutaneous immunoglobulins in autoimmune diseases, including pemphigus vulgaris though those that are published are generally positive [1084]. There has been one study investigating subcutaneous immunoglobulins in a patient with epidermolysis bullosa acquisita resistant to conventional therapies. Intravenous immunoglobulin was abandoned due to poor venous access, and subcutaneous immunoglobulins at 0.9g/kg/month divided over 5 days was successful in maintaining clinical improvement while withdrawing all immunosuppressive therapy and in reducing levels of circulating autoantibodies.

Intravenous immunoglobulin appears to be an effective therapy in autoimmune bullous diseases, being particularly useful in disease refractory to conventional therapies. It would be extremely helpful to conduct future well conducted randomised trials to allow for better definition of the role and placement of intravenous immunoglobulin in management of pemphigus.

Chapter 26

RITUXIMAB

Rituximab is a chimeric anti-CD20 monoclonal antibody constructed from a human IgG1*k* constant region fused to murine variable regions that bind with high affinity to cells expressing the CD20 antigen [1085-6]. First used to treat non-Hodgkin's B-cell lymphoma, the scope of rituximab has been expanded to include autoimmune diseases such as rheumatoid arthritis, systemic lupus erythematosus and chronic immune thrombocytopaenic purpura syndrome [826, 1087]. Its therapeutic role in dermatology has been increasing over the last decade. Deletion of B-cells responsible for pathogenic autoantibody production is surmised to result in improved symptoms and disease control. Depleting antigen presenting B-cells will also decrease the transmission of signalling pathways to other key mediators such as T-cells [62, 273].

26.1. MECHANISM OF ACTION

The B-cell antigen, CD20, is a transmembrane glycoprotein expressed on nearly all B-cells and most B-cell lymphomas [827, 1088]. Most notably, it is not found on early pre-B-cells or haemopoietic stem cells [1088]. B-cells arise from the bone marrow and afterwards mature following migration to secondary lymphoid tissues in the periphery, including the spleen and lymph nodes. In the bone marrow, they are known as plasma cells. CD20 is found only on B-cells and is expressed between the pre-B-cell and pre-plasma stages [1089-90]. Because rituximab targets CD20, plasma cells synthesising immunoglobulins within the bone marrow are spared [827]. Once rituximab binds to the CD20 protein, transmembrane signals result in altered cell cycle differentiation and activation. Direct apoptosis, cell-mediated cytotoxicity and complement-dependent cytotoxicity [1091] have been implicated in the subsequent reduction of circulating $CD20^+$ B-cells in the periphery, lymph nodes, spleen and bone marrow [1088]. The depletion of B-cell counts occurs within 3 days of rituximab administration and is reported to be reduced by about 90%, though variations occur. It is thought the variations in depletion are due to the underlying disease and polymorphisms of the receptor Fc γRIIIa [1090]. The B-cell reconstitution begins between 6 and 9 months after rituximab infusion, although the number of peripheral blood B-cells remains low up to 2 years after rituximab infusion [261, 1092]. Besides depleting B-cells, there is evidence the number of desmoglein-specific $CD4^+$ T-cells is also reduced after rituximab administration

[262]. Finally, possible mechanisms by which rituximab deplete B cells include: (1) antibody-dependent cell mediated cytotoxicity, (2) complement-mediated cytotoxicity, and (3) inhibition of cell proliferation with direct induction of B-cell apoptosis.

26.2. Dose and Route of Administration

Before rituximab is given, the patient needs to be clear of all infections, particularly tuberculosis. Their vaccination status should be updated, particularly with any live attenuated vaccines, as for other biological injectable agents [1087]. Patients should not receive live vaccines while receiving rituximab. Rituximab is typically prescribed as weekly infusions of 375 mg/m^2 (approximately 727.5 mg weekly for a 75 kg, 1.8 m tall male) for 4 weeks. Infusions are first administered over about 5h, and if well tolerated, following infusions may be managed over 3 – 5 h [1092]. Recently, there have been some studies of reducing the protocol to two intravenous infusions of 1g 2 weeks apart or even 500mg although this latter regimen seems associated with a higher rate of relapses [1093], with different outcomes for different bullous diseases.

Corticosteroids and antihistamines may reduce the intensity of adverse events and infusion-related adverse effects. Paracetamol and diphenhydramine is recommended before administration to decrease the likelihood and extent of infusion-related adverse events [1092]. Following the infusions, the full blood count and renal and hepatic functions are monitored monthly. A sharp decline in absolute numbers of B-cell counts is expected after the administration of rituximab. Failure of adequate B-cell reconstitution may potentially be clinically significant. There is no evidence that recurrent cycles of treatment confer an increased risk of adverse effects. In one report, rituximab was administered every 6–9 months for rheumatoid arthritis without significant adverse effects apart from a reduction in serum IgM levels [62].

26.3. Adverse Effects

Rituximab is generally well tolerated, with most side effects occurring at the first infusion. Acute adverse reactions are typically transient and mild to moderate in severity, transient, and mostly infusion related [1092]: which include fever, urticaria, headache, nausea, chills, orthostatic hypotension, mucocutaneous reactions and thrombocytopenia [1091]. Patients receiving rituximab for malignant disease can develop cytokine release syndrome [1094]. In such patients, the incidence of hypotension and bronchospasms can be up to 10% [1095]. Other serious side effects include Stevens-Johnson syndrome [1096], tumor lysis syndrome [1097], serious bacterial infections, herpes zoster reactivation [1098], enteroviral meningoencephalitis [1099], hepatitis B virus reactivation, autoimmune hemolytic anemia [1100], liver failure [1101], worsening of Kaposi sarcoma [1102], and late-onset neutropenia [1103] have been reported.

Polymorphisms of the receptor, FcγRIIIa, may influence the efficacy of rituximab and the extent of associated adverse effects [1091]. Serum total IgG levels do not vary significantly after rituximab treatment, whereas total IgM serum levels slightly decrease during the year after managing rituximab. Similarly, anti-pneumococcal and anti-tetanus toxoid antibodies do not vary significantly after treatment [261]. However, a few cases have reported reduced levels of immunoglobulins [1104]. Three cases of fatal pneumonia have occurred following adjuvant rituximab therapy [766, 832, 1105]. Anaemia, late onset neutropaenia and thrombocytopenia have also been reported in 1 – 7% of patients following the fourth rituximab infusion [1106]. Haemolytic anaemia following rituximab infusion has additionally been reported [1107]. Overall, the rate of severe side effects is between 5 and 10%. Given these findings, it is important to regularly monitor blood counts and for signs and symptoms of infection in patients treated with rituximab.

There have been reports of progressive multifocal leukoencephalopathy; however, this has been reported in systemic lupus erythematosus, rheumatoid arthritis and Wegener's granulomatosis, whereas this severe side effect has not been reported yet in patients with autoimmune bullous disorders [1091].

Resistance to rituximab has been reported in lymphoma patients. Possible suggested mechanisms of resistance include decrease in CD20 expression, increase in soluble CD20 level, FcRg111a polymorphisms [1108], increased tumor burden, an increase in antibody metabolism, and, most importantly, developing anti-idiotypic antibodies to rituximab by the patient [1109].

26.4. Rituximab in Pemphigus

The use of rituximab in pemphigus was first reported in 2002, and since then there has been a growing body of evidence from case reports and case series showing high efficacy, particularly in patients who have not responded to more standard treatments [828-9, 831, 1110-9]. Rituximab has additionally been used with good outcomes in paediatric patients [1120-3]. The efficacy of rituximab as an adjuvant therapy has been examined in several case series. A study in 2006 treated 11 patients with recalcitrant pemphigus with rituximab 375 mg/m^2 weekly for 3 weeks and intravenous immunoglobulin (2 g/kg) in the fourth week [1124]. This cycle was repeated in month 2. During months 3–6, patients were managed one infusion of rituximab and intravenous immunoglobulin, with 9/11 (82%) having resolution of lesions by the end of the second cycle, which was maintained for more than 20 months. The combination of intravenous immunoglobulin with rituximab was not compared with rituximab alone; therefore we cannot be certain that intravenous immunoglobulin adds any benefit to rituximab alone. Another study in 2007 treated 12 patients with recalcitrant pemphigus with rituximab, with maintenance corticosteroids and immunomodulators [1125]. The study found complete remission in 9/12 (75%) and partial remission in the remaining 3/12 (25%) by 6 months, with no relapses within a median of 12-month follow-up. An Italian study in 2012 investigated the efficacy of adjuvant rituximab at a lower dose and frequency, with two 1,000mg infusions 15 days apart in 42 patients with recalcitrant pemphigus (37 with pemphigus vulgaris, 5 with pemphigus foliaceus) [1126]. The patients were on a weaning dose of prednisone over several months beginning at 0.5 mg/kg tapered to zero. 36/42 (86%) of patients achieved a prolonged complete remission by 6 months, with all remaining patients achieving complete response at 10 months after an extra rituximab infusion (500mg) at 6 months. In the group who achieved complete remission by 6 months, the median time to remission was 70 days, with 18/36 (50%) remaining in remission in a follow-up period between 12 and 59 months. All patients who relapsed achieved complete remission following an extra 500mg infusion of rituximab. The efficacy of rituximab monotherapy was examined in a multicentre open-label French trial in 2007 [271]. Twenty-one patients (14 with pemphigus vulgaris, 7 with pemphigus foliaceus) who failed to respond, were maintained on or had a contraindication to oral corticosteroids were given a single cycle of rituximab. Each patient received one infusion (375 mg/m 2) weekly for 4 weeks, with immunologic evaluations regularly. 18/21 (86%) had complete remission at 3 months and a further 2 (95% overall) by 12 months. Of those who had a complete remission, 9/20 (45%) relapsed after a mean of 19 months, 2 of whom required a second cycle of rituximab. This study also proved the corticosteroid-sparing effect of rituximab with 8/21 (38%) patients not requiring any systemic treatment at the end of the study. An association between disease activity and antidesmoglein antibody levels was evident by reducing anti-desmoglein 1 and anti-desmoglein 3 titres in those who had experienced remission at 3 months. Rituximab does not seem to influence the immuneresponse as the mean IgG levels did not change significantly. A retrospective study in South Korea reported in 2011 included 27 patients with recalcitrant pemphigus and examined whether the number of infusions within a cycle impacted on clinical outcomes [1127]. They concluded that three or more infusions of rituximab within a cycle were more effective than two infusions. In the group receiving two rituximab infusions, complete remission was seen in 4/12 (33%) and partial remission in 5/12 (42%), with 8 having relapses within a median period of 11.5 months. In the group receiving three or more infusions, complete remission was seen in 11/15 (73%) and partial remission seen in 1/15 (7%), with none experiencing relapse within a median follow-up period of 18.0 months. Overall, complete and partial remission rates were seen in 16/27 (59%) and 5/27 (18%), respectively, with median times for complete and partial remission being 186 and 135 days. Similar positive results are seen in another study with 15 patients undergoing two infusions, with complete remissions in 8/15 (53%) and partial remissions in 7/15 (46%), with 6 (40%) relapsing within a median period of 97 weeks [1093]. A retrospective study on 24 pemphigus vulgaris and 7 pemphigus foliaceus patients showed that 58% of patients achieved complete remission off therapy or on minimal therapy after rituximab treatment and suggested that patients treated earlier in the course of disease may have better outcomes [1128]. While there occasionally have been case reports of ineffective response [1129], rituximab overall appears to be a highly efficacious tool in the treatment of pemphigus. Maintenance therapy at a lower dose may be an option which requires further evaluation [829].

In recent years, rituximab has been used off-label to successfully treat different autoimmune bullous diseases. Though traditional systemic treatments, such as corticosteroids, have been effective, they are associated with multiple adverse effects and occasionally fail to adequately control symptoms. Therefore, additional therapy in the form of weekly intravenous infusions of rituximab (375 mg/m^2) may benefit those autoimmune bullous diseases patients who are contraindicated for systemic steroids or who have recalcitrant or relapsing disease. Rituximab induces B-cell depletion and hence a decrease in pathogenic autoantibodies. Long-term monitoring is advisable, given the possibility of immunocompromise and sepsis. Exactly when to implement rituximab therapy has been debated due to the costs, potential complications and lack of data. Like other inflammatory and autoimmune diseases, the treatment of pemphigus vulgaris is at the dawn of a new era of biologic therapy. Rituximab may be an alternative, or an additional biologic agent, for those patients who fail to respond to conventional immunosuppressive corticosteroid therapies. Elimination of memory B cells that can produce autoantibodies in the future should be an essential and additional aim for any new protocol. The ultimate objective of any therapy for pemphigus vulgaris should be to treat current active disease and simultaneously to produce a prolonged sustained remission.

Chapter 27

Etanercept and Other Anti-TNF

27.1. TNFa Antagonists

The TNFα is a pro-inflammatory mediator involved in diverse cellular functions, mainly in the proliferation and cell differentiation and apoptosis [1130]. High concentrations of this cytokine are associated with exaggerated inflammation and severe organic damage [1131], also, it is involved in the pathogenesis of several autoimmune and autoinflammatory diseases, which has led to develop drugs that antagonize this molecule.

TNFα is produced by a myriad of cells including mast cells, macrophages, fibroblasts and keratinocytes [1131].

Etanercept is a fusion protein that acts as receptor inhibitor TNFα. Its structure consists of an extracellular domain of human type 2 receptor TNFα, coupled with the constant fraction of the IgG1 and can act on soluble and transmembrane TNFα [1130, 1132]. Its mechanism of action is related to competitive inhibition of TNFα receptor [1133], thus avoiding TNFα interaction on the cell surface [1134].

Etanercept also binds to soluble TNFα interacting with one of this molecule thereby producing 1: 1 complexes. The route of administration is subcutaneously and its bioavailability ranges from 58 to 63%, with an average mean-life of 70 hours [1131].

No drug interactions have been reported with the use of etanercept, because it is metabolized by peptides with amino acid recycling with bile and urine excretion [1131].

Etanercept is generally well tolerated, the most common side effect is soreness at the injection site, reported in 40% of patients [1132], others mentioned adverse effects are often prone to respiratory infections (35%) and headache (20%) [1134]. It has been also observed with continued use of etanercept, a reactivation of latent tuberculosis; developing lymphomas has also been reported but so far there are no convincing studies on the association [1132]. Other reactions reported are demyelinating disorders, aplastic anemia, pancytopenia, development or flares of lupus erythematosus and sepsis [1135]. Diaz-Lagares et al., [1136] whom studied in 344 patients with systemic autoimmune disease where they used biological treatments, found that predisposes the patient to more severe infections, being rituximab the most associated and etanercept the least associated.

Etanercept is contraindicated in patients with a history of hypersensitivity to any component of the drug and the presence of active tuberculosis at any level [1132].

27.2. Etanercept in Pemphigus

Pemphigus vulgaris is an autoimmune blistering disease characterized by autoantibodies directed to different objectives of the epidermis, mainly against desmogleins 1 and 3, which are adhesion molecules between keratinocytes and the most important constituents of the desmosome [1134]. TNFα is strongly associated with its pathogenesis [1133] since a clear relationship between clinical disease activity and circulating levels of this cytokine is found [1134].

Etanercept has been used successfully for treating pemphigus vulgaris; based on the important role of TNFα in developing acantolisis [1137].

There are many reports and case series on the use of etanercept in managing recurrent pemphigus vulgaris and/or recalcitrant, as monotherapy or in combination with systemic immunosuppressant like systemic steroids, azathioprine, methotrexate, dapsone and intravenous immunoglobulin, with improvement and control of activity disease after 3-6 weeks of use with fewer blisters and decreased risk of relapse [1132-4].

In a recent report [1133] in a double-blind, randomized trial, 6 patients with severe pemphigus vulgaris were included and treated with etanercept 50mg 2 times per week with acceptable response. In another report, we described four cases of recalcitrant pemphigus vulgaris treated with etanercept and methotrexate, also with acceptable therapeutic response [1138].

27.3. Other Anti-TNFa and Biologics in Pemphigus

TNFα has been suggested to play a role in the acantholysis of the keratinocytes in pemphigus vulgaris. Therefore, anti-TNF agents such as sulfasalazine and pentoxifylline, which are TNFα inhibitors, and infliximab, which is a fusion protein of the TNFα receptor are implicated to be effective treatments. While etanercept and infliximab are expensive and are associated with many side effects, sulfasalazine and pentoxifylline are less costly alternatives with safer drug profiles. The efficacy profile of anti-TNF agents has been unclear to date.

Adjuvant infliximab was evaluated in one study involving 20 participants [1139]. The follow-up period was 26 weeks. Outcome measures included response to treatment, adverse events, desmoglein 1 and 3 antibodies titres and B-cells levels. The study found that the infliximab group's desmoglein 1 antibody levels showed a significant decrease at week 18. No convincing differences were found in all other reported outcome measures. Limitations of the study included its small sample size and short follow-up period.

In a randomized, placebo-controlled trial [1140], infliximab therapy was not shown to be effective for treating patients with pemphigus vulgaris, although infliximab treatment may be associated with a decrease in anti-desmoglein 1 and 3 antibodies, with an acceptable safety profile. In this study, the authors showed that treatment with infliximab results in a decrease in memory B cells with an increase in the immature transitional B cells, in concordance with previous studies [1141]. This increase in transitional B cells was first observed at week 18, and persisted without additional infliximab infusions, demonstrating a biological effect in patients with pemphigus.

Adjuvant sulfasalazine (500mg three times daily) and pentoxifylline (400mg three times daily) versus placebo was evaluated in one study involving 64 participants [1142]. All patients also received conventional cyclophosphamide pulse therapy simultaneously. The follow-up period was 8 weeks. The outcome measures included clinical improvement and serum TNFα level. The study found the treatment group had superior clinical improvement than the placebo group (86 versus 18% in complete remission, P = .001). There was also a significant decrease in TNFα level in the treatment group compared to placebo group (16.81 ± 7.98 vs. 37.63 pg/mL ± 10.23, P = .001). Main limitation of the study was its short follow-up period.

Further studies of TNF blockade will be necessary to confirm these findings and determine if this treatment approach can be utilized for the benefit of this patient population.

PART 9. ADDITIONAL THERAPY AND MONITORING

Chapter 28

MANAGEMENT OF PAIN IN PEMPHIGUS VULGARIS

Pemphigus is a life-threatening autoimmune blistering disease of the skin and mucous membranes. The incidence of pemphigus varies as reported from different regions of the world, and ranges from 0.07 to 2.7/100,000 [510, 513]. Although many variants of pemphigus exist, most of pemphigus cases are pemphigus vulgaris. Clinically, the most common presentation of pemphigus vulgaris is persistent painful erosions or ulcers [502]. The primary lesions are flaccid bullae of various sizes; often the skin or mucosae simply shear off, leaving painful erosions.

Pain is a universal feature of pemphigus vulgaris, although it may vary considerably depending on the extent of the erosions and the presence of associated infection and inflammation. Care should be given to addressing underlying background pain from these lesions. It should be remembered that even older patients experience important pain from erosions, and these needs should be addressed, even with strong opioid analgesia if required.

Lesions usually occur first in the mouth, where they rupture and then remain as chronic, often painful erosions for undefined periods of time before the skin is affected. The bullae then appear, arising from healthy appearing skin, where they rapidly rupture, and leaving raw and crusting areas. Lesions usually occur in the oropharynx and upper esophagus.

The nomenclature of pemphigus vulgaris and similar blistering disease should also be briefly reviewed, as much confusion tends to occur in this area. Pemphigus vulgaris, as classically known, is characterized by flaccid bullae and erosions of the mucosa.

These areas can become hemorrhagic or seropurulent. Other sites of localization include the skin of the head, groin, and axillae. Pemphigus vegetans presents as localized plaques on the scalp. These flaccid bullae can become vegetations or proliferations. Pemphigus foliaceus consists of flaccid bullae and exfoliation. Meanwhile, pemphigus erythematosus consists of flaccid bullae and plaques that resemble those of lupus erythematosus. Understandably, owing to the life threatening nature of pemphigus vulgaris, the main focus of the peer reviewed literature has been on suppression and remission of pemphigus vulgaris.

However, remission is not instantaneous and may take over 1 month to achieve. This delay in remission, allows ample opportunity for complications to develop secondary to the pain associated with pemphigus vulgaris. This can be highlighted by cases of repeated dehydration, malnutrition, and inpatient readmission that is seen in pemphigus vulgaris patients [1143]. However, despite the pain component involved in pemphigus vulgaris, few peer reviewed works have focused on pain management in such patients. As a result, this manuscript was compiled in an attempt to compile the current reports on pemphigus vulgaris pain management and to highlight the need for further studies in this field.

Pemphigus is a serious autoimmune disease that has drawn considerable attention from academicians. Multiple peer reviewed works are in progress or have been completed in hopes of developing improved therapeutic options [774, 1144]. With few large scale randomized trials available, most management is currently based on expert opinion and clinical experience [1007]. Furthermore, the majority of reports on pemphigus focus on disease modifying therapeutic approaches. However, despite the well known pain component of pemphigus vulgaris, the pemphigus studies available rarely address the pain component directly [1145]. Interesting and novel pain control alternatives were found to include the use immunomodulating systemic and topical that is azathioprine and clobetasol respectively [1146-9].

However, in the majority of reports, the principle approach was focused on controlling acute exacerbations, with pain control to follow as a result of lesion clearing [1147]. This results in unnecessarily drawn out discomfort for patients.

It should also be noted that many pain control options are not reported, though often tried in clinical practice. Among these include the use of silver sulfadiazine, topical mixtures of 50:50 diphenhydramine and lidocaine. An initial stepwise approach using acetaminophen with or without non steroidal anti-inflammatory drugs for mild pain, adding mild opiates for moderate pain, or stronger opiates such as morphine for more severe pain.

In addition to systemic agents, topical analgesics may be helpful for a limited number of more painful ulcers. These include treatments that provide slow release of ibuprofen and the use of topical morphine (10mg morphine mixed in hydrogel) applied directly to the painful erosion twice a day.

Considering the chronic, relapsing nature of pemphigus vulgaris, an increased focus on supportive measures may be favorable. In particular, pemphigus vulgaris pain control requires a greater emphasis in both the peer reviewed literature and in clinical practice. Studies focusing on the specific comorbidities, for example pain, would be especially useful. Such studies can then lead into research focusing on classifying and management of pemphigus vulgaris pain. Further emphasis, and a stronger push to encourage large-scale studies is critical in helping these patients more quickly return to a standard pain-free lifestyle. Finally, this review should also encourage the inclusion of pain scale assessment and pain management in current studies of pemphigus.

Chapter 29

EXTENT MEASURES IN PEMPHIGUS

Pemphigus group encompasses several rare dermatoses characterized by autoantibodies against specific proteins of the skin. Due the rarity of these diseases, there is a paucity of studies in the literature to guide clinicians in the best evidence-based management of patients [1150]. A systematic review of outcome measures in pemphigus over the past 25 years identified 116 different measures across 96 articles [1151]. Most studies used outcome measures based on non-validated, subjective, or non-specific ratings of disease activity, and because of the variety of measures employed (lesion counts, quality of life scores, autoantibody titers, etc.), a significant obstacle in comparing therapeutic modalities is the absence of uniform outcome measures for correlation across studies [1151]. This is particularly relevant because the rarity of autoimmune bullous diseases results in studies often have low patient numbers, with meta-analysis combining studies only possible if uniform outcome measures are available. Many scoring systems have been developed in recent years in an attempt to provide an objective measure to assess disease activity in autoimmune bullous diseases [62]. Such measures function alongside the clinical assessment of patients, allowing objective assessment of disease activity in a patient and monitoring disease trajectory over time (Table 15). They can also be used as outcomes measures in clinical trials. The most promising extent measures for autoimmune bullous diseases are the Autoimmune Bullous Skin Disorder Intensity Score or commonly called ABSIS [1152], Pemphigus Disease Area Index, also known as PDAI [394], and the Bullous Pemphigoid Disease Area Index [836], though a range of other scoring systems have been employed in this setting.

29.1. AUTOIMMUNE BULLOUS SKIN DISORDER INTENSITY SCORE

The ABSIS was devised with the aim of developing a disease severity measure sensitive enough to capture changes in disease activity in autoimmune bullous diseases. Scoring is based on the extent of body surface area involved and the quality of the dominant skin lesions. The extent of body surface area affected is estimated using the "rule of nines" in which defined areas of the body are equivalent to 9% or multiples of 9%. This value is then multiplied by an index reflecting the most dominant lesion present: 1.5 (erosive, exudative lesions, bullae, or Nikolsky sign positivity), 1.0 (erosive, dry lesions), or 0.5 (re-epithelialized lesions). Oral involvement is evaluated using a modified version of the grading system employed by Saraswat et al. 1153 These results are tabulated to give a total score ranging from 0 to 206: 150 for skin involvement, 11 for oral involvement, and 45 for oral functional impairment. The ABSIS score has had two validity studies performed on it [395] and has been used as an outcome measure in many clinical studies in autoimmune bullous diseases [968, 1154-5].

29.2. Pemphigus Disease Area Index

The PDAI was developed by international consensus by the International Pemphigus Definitions Committee as an extent measure to objectively assess bullous disease activity. The skin and scalp are assessed for disease extent and damage, and the oral mucosa is assessed for activity alone. In the skin assessment, 12 anatomical sites (ears, nose, face, neck, chest, abdomen, back/buttocks, arms, hands, legs, feet, genitals) are reviewed and assigned a score according to disease activity (0 (no lesions), 1(1 – 3 lesions, all ≤6 cm, up to 1 >2 cm), 2 (2 – 3lesions, all ≤6 cm, at least 2 lesions >2 cm), 3(>3 lesions, all ≤6 cm), 5 (>3 lesions and/or 1lesion >6 cm), or 10 (>3 lesions and/or at least1 lesion >16 cm). When a score of 1 is given, a lesion count is also incorporated, with a score of 1 given if 1 lesion is present, 1.3 for 2 lesions, and 1.6 for 3 lesions. The 12 sites are also reviewed for the presence of post-inflammatory hyperpigmentation or erythema from resolving lesions and assigned a score of 0 (absent) or 1 (present) to assess damage. Damage scores are not included in the overall activity score, (they are there to remind graders that not all visible lesions represent activity. The scalp is assigned a score based on the presence of bullae, erosions, or new erythema of 0 (no activity), 1 (one quadrant affected), 2 (two quadrants affected), 3 (three quadrants affected), 4 (whole scalp affected), or 10 (at least 1 lesion >6 cm). A damage score of 0 or 1 is given to the entire scalp based on the presence of features previously described for the skin damage score. Mucosal activity is assessed by reviewing 12 mucosal sites (eyes, nose, buccal, hard palate, soft palate, upper gingiva, lower gingiva, tongue, floor of the mouth, labial mucosa, posterior pharynx, anogenitalia) and assigning a score based on the presence of erosions and blisters (0 (absent), 1 (1 lesion), 2 (2–3 lesions), 5 (>3 lesions or 2 lesions >2 cm), or 10 (entire area). The total possible score for the PDAI ranges from 0 to 130 for the skin score (120 points for body, 10 points for scalp) and up to 120 points for mucosal activity, with 13 points for damage. These are not combined. Validation studies, both in person and by photovalidation, have been conducted for the PDAI [395].

One study compared the two previously described index, to evaluate the inter- and intra-rater reliability of the two instruments [395]. Ten dermatologists traveled to the University of Pennsylvania and evaluated 15 pemphigus patients using the ABSIS, the PDAI, and the Physician's Global Assessment, a 10-point visual analogue scale used as a marker for convergent validity. Physicians were divided into two groups with half the physicians scoring patients with the ABSIS first, then the PDAI with the order reversed in the second group. Each physician returned to the original group 2h later and re-rated two randomly assigned patients to evaluate intra-rater reliability. Both instruments demonstrated validity when correlated against the Physician's Global Assessment with a correlation of 0.60 (0.49 – 0.71) for the PDAI and 0.43 (0.30 – 0.55) for the ABSIS. Inter-rater reliability had an overall intraclass correlation coefficient of 0.76 (0.61 – 0.91) for the PDAI and 0.77 (0.63 – 0.91) for the ABSIS. The ABSIS was slightly better in inter-rater reliability; however, for skin activity, the PDAI activity score had an intraclass correlation coefficient of 0.86 and the ABSIS 0.39, suggesting that the PDAI might be better at detecting differences in cutaneous disease. Intra-rater reliability was 0.98 (0.96 – 1.0) for the PDAI and 0.80 (0.65 – 0.96) for the ABSIS pointing out that PDAI scores were more reproducible. The results of the study demonstrated that both instruments are validated extent measures for autoimmune bullous diseases though it is possible the PDAI may be more reliable (Table 15).

29.3. Other Disease Severity Measures

A range of severity measures have been published for the objective evaluation of disease activity in autoimmune bullous diseases, though the majority have not been evaluated and have been constructed arbitrarily for use in clinical trials. One instrument which has been validated is the Index of Skin and Mucous in Pemphigus Vulgaris [1156]. Patients are scored according to the number of blisters (0 – 25 points), the size of blisters or erosions (0 – 25 points), presence of Nikolsky sign (0 – 20 points) and involving mucous membranes or sepsis (0 – 30 points). It has been validated in a small cohort of 7 patients with active disease over 76 visits and was found to have a high inter-rater reliability with a Pearson's correlation of 0.93 (0.89 – 0.95) and weighted kappa coefficient of 0.92 (0.89 – 0.96) between paired scorings of patients. The Index of Skin and Mucous in Pemphigus Vulgaris was also able to categorize patients as having mild, moderate, or severe disease to stratify disease severity. To the authors' knowledge, it is the only extent measure other than the ABSIS and PDAI to have been validated for use in autoimmune bullous diseases. One of the earliest disease activity scores employed was the Pemphigus Area and ActivityScore [1157]. The Pemphigus Area and ActivityScore divides the body into head, trunk, upper limbs, and lower limbs. Each division is assigned a score based on the number of new blisters, extension of existing blisters, and the presence of the Nikolsky sign and then multiplied by the area involved and an index, with the four scores totalled. Patients with mucosal involvement are also assigned a mucous membrane score by adding the number of mucosal sites involved to a severity score to ascertain a mucous membrane score. One scoring system employed in a study reviewing the incidence of remission in pemphigus patients graded disease activity on a score from 0 to 10 [1158]. Extent is scored from 0 to 4 depending on whether predefined areas of the body were affected and therapy was scored from 0 to 6 depending on the dose of oral corticosteroid and the need of adjuvant immunosuppression.

A retrospective case series of pemphigus patients stratified disease severity into four categories based on body surface area involvement and functional impairment [1159]. Patients are classified as having mild disease (≤10% body surface area involvement or disease limited to oral mucosa, ability to carry out activities of daily living without discomfort), moderate (10 – 25% involvement, able to carry out activities of daily living with discomfort), severe (25 – 50% involvement and oral involvement, unable to carry out activities of daily living), or extensive (>50% involvement with mucosal involvement, bedridden or has complications). Another study exploring the correlation between antibody titers and clinical severity in pemphigus used a simple scale to assess cutaneous and oral lesions [817]. Skin lesions are graded as quiescent (no lesions), mild (<5 discrete lesions), moderate (6 – 19 discrete lesions), or severe (>20 lesions or extensive confluent erosions). Oral lesions are also graded as quiescent (no lesions), mild (≤3 erosions), moderate (4 – 9 erosions or general desquamative gingivitis), or severe (≥10 lesions or extensive, confluent erosions, or generalized desquamative gingivitis with discrete erosions at other sites).

Table 15. Comparison of the Autoimmune Bullous Skin Disorder Intensity Score (ABSIS) and the Pemphigus Disease Area Index (PDAI)

Characteristic	ABSIS	PDAI
Overview	Combines quantitative (assigns weights to involve body surface area and types of lesions on the skin and oral mucosa and oropharinx) and qualitative (subjective severity scale based ability to eat and drink) components.	A quantitative measurement of the size and number of lesions on the body, scalp and mucous membranes. It incorporates both disease activity and disease damage.
Strength	Easy to use	Better inter and intra-rater reliability compared to ABSIS; might better detect changes in mild-moderate disease.
Weakness	The majority of its inter-rater reliability comes from its subjective component. Not able to detect clinically significant disease, since it depends on having at least 1% involvement in any body areas measured, which is frequently not the case. It is difficult to incorporate into daily practice.	Difficult to incorporate into daily practice.

The Pemphigus Activity Score is an extent measure evaluating skin lesion area, oral mucosal lesions, and number of new blisters daily with each domain graded from 0 to 3 [1160]. Skin lesions are stratified as none (0), <5% (1), 6 – 15% (2), or ≥15% (3); mucosal lesions as none (0), <5% (1), 6–30% (2) or ≥30% (3); and daily blisters as none (0), occasionally (1), 1–4 (2), and ≥5 (3). Scores across each domain were summed to yield a final Pemphigus Activity Score out of 12. A novel approach to assessing disease activity in oral pemphigus was devised by Saraswat et al. [1153]. The scoring system is divided into two parts assessing the extent of disease and the consequent functional impairment. Eleven sites in the oral cavity (the upper and lower labial mucosa, upper and lower gingival mucosa, left and right buccal mucosa, dorsal and ventral lingual mucosa, hard and soft palate, and uvula) are assigned a score of 0 or 1 depending on the presence or absence of lesions, regardless of severity. A functional assessment is then determined using a modified version of the validated grading system employed in gastroenterology [1161], which utilizes information about the frequency of pain and bleeding with nine different food groups to evaluate functional impairment. Most of these extent measures were not validated before use as endpoints in clinical trials and devised arbitrarily. The diversity of extent measures employed in the past highlights the need for a unifying disease severity measure in a specific autoimmune bullous disease, to allow comparisons between the effectiveness of different interventions.

Objectively evaluating disease activity in autoimmune bullous diseases is important in terms of the clinical assessment of patients and as an outcome measure for clinical trials. Extent measures need to be general enough to capture the specific issues for the differing bullous dermatoses but specific enough to capture any changes to disease status for a patient.

Different tools have been put forward over the last 15 years, but presently the PDAI and ABSIS seem to be the most promising tools to assess disease activity in autoimmune bullous diseases. Further studies need to be performed to validate such measures, with correlations with autoantibody titers and quality of life instruments possible avenues in the future. Work has already been done to make these tools easier to utilize clinically, such as the development of a software program to facilitate electronic completion of the PDAI and ABSIS and software to capture these scores and convert these into decision making tools for clinicians [1162]. Assessing disease activity in autoimmune bullous diseases will continue to be an important area of research in the future, as it will function as the cornerstone for future clinical trials to help physicians decide the best evidence-based approach to management in this setting.

Chapter 30

QUALITY OF LIFE IN PEMPHIGUS

Skin diseases are rarely life-threatening; however, they are capable of a massive impact on quality of life; for instance, psoriasis has been found to affect quality of life in a comparable way to heart failure [1163]. Contributing factors encompass physical discomfort, time spent on treatment, staining of linen and clothes with skin scales or blood, and the obvious nature of skin disease, with its adverse impact on body image and its consequences on social function, which may be not commensurate with clinical severity. Physical symptoms such as pain and itching can strongly affect quality of life [1164]; related problems such as functional limitations, financial burden, and side effects of treatment all contribute to a poor quality of life [1165]. Accordingly, an assessment of quality of life helps evaluate the impact of a patient's dermatosis on well-being. Quantification of this impact is a relatively recent endeavor prompted by the desire to gauge the outcomes of medical intervention. Several quality of life measurement tools have been developed to assess disease impact on patient well-being in a reliable, statistically validated way. The literature shows that patients and dermatologists often have different perceptions of a patient's quality of life and that this inconsistency is associated to a lower degree of satisfaction with medical care [1166]. The findings of the application of quality of life tools can be used with clinical assessment and disease activity parameters to score disease severity objectively. Indeed, some tools afford analysis of the aspects of disease that distress a patient the most (for example, symptoms such as itching or pain, the esthetic problem, the financial burden), simplifying to provide personalized care [62]. Quality of life assessments can also be used to evaluate the effectiveness of therapeutic interventions and monitor disease course over time, besides providing a valuable patient-based endpoint for clinical trials, to quantify changes in the disease process that may not correlate with changes in clinical disease activity [1167]. Quantifying the burden of disease is also important for its patient advocacy implications, given its influence on allocating research support and clinical resources as well as the public perception of dermatological conditions [1168]. Moreover, a greater awareness of quality of life may enhance communication and shared decision making between physician and patient. Greater patient satisfaction involves greater adherence to treatment, a more stable relationship with the physician, relief from anxiety, and an increased sense of personal control on events, all of which contribute to the recovery process [1169]. However, quality of life assessments are not routinely implemented by a number of healthcare professionals. The reasons include inadequate resources, limited time, or lack of appropriate instruments. Many clinicians are less familiar with quality of life assessment administration or evaluation than with other diagnostic tests; quality of life is sometimes viewed as providing "soft" data as opposed to "hard" laboratory data. Many practitioners report that it is more difficult to conduct quality of life assessments on the elderly, because of higher rates of illiteracy, lower completion rates, cognitive disorders, and comorbidities. Patients find quality of life questionnaires more acceptable if they offer fewer answer options and if questions/answers are in the form of words rather than numbers. Questionnaires that did not ask overly personal, sensitive, or irrelevant questions also seem to be favored. Quality of life assessments are not yet widely used in dermatology, although the interest in them is growing. Studies exploring quality of life in autoimmune bullous dermatosis have focused mainly on pemphigus (i.e., pemphigus vulgaris and pemphigus foliaceus) and bullous pemphigoid. Studies regarding other forms of pemphigus as well as other acquired bullous diseases such as mucous membrane pemphigoid, epidermolysis bullosa acquisita, and linear IgA bullous dermatosis are few and sparse.

The earliest paper exploring quality of life in autoimmune bullous diseases involved 380 pemphigus patients in Japan [1170]. Participants were stratified into those with mild (67.7%), moderate (25.9%), or severe (6.3%) disease and were asked to complete a questionnaire regarding activities of daily living and the financial implications of their condition. The survey found that patients retained good activities of daily living independence, since 99.7% were able to feed themselves and use the toilet unaided, 97% were able to shave or apply makeup, 96.5% were able to bathe, 90.8% were able to use public transport, 85.2% could cook, and 82.3% could drive without help. However, the economic burden was considerable, as 41.9% (60% of those with severe disease) reported a reduced income due to lost work time, and 41.3% (57.9% of those with severe disease) described their financial status as poverty. Since only 2.2% of patients were experiencing active disease (the rest being in varying phases of remission), the data show that pemphigus does not significantly impair activities of daily living if appropriately treated. In contrast, its financial burden may be heavy despite clinical improvement, something that should be considered when assessing these patients. Another study of quality of life in pemphigus used the SF-36 to compare patients with pemphigus and the wider population in Morocco [1171]. The study cohort included 30 consecutive pemphigus patients presenting to dermatology clinics or admitted to hospital; the control cohort consisted of 60 patients presenting with non-debilitating conditions such as verrucous warts or benign cutaneous tumors. Patient inclusion criteria were bullous dermatitis with fluid-filled bullae and intraepidermal division on a cutaneous biopsy, presence of acantholytic cells, and immunoglobulin deposition in the epidermis under direct immunofluorescence. Because of the high illiteracy rate, the questionnaires were completed by the investigators, although they had originally been designed either for self-administration or for administration by a trained examiner in person or by telephone. To minimize biases, a single interviewer completed the questionnaires for all participants, whether literate or illiterate. The authors identified significant differences between cohorts, with the pemphigus group displaying lower mean scores across all dimensions but "Physical pain" and "Change compared to the previous year." Physical status and emotional status were the most affected domains, with facial involvement and lesion extent correlating well with overall scores. As many as 70% reported being deeply ashamed of their appearance; 60% were anxious about what others thought of their disease, and 63% reported a significant loss of self-confidence. Repercussions on sexual function were also extensive, 81% of patients reporting concern. Cultural factors were noted to play a large role in quality of life decline due to misconceptions associating skin conditions to poor hygiene or improper sexual practices. Further considerations were the high cost of disease management and social issues such as the impairment of young women's marriage prospects. The use of a generic quality of life tool therefore identified a significant impact of pemphigus on quality of life and highlighted that besides the functional aspects of disease burden, the SF-36 also explores social domains and self-image, which are very significant in this disease [62].

Quality of life was evaluated in 27 German patients with pemphigus vulgaris using a dermatology-specific tool [1172]. Their mean Dermatology Life Quality Index was 10.1 ± 6.6 compared to healthy individuals, whose mean score was 0.5 ± 1.1, leading the authors to conclude that the disease greatly impairs quality of life. The mean Dermatology Life Quality Index of patients with mucosal involvement was 10.4 ± 7.3, while that of patients whose mucosa was spared was 9.3 ± 5.1, indicating a poorer quality of life in the former individuals. Itching was also associated to quality of life deterioration, as these patients scored 11.5 ± 7.5 vs 7.9 ± 4.8 of those without itching. Burning was also found to impair quality of life, since the index score of patients who suffered from it was almost double that of patients who did not (10.8 ± 6.6. vs 5.5 ± 5.7). None of these differences achieved statistical significance, possibly due to the small cohort size. Notably, 22.2% of participants reported that their quality of life was unchanged. The mean Dermatology Life Quality Index of pemphigus was higher than the mean scores of similar autoimmune bullous diseases, such as bullous pemphigoid (6.92 ± 3.80), perhaps because of the low frequency of mucosal involvement in bullous pemphigoid or because its good response to lower drug doses entails fewer and less unpleasant adverse effects. For example, bullous pemphigoid typically responds to prednisone doses not exceeding 0.5 mg/kg/day, whereas pemphigus usually requires a starting dose of at least 1 mg/kg/day [1173]. The authors concluded that the Dermatology Life Quality Index may be useful as an additional measure of treatment response in patients with pemphigus. The mean Dermatology Life Quality Index of pemphigus was also higher than those of other dermatological conditions, such as basal cell carcinoma (2.0 ± 2.2), but it was lower than that of atopic eczema (12.5 ± 5.8), an evaluation facilitated by the use of a skin-specific quality of life instrument to compare severity. However, quality of life is a complex area influenced by several factors, and the Dermatology Life Quality Index does not appear to be an optimal tool to assess pemphigus patients. Indeed the questionnaire was devised using data from 120 patients, only one of whom had blisters, whereas there were at least 10 with eczema, 14 with psoriasis, and 15 with acne [1174-5]. Therefore, the Dermatology Life Quality Index is likely more appropriate to assess patients with these conditions than individuals with pemphigus. In addition, given that scores reflect tool construction, these patients may quite possibly place emphasis on aspects of their handicap that are not covered by the Dermatology Life Quality Index, and no emphasis at all on some that are. Moreover, questions regard only the previous week, which may miss flares in chronic disease.

A study reviewing the health status of 58 Italian in patients undergoing treatment for pemphigus also demonstrated a significantly decreased quality of life compared to the general population [1176]. Participants were asked to complete the SF-36, the Institute for Personality and Aptitude Testing Anxiety Scale Questionnaire (ASQ), and the Clinical Depression Questionnaire (CDQ). As expected, pemphigus had a stronger impact on SF-36 scores compared to normative data. No significant difference was seen between patients with pemphigus vulgaris (n = 51) and those with pemphigus foliaceus (n = 7); however, individuals with disease duration ≥5 years, recent disease onset, disease that had worsened compared to the previous year, mucocutaneous involvement, higher anti-desmoglein 3 antibodies, or with more severe disease all had subjectively worse SF-36 scores. ASQ and CDQ values had a strong negative correlation with SF-36 scores, indicating that poorer quality of life scores were associated to higher levels of anxiety and depression. A study from Italy used generic and dermatology-specific instruments to assess quality of life in 126 in patients with pemphigus [1177]. Most had pemphigus vulgaris (112), although the cohort also comprised patients with pemphigus foliaceus [1178], paraneoplastic pemphigus, and IgA pemphigus. Patients received the SF-36, the Skindex-29, and the GHQ-12 to assess quality of life; the Ikeda index, the PGA, and autoantibody titers were used to measure disease severity. Comparison to normative scores for the general Italian population showed that pemphigus adversely affected SF-36 and Skindex-29 scores ($P < .05$). Disease severity was significantly associated to poorer quality of life scores as was female sex, a finding that had not emerged from previous quality of life studies of pemphigus patients although it has been described in other dermatological conditions. Anti-desmoglein antibody titers correlated neither with clinical severity nor with quality of life scores. GHQ positivity (suggesting the possible presence of minor non-psychotic psychiatric conditions) was found in 39.7% of participants, compared to 10 – 12% in the general population, and correlated with clinical severity. Patients with pemphigus foliaceus had slightly worse quality of life than those with pemphigus vulgaris on the Skindex-29, with a significant difference in symptom scale; 70% of pemphigus foliaceus patients were GHQ positive. However, there were only ten patients with pemphigus foliaceus and 112 with pemphigus vulgaris in this study; given the in patient setting, subjects with pemphigus foliaceus likely had more severe disease at presentation. The authors suggest that psychological distress and personality disorders may have a role in disease development, maintenance, and progression, which in turn are likely to affect quality of life. They conclude that proper assessment of patients' health status would require a generic and a dermatology-specific quality of life tool, with a psychiatric-oriented questionnaire to help select patients who would benefit from psychological support in addition to the standard treatment. Another cross-sectional study from Iran compared quality of life in 76 patients who had had pemphigus for at least 3 months and in 86 healthy controls who accompanied them to clinic appointments, most likely relatives (which ensured a similar environment and social status) [1179]. The study used Farsi translations of the SF-36 and the Goteborg Quality of Life (GQL) instrument. The authors do not clarify whether they employed validated Farsi translations of the instruments, or the degree of Farsi proficiency of patients, given ethnic diversity in Iran. As expected, patients had significantly lower quality of life scores across all parameters, with a mean score of 69.38 compared to the control mean (85.43; $P < .0001$). Factors associated to worse quality of life scores were age >50 years ($P < .04$), longer disease duration ($P < .01$), repeated hospitalization ($P < .001$), and treatment protocol (steroid and adjuvant, $P < .001$). Of note, patients with a university education ($P < .01$) and those in some particular professions had better quality of life scores. Housekeepers had a very large number of poor quality of life scores; this may have been due to confounding factors, because all housekeepers in the study were women and this factor was associated to worse quality of life scores. Patients with higher and lower incomes had no significantly different quality of life scores, although the latter had slightly better scores; this may be due to the small number of patients with high incomes. The importance of quality of life in autoimmune bullous diseases is increasingly being recognized, and several studies are now including it as an important outcome measure. For instance, a small study of Brazilian pemphigus patients recently investigated the effects of physiotherapy with quality of life, the only outcome of interest [1180]. Seven patients received 25 physiotherapy sessions over a 4-month period; quality of life was measured with the SF-36 at baseline and at completion. Patients who participated in the physical therapy sessions exhibited a tendency toward improvement in the symptom component of the SF-36, but not in the social or psychological aspects. The sole significant improvement was in the pain score ($P < .005$). Further studies of larger samples are required to establish the effects of physiotherapy on quality of life in pemphigus. Since quality of life is being included with increasing frequency as an outcome in clinical trials, it would be important to have reliable validated instruments to measure it. Another recent Iranian study assesses the effect on quality of life of the disease per se before treatment and evaluates psychological status and its effect [1181]. Participants were 61 patients with newly diagnosed, non-treated pemphigus vulgaris. The Persian version of the Dermatology Life Quality Index was used to measure quality of life and the 28-item GHQ (GHQ-28) to evaluate psychological status. The mean Dermatology Life Quality Index score was 10.9 ± 6.9; quality of life was worse in patients with nasal and pharyngeal involvement, in those with a positive Nikolsky sign, severe skin involvement, and itching. The Dermatology Life Quality Index score exhibited a negative correlation with disease duration. More than 77% of patients experienced anxiety and depression, resulting in a worse quality of life. The authors concluded by highlighting the well-known strong impact of severe pemphigus on quality of life, its greater influence in early disease, and the need for clinicians to consider quality of life impairment in disease management right from the start of treatment.

Autoimmune bullous diseases have the potential to impose a significant disease burden, and the impact exerted on quality of life is often multifaceted [1182]. As expected, the qualitative and quantitative studies assessing quality of life in patients with bullous disease have all reported a significantly impaired quality of life compared to the greater population, using a range of patient-based measures [1183-4]. These findings have been obtained through the use of generic and dermatology-specific quality of life instruments. To our knowledge, no autoimmune bullous diseases-specific quality of life instrument has yet been devised despite efforts by several researchers to develop the Autoimmune Bullous Disease Quality of Life Questionnaire [1185]. Following a comprehensive item-generation process, a pilot instrument was established and administered, along with the Dermatology Life Quality Index, to 73 autoimmune bullous diseases patients across Australia. The results were evaluated using factor analysis and review by experts in bullous disease to refine it to the current 17-item Autoimmune Bullous Disease Quality of Life questionnaire. Psychometric evaluation of the Autoimmune Bullous Disease Quality of Life Questionnaire has shown it to be a valid and reliable tool that may be used to monitor disease activity and serve as an end point in clinical trials [1186-7].

A range of instruments, usually classified into generic, dermatology-specific, and disease-specific, have been used to assess quality of life in clinical settings [1178, 1188-9]. Generic quality of life measures have been used by the greater medical community to assess life quality across general medical problems [1190]. The benefits of generic tools include their breadth and applicability across different conditions and interventions; however, assessment of quality of life requires instruments capable of detecting even minor changes in patient distress. Generic quality of life instruments are not endowed with this degree of sensitivity, but are used nonetheless, because they provide a suitable means to compare cohorts across the greater community [1191]. Generic tools make it possible to conduct comparisons across all diseases; for instance, the Medical Outcome Study 36-item Short-form Survey (SF-36) measures health-related quality of life and is thus used to compare quality of life in autoimmune bullous diseases patients and in the general population [1192]. Albeit devised as a generic health status indicator for use in population surveys and health policy studies, the SF-36 can also be combined with disease-specific tools as an outcome measure. It includes 36 items in a Likert-type or forced-choice format and measures eight dimensions: physical functioning (limitations in performing physical activities, e.g., bathing or dressing), role-physical (RP) (limitations in work and other daily activities connected with physical health), bodily pain (BP) (how severe and limiting pain is), GH (how general personal health is perceived by the patient), vitality (feeling tired and worn out vs energetic), social functioning (interference of physical or emotional problems with normal social activities), role-emotional (RE) (limitations in work and other daily activities due to emotional problems), and mental health (feeling nervous and depressed vs peaceful, happy, and calm). In addition, question 2 covers changes in health status during the past year; this is not counted in scoring the eight dimensions, but is used to estimate change in health from a cross-sectional administration of the SF-36. Scores for each domain range from 0 to 100, higher scores indicating better health. Skin-specific measures used in dermatology allow for comparisons across cutaneous diseases. Several skin-specific quality of life instruments have also been developed and have the advantage of being more sensitive and responsive than generic measures [1193]. Although generic tools have been tested and validated repeatedly for their psychometric properties, it has been claimed that they do not necessarily highlight issues that are specific to patients with skin conditions. Dermatology-specific instruments generally explore a given domain more thoroughly than a generic measure, resulting in greater responsiveness to change, thus allowing comparison of patients with different skin conditions within dermatology. The Dermatology Life Quality Index was derived from patients with a variety of skin diseases and provides a simple tool to score the influence of skin disease on quality of life [1194]. It evaluates questions addressing symptoms and feelings (items 1 and 2), daily activities (items 3 and 4), leisure (items 5 and 6), work and school (item 7), personal relationships (items 8 and 9), and treatment (item 10). Each question has four possible responses ("not at all," "a little," "a lot," or "very much") that are assigned a score of 0, 1,2, or 3 respectively; "not relevant" is also assigned a score of 0. The sum of the scores of all responses gives a Dermatology Life Quality Index score that ranges from 30 to 0 points. Higher scores reflect greater quality of life impairment; healthy subjects have an average score of 0.5 [1195].

The Skindex, another skin-specific measure, was designed to assess the effect of symptoms and the burden on social function and emotional state. The original Skindex consisted of 61 items, but it has now been reduced to questionnaires of 29, 17, and 16 items (Skindex-29, Skindex-17, and Skindex-16, respectively), to decrease respondent burden and improve discrimination and evaluation. Higher values correspond to a worse quality of life [1196-8]. Used with dermatological measures focusing specifically on skin-related issues, they are useful, for instance, in comparing patients with different skin diseases or in detecting changes in the effects of skin disease on patients in clinical trials or longitudinal studies [1199].

Psychiatric-related measures are also used to investigate quality of life in autoimmune bullous diseases. Psychiatric morbidity is quite common among patients with skin diseases, and the prevalence of depression ranges between 25 and 40% compared to only 2 – 5% in the general population [1200]. The GHQ-12 is a self-administered 12-item questionnaire designed to measure psychological distress and to detect current non-psychotic or psychiatric disorders, such as depression and anxiety [1201-2]. The reliability and validity of the Italian version have been tested in several diseases, including dermatological conditions [1203-4]. Answers are scored on a four-point scale; for instance, the question "in the last weeks, did you feel under strain?" can be answered as "no," "no more than usual," "more than usual," and "much more than usual." When scored with the binary method (0 – 0 – 1 – 1), the GHQ-12 can be used as a screening tool to detect minor non-psychotic or psychiatric disorders, yielding final scores that range from 0 to 12. Patients scoring 4 or more are considered to be GHQ positive.

The Japanese Ministry of Health, Labor, and Welfare applies its own measure of disease burden. The questionnaire inquires about the respondent's ability to perform common activities of daily living unaided, including bathing, eating, cooking, shaving or applying makeup, using the toilet, using public transportation, and driving. Disease-specific quality of life instruments are even more perceptive than skin-specific tools, because they are sensitive to specific issues associated to a particular disease. The advantages of disease specific instruments are that questions are perceived as being of direct relevance to the patient, having a high face validity, and that question specificity maximizes the ability to detect any changes in the disease process [1205-6]. However, the fact that investigators cannot apply the more specific instruments across diverse populations or different conditions hampers comparisons between groups [1207-8]. An autoimmune bullous disease-specific measure would greatly benefit both patients and health practitioners. Researchers often use a combination of specific and generic quality of life instruments to maximize responsiveness and comparability; a recent systematic review has suggested that harnessing a generic and a dermatology-specific tool may be the best combination of quality of life instruments in dermatology [1209]. Investigations into the adverse impact of autoimmune bullous diseases on patients' quality of life have addressed primarily pemphigus, in particular pemphigus vulgaris. As a consequence, data regarding quality of life in other forms of pemphigus and in other acquired bullous diseases, such as bullous pemphigoid, mucous membrane pemphigoid, epidermolysis bullosa acquisita, and linear IgA bullous dermatosis, are quite scanty [1210-2]. However, very few studies, using a variety of instruments, have explored quality of life in patients with pemphigus [62].

In a study performed by our group in Mexico, we found that quality of life was significantly affected in patients with pemphigus vulgaris. This asseveration is explained on the basis of pain and functional limitation, medication and treatment and social and emotional status of the patient.

With increasing disease severity, we observed a worse quality of life that was attributed mainly to worsening pain and functional limitation, characteristic in pemphigus vulgaris. After one month of treatment, the worse quality of life was attributable to disease severity, and also to the treatment side effects. Social and emotional status is an important factor that affects quality of life independent of disease severity and disability related and treatment; moreover, proper education about pemphigus vulgaris, patient counseling, and assurance about the success of available treatment modalities must be included in managing pemphigus vulgaris as recommended on literature consulted [1213-4].

Ghodsi et al., [1215] studied quality of life in 61 patients with pemphigus vulgaris using a version of the Dermatology Life Quality Index. They observed a negative correlation between the index and duration of the disease and concluded that pemphigus vulgaris is responsible for great alteration of quality of life, especially on its severe stage.

In our study, we found that pain and functional limitation secondary to disease is an important element that impact on quality of life with or without treatment, moreover, it should be properly evaluated and treated when possible to help improve the patient's quality of life.

Rajan et al., [1216] found that questionnaires, like Chronic Oral Mucosal Diseases Questionnaire, provide a detailed picture of the impact of oral diseases, including pemphigus vulgaris, on patients, which add information that may be useful in clinical practice. This questionnaire may help give a greater focus to the limited time available at follow-up appointments. Furthermore, the Chronic Oral Mucosal Diseases Questionnaire may allow the patient to assist in the evaluation and assessment of treatment effectiveness and it could supply valuable information regarding the patient's perspective on quality of life, which helps the clinician to modify the strategy for managing pemphigus vulgaris.

Limitations of our study include that long-term use of therapy was not evaluated; there was a lack of uniformity in treatment schemes, there was not a control group and finally, psychiatric morbidity was not evaluated, which is known to impact on quality of life, however, none of the patients had previous reports of psychiatric diseases or related treatment.

The clinical evaluation of quality of life, may give information about the cause, can help to choose a specific treatment, and can also provide clues about the prognosis, although it can´t reflect the resulting level of impairment. These measurements must be simple and practical enough for the clinician and patient to use and interpret. We found the test reliable, simple to use, and sensitive to clinical parameters and treatment modalities.

Finally, the first and successive evaluations and management of pemphigus vulgaris must consider the impact of quality of life on patient outcome.

REFERENCES

[1] Müller, EJ; Galichet, A; Wiener, D; et al. Keratinocyte biology and pathology. *Vet Dermatol*, 2014, 25, 236-8.

[2] Nishifuji, K; Yoon, JS. The stratum corneum: the rampart of the mammalian body. *Vet Dermatol*, 2013, 24, 60–72.

[3] Suter, MM; Schulze, K; Bergman, W; et al. The keratinocyte in epidermal renewal and defence. *Vet Dermatol*, 2009, 20, 515–32.

[4] Drögemüller, M; Jagannathan, V; Becker, D; et al. A mutation in the FAM83G gene in dogs with hereditary footpad hyperkeratosis (HFH). *PLoS Genet*, 2014, 10, e1004370.

[5] Jagannathan, V; Bannoehr, J; Plattet, P; et al. A mutation in theSUV39H2 gene in Labrador Retrievers with hereditary nasalparakeratosis (HNPK) provides insights into the epigenetics of keratinocyte differentiation. *PLoS Genet*, 2013, 9, e1003848.

[6] Müller, EJ; Caldelari, R; Kolly, C; et al. Consequences of depleted SERCA2-gated calcium stores in the skin. *J Invest Dermatol*, 2006, 126, 721–31.

[7] Klukowska-Rötzler, J; Chervet, L; Müller, EJ; et al. Expression of thymic stromal lymphopoiet in in canine atopic dermatitis. *Vet Dermatol*, 2013, 24, 54–9.

[8] Chervet, L; Galichet, A; McLean, WH; et al. Missing C-terminal filaggrin expression, NFkappaB activation and hyperproliferation identify the dog as a putative model to study epidermal dysfunction in atopic dermatitis. *Exp Dermatol*, 2010, 19, e343–e346.

[9] Owczarek-Lipska, M; Lauber, B; Molitor, V; et al. Two loci on chromosome 5 are associated with serum IgE levels in Labrador retrievers. *PLoS One*, 2012, 7, e39176.

[10] Lauber, B; Molitor, V; Meury, S; et al. Total IgE and allergen-specific IgE and IgG antibody levels in sera of atopic dermatitis affected and non-affected Labrador- and Golden retrievers. *Vet Immunol Immunopathol*, 2012, 149, 112–118.

[11] Williamson, L; Raess, NA; Caldelari, R; et al. Pemphigus vulgaris identifies plakoglobin as key suppressor of c-Myc in the skin. *EMBO J*, 2006, 25(14), 3298–309.

[12] Muller, EJ; Williamson, L; Kolly, C; Suter, MM. Outside-in signaling through integrins and cadherins, a central mechanism to control epidermal growth and differentiation? *J Invest Dermatol*, 2008, 128(3), 501–16.

[13] Galichet, A; Borradori, L; Müller, EJ. A new light on an old disease: adhesion signaling in pemphigus vulgaris. *J Invest Dermatol*, 2014, 134, 8–10.

[14] Getsios, S; Waschke, J; Borradori, L; et al. From cell signaling to novel therapeutic concepts: international pemphigus meeting on advances in pemphigus research and therapy. *J Invest Dermatol*, 2010, 130, 1764–8.

[15] Blanpain, C; Horsley, V; Fuchs, E. Epithelial stem cells: turning over new leaves. *Cell*, 2007, 128, 445–58.

[16] Kolly, C; Suter, MM; Müller, EJ. Proliferation, cell cycle exit, and onset of terminal differentiation in cultured keratinocytes: pre-programmed pathways in control of C-Myc and Notch1 prevailover extracellular calcium signals. *J Invest Dermatol*, 2005, 124, 1014–25.

[17] Caldelari, R; Müller, EJ. Short- and long-term cultivation of embryonic and neonatal murine keratinocytes. *Methods Mol Biol*, 2010, 633, 125–38.

[18] Sasai, Y. Cytosystems dynamics in self-organization of tissue architecture. *Nature*, 2013, 493, 318–26.

[19] Bos, JD; Kapsenberg, ML. The skin immune system: progress in cutaneous biology. *Immunol Today*, 1993, 14(2), 75–8.

[20] Streilein, JW. Skin-associated lymphoid tissues (SALT): origins and functions. *J Invest Dermatol*, 1983, 80(Suppl), 12–6.

[21] Egawa, G; Kabashima, K. Skin as a peripheral lymphoid organ: revisiting the concept of skin- associated lymphoid tissues. *J Invest Dermatol*, 2011, 131(11), 2178–85.

[22] Nestle, FO; Di Meglio, P; Qin, JZ; Nickoloff, BJ. Skin immune sentinels in health and disease. *Nat Rev Immunol*, 2009, 9(10), 679–91.

[23] Gorelik, M; Frischmeyer-Guerrerio, PA. Innate and adaptive dendritic cell responses to immunotherapy. *Curr Opin Allergy Clin Immunol*, 2015, 15(6), 575-80.

[24] Schakel, K; Hansel, A. News from dendritic cells in atopic dermatitis. *Curr Opin Allergy Clin Immunol.*, 2011, 11(5), 445–50.

[25] Di Meglio, P; Perera, GK; Nestle, FO. The multitasking organ: recent insights into skin immune function. *Immunity*, 2011, 35(6), 857–69.

[26] Tomura, M; Honda, T; Tanizaki, H; et al. Activated regulatory T cells are the major T cell type emigrating from the skin during a cutaneous immune response in mice. *J Clin Invest*, 2010, 120(3), 883–93.

[27] Machado, I; González, P; Schiöth, HB; Lasaga, M; Scimonelli, TN. α-Melanocyte-stimulating hormone (α-MSH) reverses impairment of memory reconsolidation induced by interleukin-1 beta (IL-1 beta) hippocampal infusions. *Peptides*, 2010, 31(11), 2141-4.

[28] Piskin, G; Sylva-Steenland, RMR; Bos, JD; et al. *In vitro* and *in vivo* expression of IL-23 by keratinocytes in healthy skin and psoriasis lesions: enhanced expression in psoriatic skin. *J Immunol*, 2006, 176, 1908–15.

[29] Soumelis, V; Reche, PA; Kanzler, H; et al. Human epithelial cells trigger dendritic cell-mediated allergic inflammation by producing TSLP. *Nat Immunol*, 2002, 3, 673–80.

[30] Akira, S; Uematsu, S; Takeuchi, O. Pathogen recognition and innate immunity. *Cell*, 2006, 124, 783–801.

[31] Ting, JPY; Kastner, DL; Hoffman, HM. Caterpillers, pyrin and hereditary immunological disorders. *Nat Rev Immunol*, 2006, 6, 183–95.

[32] Robinson, MJ; Sancho, D; Slack, EC; et al. Myeloid C-type lectins in innate immunity. *Nat Immunol*, 2006, 12, 1258–65.

[33] van der Aar, AMG; Sylva-Steenland, RMR; Bos, JD; et al. Cutting edge: loss of TLR2, TLR4, and TLR5 on Langerhans cells abolishes bacterial recognition. *J Immunol*, 2007, 178, 1986–900.

[34] Medzhitov, R; Janeway, CA. Innate immunity. *N Engl J Med*, 2000, 343, 338–44.

[35] Esche, C; Stellato, C; Beck, LA. Chemokines: key players in innate and adaptive immunity. *J Invest Dermatol*, 2005, 125, 615–28.

[36] McGirt, LY; Beck, LA. Innate immune defects in atopic dermatitis. *J Allergy Clin Immunol*, 2006, 118, 202–8.

[37] Bos, JD; De Rie, MA; Teunissen, MBM; et al. Psoriasis: activation of innate immunity. *Br J Dermatol*, 2005, 152, 1098–107.

[38] Mihai, S; Sitaru, C. Immunopathology and molecular diagnosis of autoimmune bullous diseases. *J Cell Mol Med*, 2007, 11(3), 462–81.

[39] Amagai, M; Stanley, JR. Desmoglein as a target in skin disease and beyond. *J Invest Dermatol*, 2012, 132(3 Pt 2), 776–84.

[40] Tsuruta, D; Dainichi, T; Hamada, T; Ishii, N; Hashimoto, T. Molecular diagnosis of autoimmune blistering diseases. *Methods Mol Biol*, 2013, 961, 17–32.

[41] Kneisel, A; Hertl, M. Autoimmune bullous skin diseases. Part 1: clinical manifestations. *J Dtsch Dermatol Ges*, 2011, 9(10), 844–56.

[42] Kneisel, A; Hertl, M. Autoimmune bullous skin diseases. Part 2: diagnosis and therapy. *J Dtsch Dermatol Ges*, 2011, 9(11), 927–47.

[43] Amagai, M; Matsuyoshi, N; Wang, ZH; Andl, C; Stanley, JR. Toxin in bullous impetigo and staphylococcalscalded-skin syndrome targets desmoglein 1. *Nat Med*, 2000, 6(11), 1275–7.

[44] Sitaru, C; Mihai, S; Otto, C; et al. Induction of dermal-epidermal separation in mice by passive transfer of antibodies specific to type VII collagen. *J Clin Invest*, 2005, 115(4), 870–8.

[45] Nishie, W; Sawamura, D; Goto, M; et al. Humanization of autoantigen. *Nat Med*, 2007, 13(3), 378–83.

[46] Eming, R; Hennerici, T; Backlund, J; et al. Pathogenic IgG antibodies against desmoglein 3 in pemphigus vulgaris are regulated by HLA-DRB1*04: 02-restricted T cells. *J Immunol*, 2014, 193(9), 4391–9.

[47] Anhalt, GJ; Labib, RS; Voorhees, JJ; Beals, TF; Diaz, LA. Induction of pemphigus in neonatal mice by passive transfer of IgG from patients with the disease. *N Engl J Med*, 1982, 306(20), 1189–96.

[48] Gushi, M; Yamamoto, Y; Mine, Y; et al. Neonatal pemphigus vulgaris. *J Dermatol*, 2008, 35(8), 529–35.

[49] Grando, SA. Pemphigus autoimmunity: hypotheses and realities. *Autoimmunity*, 2012, 45(1), 7–35.

[50] Cirillo, N; Cozzani, E; Carrozzo, M; Grando, SA. Urban legends: pemphigus vulgaris. *Oral Dis*, 2012, 18(5), 442–58.

[51] Marchenko, S; Chernyavsky, AI; Arredondo, J; Gindi, V; Grando, SA. Antimitochondrial autoantibodies in pemphigus vulgaris: a missing link in disease pathophysiology. *J Biol Chem*, 2010, 285(6), 3695–704.

[52] Hacker, MK; Janson, M; Fairley, JA; Lin, MS. Isotypes and antigenic profiles of pemphigus foliaceus and pemphigus vulgaris autoantibodies. *Clin Immunol*, 2002, 105(1), 64–74.

[53] Funakoshi, T; Lunardon, L; Ellebrecht, CT; Nagler, AR; O'Leary, CE; Payne, AS. Enrichment of total serum IgG4 in patients with pemphigus. *Br J Dermatol*, 2012, 167(6), 1245–53.

[54] Amagai, M; Ahmed, AR; Kitajima, Y; et al. Are desmoglein autoantibodies essential for the immunopathogenesis of pemphigus vulgaris, or just "witnesses of disease"? *Exp Dermatol*, 2006, 15(10), 815–31.

[55] Saito, M; Stahley, SN; Caughman, CY; et al. Signaling dependent and independent mechanisms in pemphigus vulgaris blister formation. *PLoS One*, 2012, 7(12), e50696.

[56] Yamamoto, Y; Aoyama, Y; Shu, E; Tsunoda, K; Amagai, M; Kitajima, Y. Anti-desmoglein 3 (Dsg3) monoclonal antibodies deplete desmosomes of Dsg3 and differ in their Dsg3-depleting activities related to pathogenicity. *J Biol Chem*, 2007, 282(24), 17866–76.

[57] Bektas, M; Runager, K; Petersen, JS; Rubenstein, DS. Advances in pemphigus research, signaling, and acantholysis. *G Ital Dermatol Venereol*, 2010, 145(5), 675–87.

[58] Lotti, R; Marconi, A; Pincelli, C. Apoptotic pathways in the pathogenesis of pemphigus: targets for new therapies. *Curr Pharm Biotechnol*, 2012, 13(10), 1877–81.

[59] van der Wier, G; Jonkman, MF; Pas, HH; Diercks, GF. Ultrastructure of acantholysis in pemphigus foliaceus re-examined from the current perspective. *Br J Dermatol*, 2012, 167(6), 1265–71.

[60] Mahoney, MG; Wang, Z; Rothenberger, K; Koch, PJ; Amagai, M; Stanley, JR. Explanations for the clinical and microscopic localization of lesions in pemphigus foliaceus and vulgaris. *J Clin Invest*, 1999, 103(4), 461–8.

[61] Tsuruta, D; Ishii, M; Hashimoto, T. The diagnosis and treatment of pemphigus. *Immunotherapy*, 2012, 4(7), 735–45.

[62] Murell, D Ed. Blistering diseases. Springer Ed. *Berlin*, 2015. ISBN 978-3-662-45697-2.

[63] Serrano-Osuna, R; López-López, RM; Brito-Zurita, OR; Sabag-Ruiz, E; Pérez-Fernández, H; Ornelas-Aguirre, JM. Seroprevalence of antinuclear antibodies in blood donors in the Yaqui Valley. *Cir Cir*, 2014, 82(6), 619-27.

[64] Kretz-Rommel, A; Rubin, RL. Disruption of positive selection of thymocytes causes autoimmunity. *Nat Med*, 2000, 6, 298–305.

[65] Stockinger, B. T lymphocyte tolerance: from thymic deletion to peripheral control mechanisms. *Adv Immunol*, 1999, 71, 229–65.

[66] Bouneaud, C; Kourilsky, P; Bousso, P. Impact of Negative Selection on the T Cell RepertoireReactive to a Self-Peptide. A Large Fraction of T Cell Clones Escapes Clonal Deletion. *Immunity*, 2000, 13, 829–840.

[67] Kisielow, P; Teh, HS; Bluthmann, H; von Boehmer, H. Positive selection of antigen specific T cells in thymus by restricting MHC molecules. Nature 1988, 335, 730–733.

[68] Rocha, B; von Boehmer, H. Peripheral selection of the T cell repertoire. *Science*, 1991, 251, 1225–1228.

[69] Leventhal, J; Miller, J; Abecassis, M; Tollerud, DJ; Ildstad, ST. Evolving approaches of hematopoietic stem cell-based therapies to induce tolerance to organ transplants: the long road to tolerance. *Clin Pharmacol Ther*, 2013, 93(1), 36-45.

[70] Blackman, M; Kappler, J; Marrack, P. The role of the T cell receptor in positive andnegative selection of developing T cells. *Science*, 1990, 248, 1335–41.

[71] Bonomo, A; Matzinger, P. Thymus epithelium induces tissue-specific tolerance. *J Exp Med*, 1993, 177, 1153–64.

[72] Arnold, B; Schonrich, G; Hammerling, GJ. Multiple levels of peripheral tolerance. *Immunol Today*, 1993, 14, 12–4.

[73] Rocken, M; Shevach, EM. Immune deviation – the third dimension of non deletional T cell tolerance. *Immunol Rev*, 1996, 149, 175–94.

[74] Moskophidis, D; Lechner, F; Pircher, H; Zinkernagel, RM. Virus persistence inacutely infected immunocompetent mice by exhaustion of antiviral cytotoxic effector T cells. *Nature*, 1993, 362, 758–61.

[75] Webb, S; Morris, C; Sprent, J. Extrathymic tolerance of mature T cells: clonal elimination as a consequence of immunity. *Cell*, 1990, 63, 1249–56.

[76] Alferink, J; Tafuri, A; Vestweber, D; Hallmann, R; Hammerling, GJ; Arnold, B. Control of neonatal tolerance to tissue antigens by peripheral T cell trafficking. *Science*, 1998, 282, 1338–41.

[77] Schonrich, G; Kalinke, U; Momburg, F; et al. Down-regulation of T cell receptors on self-reactiveT cells as a novel mechanism for extrathymic tolerance induction. *Cell*, 1991, 65, 293–304.

[78] Ohashi, PS; Oehen, S; Buerki, K; et al. Ablation of "tolerance" and induction of diabetes by virusinfection in viral antigen transgenic mice. *Cell*, 1991, 65, 305–17.

[79] Oldstone, MB; Nerenberg, M; Southern, P; Price, J; Lewicki, H. Virus infection triggersinsulin-dependent diabetes mellitus in a transgenic model: role of anti-self (virus) immuneresponse. *Cell*, 1991, 65, 319–31.

[80] von Herrath, MG; Guerder, S; Lewicki, H; Flavell, RA; Oldstone, MB. Coexpression of B7-1 and viral ("self") transgenes in pancreatic beta cells can break peripheral ignorance and lead to spontaneous autoimmune diabetes. *Immunity*, 1995, 3, 727–38.

[81] Weinberg, AD; English, M; Swain, SL. Distinct regulation of lymphokine production is found in fresh versus *in vitro* primed murine helper T cells. *J Immunol*, 1990, 144, 1800–7.

[82] Mosmann, TR; Sad, S. The expanding universe of T-cell subsets: Th1, Th2 and more. *Immunol Today*, 1996, 17, 138–46.

[83] Rocken, M; Racke, M; Shevach, EM. IL-4-induced immune deviation as antigen specific therapy for inflammatory autoimmune disease. *Immunol Today*, 1996, 17, 225–31.

[84] Rocken, M; Saurat, JH; Hauser, C. A common precursor for CD4+ T cells producingIL-2 or IL-4. *J Immunol*, 1992, 148, 1031–6.

[85] Adorini, L; Sinigaglia, F. Pathogenesis and immunotherapy of autoimmune diseases. *Immunol Today*, 1997, 18, 209–11.

[86] Katz, JD; Benoist, C; Mathis, D. T helper cell subsets in insulin-dependent diabetes. *Science*, 1995, 268, 1185–8.

[87] Kolb, H; Kolb-Bachofen, V; Roep, BO. Autoimmune versus inflammatory type Idiabetes: a controversy? *Immunol Today*, 1995, 16, 170–2.

[88] Powrie, F. T cells in inflammatory bowel disease: protective and pathogenic roles. *Immunity*, 1995, 3, 171–4.

[89] Racke, MK; Bonomo, A; Scott, DE; et al. Cytokine-induced immune deviation as a therapy for inflammatory autoimmunedisease. *J Exp Med*, 1994, 180, 1961–6.

[90] Budinger, L; Borradori, L; Yee, C; et al. Identification and characterization of autoreactive T cell responses tobullous pemphigoid antigen 2 in patients and healthy controls. *J Clin Invest*, 1998, 102, 2082–9.

[91] Mosmann, TR. Coffman RL. TH1 and TH2 cells: different patterns of lymphokinesecretion lead to different functional properties. *Annu Rev Immunol*, 1989, 7, 145–73.
[92] Goldman, M; Druet, P; Gleichmann, E. TH2 cells in systemic autoimmunity: insightsfrom allogeneic diseases and chemically-induced autoimmunity. *Immunol Today*, 1991, 12, 223–7.
[93] Hertl, M; Karr, RW; Amagai, M; Katz, SI. Heterogeneous MHC II restriction pattern of autoreactive desmoglein 3 specific T cell responses in pemphigus vulgarispatients and normals. *J Invest Dermatol*, 1998, 110(4), 388–92.
[94] Biedermann, T; Zimmermann, S; Himmelrich, H; et al. IL-4 instructs TH1 responses and resistance to Leishmania major in susceptible BALB/c mice. *Nat Immunol*, 2001, 2, 1054–60.
[95] Ghoreschi, K; Thomas, P; Breit, S; et al. Interleukin-4 therapy of psoriasis induces Th2 responses and improves human autoimmune disease. *Nat Med*, 2003, 9, 40–6.
[96] Luger, D; Silver, PB; Tang, J; et al. Either a Th17 or a Th1 effector response can drive autoimmunity: conditions of disease induction affect dominant effector category. *J Exp Med*, 2008, 205, 799–810.
[97] Nestle, FO; Kaplan, DH; Barker, J. Psoriasis. *N Engl J Med*, 2009, 361, 496–509.
[98] Akdis, CA; Joss, A; Akdis, M; Faith, A; Blaser, K. A molecular basis for T cell suppression by IL-10, CD28-associated IL-10 receptor inhibits CD28 tyrosine phosphorylation and phosphatidylinositol 3-kinase binding. *Faseb J*, 2000, 14, 1666–8.
[99] Groux, H; O'Garra, A; Bigler, M; et al. A CD4+ T-cell subset inhibits antigen-specific T-cell responses and prevents colitis. *Nature*, 1997, 389, 737–42.
[100] Bluestone, JA; Tang, Q. Therapeutic vaccination using CD4+CD25+ antigen-specific regulatory T cells. *Proc Natl Acad Sci U S A*, 2004, 101 Suppl 2, 14622-6.
[101] Walker, MR; Kasprowicz, DJ; Gersuk, VH; et al. Induction of FoxP3 and acquisition of T regulatory activity by stimulatedhuman CD4+CD25- T cells. *J Clin Invest*, 2003, 112, 1437–1443.
[102] Fontenot, JD; Gavin, MA; Rudensky, AY. Foxp3 programs the development and function of CD4+CD25+ regulatory T cells. *Nat Immunol*, 2003, 4, 330–6.
[103] Kriegel, MA; Lohmann, T; Gabler, C; Blank, N; Kalden, JR; Lorenz, HM. Defective suppressor function of human CD4+ CD25+ regulatory T cells in autoimmune polyglandular syndrome type II. *J Exp Med*, 2004, 199, 1285–91.
[104] Xing, Y; Hogquist, KA. T-cell tolerance: central and peripheral. *Cold Spring Harb Perspect Biol*, 2012, 4(6), 1–15.
[105] Guerder, S; Picarella, DE; Linsley, PS; Flavell, RA. Costimulator B7-1 confers antigen-presenting cell function to parenchymal tissue and in conjunction with tumor necrosis factor alpha leads to autoimmunity in transgenic mice. *Proc Natl Acad Sci U S A*, 1994, 91, 5138–42.
[106] Sakaguchi, S; Sakaguchi, N; Asano, M; Itoh, M; Toda, M. Immunologic self-tolerance maintained by activated T cells expressing IL-2 receptor alpha-chains (CD25). Breakdown of a single mechanism of self-tolerance causes various autoimmune diseases. *J Immunol*, 1995, 155, 1151–64.
[107] Sakaguchi, S; Takahashi, T; Nishizuka, Y. Study on cellular events in post-thymectomy autoimmune oophoritis in mice. II. Requirement of Lyt-1 cells in normal female mice for the prevention of oophoritis. *J Exp Med*, 1982, 156, 1577–86.

[108] Smith, H; Sakamoto, Y; Kasai, K; Tung, KS. Effector and regulatory cells in autoimmune oophoritis elicited by neonatal thymectomy. *J Immunol*, 1991, 147, 2928–33.

[109] Suri-Payer, E; Amar, AZ; Thornton, AM; Shevach, EM. CD4+CD25+ T cells inhibit both the induction and effector function of autoreactive T cells and represent a unique lineage of immunoregulatory cells. *J Immunol*, 1998, 160, 1212–8.

[110] Chatila, TA; Blaeser, F; Ho, N; Lederman, HM; Voulgaropoulos, C; Helms, C; Bowcock, AM. JM2, encoding a fork head-related protein, is mutated in X-linked autoimmunity-allergic disregulation syndrome. *J Clin Invest*, 2000, 106, R75–81.

[111] Brunkow, ME; Jeffery, EW; Hjerrild, KA; et al. Disruption of a new forkhead/winged-helix protein, scurfin, results in the fatal lymphoproliferative disorder of the scurfy mouse. *Nat Genet*, 2001, 27, 68–73.

[112] Fontenot, JD; Rasmussen, JP; Williams, LM; Dooley, JL; Farr, AG; Rudensky, AY. Regulatory T cell lineage specification by the forkhead transcription factor foxp3. *Immunity*, 2005, 22, 329–41.

[113] Hori, S; Nomura, T; Sakaguchi, S. Control of regulatory T cell development by the transcription factor Foxp3. *Science*, 2003, 299, 1057–61.

[114] Khattri, R; Cox, T; Yasayko, SA; Ramsdell, F. An essential role for Scurfin in CD4+CD25+ T regulatory cells. *Nat Immunol*, 2003, 4, 337–42.

[115] Wan, YY; Flavell, RA. Identifying Foxp3-expressing suppressor T cells with a bicistronic reporter. *Proc Natl Acad Sci U S A*, 2005, 102, 5126–31.

[116] Wing, JB; Sakaguchi, S. Multiple treg suppressive modules and their adaptability. *Front Immunol*, 2012, 3, 178.

[117] Shevach, EM. Mechanisms of foxp3+ T regulatory cell-mediated suppression. *Immunity*, 2009, 30, 636–45.

[118] Yamaguchi, T; Wing, JB; Sakaguchi, S. Two modes of immune suppression by Foxp3(+) regulatory T cells under inflammatory or non-inflammatory conditions. *Semin Immunol*, 2011, 23, 424–30.

[119] Takahashi, T; Tagami, T; Yamazaki, S; et al. Immunologic self-tolerance maintained by CD25(+)CD4(+) regulatory T cells constitutively expressing cytotoxic T lymphocyte-associated antigen 4. *J Exp Med*, 2000, 192, 303–10.

[120] Tang, Q; Henriksen, KJ; Bi, M; et al. *In vitro*-expanded antigen-specific regulatory T cells suppress autoimmune diabetes. *J Exp Med*, 2004, 199, 1455–65.

[121] Tarbell, KV; Yamazaki, S; Olson, K; Toy, P; Steinman, RM. CD25+ CD4+ T cells, expanded with dendritic cells presenting a single autoantigenic peptide, suppresses autoimmune diabetes. *J Exp Med*, 2004, 199, 1467–77.

[122] Chen, Z; Herman, AE; Matos, M; Mathis, D; Benoist, C. Where CD4+CD25+ T reg cells impinge on autoimmune diabetes. *J Exp Med*, 2005, 202, 1387–97.

[123] Atarashi, K; Tanoue, T; Shima, T; et al. Induction of colonic regulatory T cells by indigenous Clostridium species. *Science*, 2011, 331, 337–41.

[124] Di Ianni, M; Falzetti, F; Carotti, A; et al. Tregs prevent GVHD and promote immune reconstitution in HLA-haploidentical transplantation. *Blood*, 2011, 117, 3921–8.

[125] Lathrop, SK; Bloom, SM; Rao, SM; et al. Peripheral education of the immune system by colonic commensal microbiota. *Nature*, 2011, 478, 250–4.

[126] Sagoo, P; Lombardi, G; Lechler, RI. Relevance of regulatory T cell promotion of donor-specific tolerance in solid organ transplantation. *Front Immunol*, 2012, 3, 184.

[127] Geiger, TL; Tauro, S. Nature and nurture in Foxp3(+) regulatory T cell development, stability, and function. *Hum Immunol*, 2012, 73, 232–9.

[128] Apostolou, I; von Boehmer, H. *In vivo* instruction of suppressor commitment in naive T cells. *J Exp Med*, 2004, 199, 1401–8.

[129] Kretschmer, K; Apostolou, I; Hawiger, D; Khazaie, K; Nussenzweig, MC; von Boehmer, H. Inducing and expanding regulatory T cell populations by foreign antigen. *Nat Immunol*, 2005, 6, 1219–27.

[130] Haribhai, D; Williams, JB; Jia, S; et al. A requisite role for induced regulatory T cells in tolerance based on expanding antigen receptor diversity. *Immunity*, 2011, 35, 109–22.

[131] Daniel, BS; Murrell, DF. The actual management of pemphigus. *G Ital Dermatol Venerol*, 2010, 145, 689–702.

[132] Chen, W; Jin, W; Hardegen, N; Lei, KJ; Li, L; Marinos, N; McGrady, G; Wahl, SM. Conversion of peripheral CD4+CD25- naive T cells to CD4+CD25+ regulatory T cells by TGF-beta induction of transcription factor Foxp3. *J Exp Med*, 2003, 198, 1875–86.

[133] Peng, Y; Laouar, Y; Li, MO; Green, EA; Flavell, RA. TGF-beta regulates *in vivo* expansion of Foxp3-expressing CD4+CD25+ regulatory T cells responsible for protection against diabetes. *Proc Natl Acad Sci U S A*, 2004, 101, 4572–7.

[134] Banchereau, J; Steinman, RM. Dendritic cells and the control of immunity. *Nature*, 1998, 392, 245–52.

[135] Schuler, G; Steinman, RM. Dendritic cells as adjuvants for immune-mediated resistance to tumors. *J Exp Med*, 1997, 186, 1183–7.

[136] Schuler, G; Thurner, B; Romani, N. Dendritic cells: from ignored cells to major playersin T-cell-mediated immunity. *Int Arch Allergy Immunol*, 1997, 112, 317–22.

[137] Chung, CY; Ysebaert, D; Berneman, ZN; Cools, N. Dendritic cells: cellular mediators for immunological tolerance. *Clin Dev Immunol*, 2013, 2013, 972865.

[138] Kalinski, P; Hilkens, CM; Wierenga, EA; Kapsenberg, ML. T-cell priming by type-1 and type-2 polarized dendritic cells, the concept of a third signal. *Immunol Today*, 1999, 20, 561–567.

[139] Moser, M; Murphy, KM. Dendritic cell regulation of TH1-TH2 development. *Nat Immunol*, 2000, 1, 199–205.

[140] Korn, T; Bettelli, E; Oukka, M; Kuchroo, VK. IL-17 and Th17 Cells. *Annu Rev Immunol*, 2009, 27, 485–517.

[141] Abraham, C; Cho, JH. IL-23 and Autoimmunity: New Insights into the Pathogenesis of Inflammatory Bowel Disease. *Annu Rev Med*, 2009, 60, 97–110.

[142] Jonuleit, H; Schmitt, E; Schuler, G; Knop, J; Enk, AH. Induction of interleukin10-producing, nonproliferating CD4(+) T cells with regulatory properties by repetitive stimulationwith allogeneic immature human dendritic cells. *J Exp Med*, 2000, 192, 1213–22.

[143] Volz, T; Nega, M; Buschmann, J; et al. Natural Staphylococcus aureus-derived peptidoglycan fragments activate NOD2 and act as potent costimulators of the innate immune system exclusively in the presence of TLR signals. *FASEB J*, 2010, 24(10), 4089-102.

[144] Koch, KN; Hartung, ML; Urban, S; et al. Helicobacter urease-induced activation of the TLR2/NLRP3/IL-18 axis protects against asthma. *J Clin Invest*, 2015, 125(8), 3297-302.

[145] Iwasaki, A; Medzhitov, R. Regulation of Adaptive Immunity by the Innate Immune System. *Science*, 2010, 5963, 291–5.
[146] Schroder, K; Tschopp, J. The inflammasomes. *Cell*, 2009, 140, 821–32.
[147] Nagata, S; Hanayama, R; Kawane, K. Autoimmunity and the clearance of dead cells. *Cell*, 2010, 140, 619–30.
[148] Mocikat, R; Braumuller, H; Gumy, A; et al. Natural killer cells activatedby MHC class I(low) targets prime dendritic cells to induce protective CD8 T cell responses. *Immunity*, 2003, 19, 561–9.
[149] Rocken, M; Urban, JF; Shevach, EM. Infection breaks T-cell tolerance. *Nature*, 1992, 359, 79–82.
[150] Harrison, LC; Honeyman, MC; De Aizpurua, HJ; et al. Inverse relation between humoral and cellular immunity to glutamicacid decarboxylase in subjects at risk of insulin-dependent diabetes. *Lancet*, 1993, 341, 1365–9.
[151] Albert, ML; Sauter, B; Bhardwaj, N. Dendritic cells acquire antigen from apoptotic cells and induce class I-restricted CTLs. *Nature*, 1998, 392, 86–9.
[152] Matzinger, P; Anderson, CC. Immunity or tolerance: Opposite outcomes of microchimerism from skin grafts. *Nat Med*, 2001, 7, 80–7.
[153] Naucler, CS; Larsson, S; Moller, E. A novel mechanism for virus-induced autoimmunity in humans. *Immunol Rev*, 1996, 152, 175–92.
[154] Matzinger, P. Tolerance, danger, and the extended family. *Annu Rev Immunol*, 1994, 12, 991–1045.
[155] Sinha, AA; Lopez, MT; McDevitt, HO. Autoimmune diseases: the failure of self tolerance. *Science*, 1990, 248, 1380–8.
[156] Goodnow, CC; Brink, R; Adams, E. Breakdown of self-tolerance in anergic B lymphocytes. *Nature*, 1991, 352, 532–6.
[157] Louis, JA; Chiller, JM; Weigle, WO. The ability of bacterial lipopolysaccharide tomodulate the induction of unresponsiveness to a state of immunity. Cellular parameters. *J Exp Med*, 1973, 138, 1481–95.
[158] Limmer, A; Sacher, T; Alferink, J; et al. Failure to induce organ-specific autoimmunity by breaking of tolerance: importance of the microenvironment. *Eur J Immunol*, 1998, 28, 2395–406.
[159] Gautam, AM; Lock, CB; Smilek, DE; Pearson, CI; Steinman, L; McDevitt, HO. Minimum structural requirements for peptide presentation by major histocompatibility complexclass II molecules: implications in induction of autoimmunity. *Proc. Natl. Acad. Sci. U.S.A*, 1994, 91, 767–71.
[160] Wucherpfennig, KW; Strominger, JL. Molecular mimicry in T cell-mediated autoimmunity: viral peptides activate human T cell clones specific for myelin basic protein. *Cell*, 1995, 80, 695–705.
[161] Prinz, JC. Which T cells cause psoriasis? *Clin Exp Dermatol*, 1999, 24, 291–5.
[162] Chuang, TY; Stitle, L; Brashear, R; Lewis, C. Hepatitis C virus and lichen planus: Acase-control study of 340 patients. *J Am Acad Dermatol*, 1999, 41, 787–9.
[163] Lefort, A; Dachary, D; Vergier, B; Boiron, G. Lichen planus and vaccination against hepatitis B. *Ann Dermatol Venereol*, 1995, 122(10), 701-3.
[164] Tessari, G; Barba, A; Schena, D. Lichen ruber planus following the administration ofhuman anti-hepatitis B virus immunoglobulins [letter]. *Acta Derm. Venereol*, 1996, 76, 154.

[165] Berg, PA; Klein, R; Rocken, M. Cytokines in primary biliary cirrhosis. *Semin Liver Dis*, 1997, 17, 115–23.

[166] Gerlach, JT; Diepolder, HM; Jung, MC; et al. Recurrence of hepatitis C virus after loss of virus-specific CD4(+) T-cell response in acute hepatitis C. *Gastroenterology*, 1999, 117, 933–41.

[167] Moradpour, D; Blum, HE. Current and evolving therapies for hepatitis C. *Eur. J Gastroenterol Hepatol*, 1999, 11, 1199–202.

[168] Rocken, M; Urban, J; Shevach, EM. Antigen-specific activation, tolerization, and reactivation of the interleukin 4 pathway *in vivo*. *J Exp Med*, 1994, 179, 1885–93.

[169] Nemazee, D; Buerki, K. Clonal deletion of autoreactive B lymphocytes in bone marrow chimeras. *Proc Natl Acad Sci USA*, 1989, 86, 8039–43.

[170] Menard, L; Saadoun, D; Isnardi, I; et al. The PTPN22 allele encoding an R620W variant interferes with the removal of developing autoreactive B cells in humans. *J Clin Invest*, 2011, 121, 3635–44.

[171] Smilek, DE; Ehlers, MR; Nepom, GT. Restoring the balance: immunotherapeutic combinations for autoimmune disease. *Dis Model Mech*, 2014, 7(5), 503-13.

[172] Hartley, SB; Crosbie, J; Brink, R; Kantor, AB; Basten, A; Goodnow, CC. Elimination fromperipheral lymphoid tissues of self reactive B lymphocytes recognizing membrane bound antigens. *Nature*, 1991, 353, 765–9.

[173] Quách, TD; Manjarrez-Orduño, N; Adlowitz, DG; et al. Anergic responses characterize a large fraction of human autoreactive naive B cells expressing low levels of surface IgM. *J Immunol*, 2011, 186, 4640–8.

[174] Gauld, SB; Benschop, RJ; Merrell, KT; Cambier, JC. Maintenance of B cell anergy requires constant antigen receptor occupancy and signaling. *Nat Immunol*, 2005, 6, 1160–7.

[175] Cambier, JC. Autoimmunity risk alleles: hotspots in B cell regulatory signaling pathways. *J Clin Invest*, 2013, 123, 1928–31.

[176] Oropallo, MA; Kiefer, K; Marshak-Rothstein, A; Cancro, MP. Beyond transitional selection: New roles for BLyS in peripheral tolerance. *Drug Dev Res*, 2011, 72, 779–87.

[177] Treml, LS; Carlesso, G; Hoek, KL; et al. TLR stimulation modifies BLyS receptor expression in follicular and marginal zone B cells. *J Immunol*, 2007, 178, 7531–9.

[178] Rawlings, DJ; Schwartz, MA; Jackson, SW; Meyer-Bahlburg, A. Integration of B cell responses through Toll-like receptors and antigen receptors. *Nat Rev Immunol*, 2012, 12, 282–94.

[179] Amagai, M. The molecular logic of pemphigus and impetigo: the desmoglein story. *Vet Dermatol*, 2009, 20(5–6), 308–12.

[180] Rock, B; Martins, CR; Theofilopoulos, AN; et al. The pathogenic effect of IgG4 autoantibodies in endemicpemphigus foliaceus (fogo selvagem). *N Engl J Med*, 1989, 320, 1463–9.

[181] Hertl, M; Eming, R; Veldman, C. T cell control inautoimmune bullous skin disorders. *J Clin Invest*, 2006, 116(5), 1159–66.

[182] Liu, Z; Shapiro, SD; Zhou, X; et al. A critical role for neutrophil elastase in experimental bullous pemphigoid. *J Clin Invest*, 2000, 105, 113–23.

[183] Liu, Z; Shipley, JM; Vu, TH; et al. GelatinaseB-deficient mice are resistant to experimental bullous pemphigoid. *J Exp Med*, 1998, 188, 475–82.

[184] Liu, Z; Giudice, GJ; Swartz, SJ; et al. The role of complement in experimental bullous pemphigoid. *J Clin Invest*, 1995, 95, 1539–44.

[185] Stenger, S; Modlin, RL. T cell mediated immunity to Mycobacterium tuberculosis. *Curr Opin Microbiol*, 1999, 2, 89–93.

[186] Zinkernagel, RM. Immunology taught by viruses. *Science*, 1996, 271, 173–8.

[187] Krueger, GG; Langley, RG; Leonardi, C; et al. A human interleukin-12/23 monoclonalantibody for the treatment of psoriasis. *N Engl J Med*, 2007, 356, 580–92.

[188] Biedermann, T; Kneilling, M; Mailhammer, R; et al. Mast Cells Control Neutrophil Recruitment during TCell-mediated Delayed-type Hypersensitivity Reactions through Tumor Necrosis Factor and Macrophage Inflammatory Protein 2. *J Exp Med*, 2000, 192, 1441–52.

[189] Kneilling, M; Mailhammer, R; Hultner, L; et al. Direct cross talk between mast cell-TNF and TNFR1-expressing endothelia mediates local tissue inflammation. *Blood*, 2009, 114, 1696–706.

[190] Chen, R; Diaz L; Giudice G; Liu Z. The role of C5a in mast cell activation during sub epidermal blistering in experimetnal bullous pemphigoid. *J Invest Dermatol*, 2000, 114, 762.

[191] Green, EA; Flavell, RA. The temporal importance of TNFalpha expression in the development of diabetes. *Immunity*, 2000, 12, 459–69.

[192] Bendelac, A; Carnaud, C; Boitard, C; Bach, JF. Syngeneic transfer of autoimmunediabetes from diabetic NOD mice to healthy neonates. Requirement for both L3T4+ and Lyt-2+T cells. *J Exp Med*, 1987, 166, 823–32.

[193] Martin, R; McFarland, HF; McFarlin, DE. Immunological aspects of demyelinatingdiseases. *Annu Rev Immunol*, 1992, 10, 153–87.

[194] Salou, M; Nicol, B; Garcia, A; Laplaud, DA. Involvement of CD8(+) T Cells in Multiple Sclerosis. *Front Immunol*, 2015, 6, 604.

[195] Austin, LM; Ozawa, M; Kikuchi, T; Walters, IB; Krueger, JG. The majority of epidermalT cells in Psoriasis vulgaris lesions can produce type 1 cytokines, interferon-γ, interleukin-2, and tumor necrosis factor-alpha, defining TC1 (cytotoxic T lymphocyte) and TH1effector populations: a type 1 differentiation bias is also measured in circulating blood T cells in psoriatic patients. *J Invest Dermatol*, 1999, 113, 752–9.

[196] Vollmer, S; Menssen, A; Trommler, P; Schendel, D; Prinz, JC. T lymphocytes derived from skin lesions of patients with psoriasis vulgaris express a novel cytokine pattern that is distinct from that of T helper type 1 and T helper type 2 cells. *Eur J Immunol*, 1994, 24, 2377–82.

[197] Feldmann, M; Brennan, FM; Maini, RN. Role of cytokines in rheumatoid arthritis. *Annu Rev Immunol*, 1996, 14, 397–440.

[198] Mease, PJ; Goffe, BS; Metz, J; VanderStoep, A; Finck, B; Burge, DJ. Etanercept inthe treatment of psoriatic arthritis and psoriasis: a randomised trial. *Lancet*, 2000, 356, 385–90.

[199] Tirado-Sánchez, A; Ponce-Olivera, RM; Vazquez-González, D; Bonifaz, A. Th-17 and the lack of efficacy of ustekinumab in pemphigus vulgaris. *Dermatol Online J*, 2013 15, 19(3), 15.

[200] Abrams, JR; Kelley, SL; Hayes, E; et al. Blockade of T lymphocyte costimulation with cytotoxic T lymphocyte-associated antigen 4-immunoglobulin (CTLA4Ig) reverses the

cellular pathology of psoriatic plaques, including the activation of keratinocytes, dendritic cells, and endothelial cells. *J Exp Med*, 2000, 192, 681–94.

[201] Krueger, GG; Ellis, CN. Alefacept therapy produces remission for patients with chronicplaque psoriasis. *Br J Dermatol*, 2003, 148, 784–8.

[202] Biedermann, T; Mailhammer, R; Mai, A; et al. Reversal of established delayed type hypersensitivity reactionsfollowing therapy with IL-4 or antigen-specific Th2 cells. *Eur J Immunol*, 2001, 31, 1582–91.

[203] Amagai, M. Adhesion molecules. I: keratinocytekeratinocyteinteractions; cadherins and pemphigus. *J Invest Dermatol*, 1995, 104(1), 146–52.

[204] Gniadecki, R. Desmoglein autoimmunity in the pathogenesis of pemphigus. *Autoimmunity*, 2006, 39(7), 541-7.

[205] Patel, SD; Chen, CP; Bahna, F; Honig, B; Shapiro, L. Cadherin-mediated cell-cell adhesion, sticking togetheras a family. *Curr Opin Struct Biol*, 2003, 13(6), 690–8.

[206] Blaschuk, OW; Sullivan, R; David, S; Pouliot, Y. Identification of a cadherin cell adhesion recognitionsequence. *Dev Biol*, 1990, 139(1), 227–9.

[207] Runswick, SK; O'Hare, MJ; Jones, L; Streuli, CH; Garrod, DR. Desmosomal adhesion regulates epithelialmorphogenesis and cell positioning. *Nat Cell Biol*, 2001, 3(9), 823–30.

[208] Tselepis, C; Chidgey, M; North, A; Garrod, D. Desmosomal adhesion inhibits invasive behavior. *Proc Natl Acad Sci U S A*, 1998, 95(14), 8064–9.

[209] Garrod, D; Chidgey, M; North, A. Desmosomes: differentiation, development, dynamics and disease. *Curr Opin Cell Biol*, 1996, 8(5), 670–8.

[210] Hirano, S; Nose, A; Hatta, K; Kawakami, A; Takeichi, M. Calcium-dependent cell-cell adhesion molecules (cadherins), subclass specificities and possible involvement of actin bundles. *J Cell Biol*, 1987, 105(6 Pt 1), 2501–10.

[211] Yap, AS; Brieher, WM; Gumbiner, BM. Molecular andfunctional analysis of cadherin-based adherens junctions. *Annu Rev Cell Dev Biol*, 1997, 13, 119–46.

[212] Green, KJ; Gaudry, CA. Are desmosomes more thantethers for intermediate filaments? *Nat Rev Mol Cell Biol*, 2000, 1(3), 208–16.

[213] Bornslaeger, EA; Corcoran, CM; Stappenbeck, TS; Green, KJ. Breaking the connection: displacement ofthe desmosomal plaque protein desmoplakin fromcell-cell interfaces disrupts anchorage of intermediatefilament bundles and alters intercellular junctionassembly. *J Cell Biol*, 1996, 134(4), 985–1001.

[214] Hirai, Y; Nose, A; Kobayashi, S; Takeichi, M. Expression and role of E- and P-cadherin adhesion molecules inembryonic histogenesis. II. Skin morphogenesis. *Development*, 1989, 105(2), 271–7.

[215] Delva, E; Tucker, DK; Kowalczyk, AP. The desmosome. *Cold Spring Harb Perspect Biol*, 2009, 1(2), a002543.

[216] Franke, WW. Discovering the molecular componentsof intercellular junctions—a historical view. *Cold Spring Harb Perspect Biol*, 2009, 1(3), a003061.

[217] Skerrow, CJ; Matoltsy, AG. Isolation of epidermal desmosomes. *J Cell Biol*, 1974, 63(2 Pt 1), 515–23.

[218] Koch, PJ; Walsh, MJ; Schmelz, M; Goldschmidt, MD; Zimbelmann, R; Franke, WW. Identification of desmoglein, a constitutive desmosomal glycoprotein, as amember of the cadherin family of cell adhesionmolecules. *Eur J Cell Biol*, 1990, 53(1), 1–12.

[219] Dusek, RL; Godsel, LM; Green, KJ. Discriminating roles of desmosomal cadherins: beyond desmosomal adhesion. *J Dermatol Sci*, 2007, 45(1), 7–21.

[220] Cowley, CM; Simrak, D; Marsden, MD; King, IA; Arnemann, J; Buxton, RS. A YAC contig joiningthe desmocollin and desmoglein loci on human. Chromo some 18 and ordering of the desmocollingenes. *Genomics*, 1997, 42(2), 208–16.

[221] Al-Amoudi, A; Diez, DC; Betts, MJ; Frangakis, AS. Themolecular architecture of cadherins in native epidermaldesmosomes. *Nature*, 2007, 450(7171), 832–7.

[222] Boggon, TJ; Murray, J; Chappuis-Flament, S; Wong, E; Gumbiner, BM; Shapiro, L. C-cadherin ectodomain structure and implications for cell adhesion mechanisms. *Science*, 2002, 296(5571), 1308–13.

[223] Amagai, M; Karpati, S; Klaus-Kovtun, V; Udey, MC; Stanley, JR. Extracellular domain of pemphigus vulgarisantigen (desmoglein 3) mediates weak hemophilic adhesion. *J Invest Dermatol*, 1994, 102(4), 402–8.

[224] Syed, SE; Trinnaman, B; Martin, S; Major, S; Hutchinson, J; Magee, AI. Molecular interactionsbetween desmosomal cadherins. *Biochem J*, 2002, 362(Pt 2), 317–27.

[225] Waschke, J; Bruggeman, P; Baumgartner, W; Zillikens, D; Drenckhahn, D. Pemphigus foliaceus IgG causes dissociationof desmoglein 1-containing junctions without blocking desmoglein 1 transinteraction. *J Clin Invest*, 2005, 115(11), 3157–65.

[226] Nie, Z; Merritt, A; Rouhi-Parkouhi, M; Tabernero, L; Garrod, D. Membrane-impermeable cross-linkingprovides evidence for hemophilic, isoform-specific binding of desmosomal cadherins in epithelial cells. *J Biol Chem*, 2011, 286(3), 2143–54.

[227] Spindler, V; Heupel, WM; Efthymiadis, A; et al. Desmocollin 3-mediated binding is crucial for keratinocyte cohesion and is impaired in pemphigus. *J Biol Chem*, 2009, 284(44), 30556–64.

[228] Chitaev, NA; Troyanovsky, SM. Direct Ca2+-dependent heterophilic interaction between desmosomalcadherins, desmoglein and desmocollin, contributes to cell-cell adhesion. *J Cell Biol*, 1997, 138(1), 193–201.

[229] Pokutta, S; Weis, WI. Structure and mechanism of cadherins and catenins in cellecell contacts. *Annu Rev Cell Dev Biol*, 2007, 23, 237e61.

[230] Aberle, H; Bierkamp, C; Torchard, D; et al. The humanplakoglobin gene localizes on chromosome 17q21 and is subjected to loss of heterozygosity in breast and ovarian cancers. *Proc Natl Acad Sci U S A*, 1995, 92(14), 6384–8.

[231] Palka, HL; Green, KJ. Roles of plakoglobin end domains in desmosome assembly. *J Cell Sci*, 1997, 110(Pt 19), 2359–71.

[232] Peifer, M; McCrea, PD; Green, KJ; Wieschaus, E; Gumbiner, BM. The vertebrate adhesive junction proteins beta-catenin and plakoglobin and the Drosophilasegment polarity gene armadillo form a multi gene family with similar properties. *J Cell Biol*, 1992, 118(3), 681–91.

[233] Choi, HJ; Gross, JC; Pokutta, S; Weis, WI. Interactions of plakoglobin and beta-catenin with desmosomal cadherins: basis of selective exclusion of alpha- andbeta-catenin from desmosomes. *J Biol Chem*, 2009, 284(46), 31776–88.

[234] Kowalczyk, AP; Bornslaeger, EA; Borgwardt, JE; et al. The amino-terminal domain of desmoplakin binds to plakoglobin and clusters desmosomal cadherin plakoglobin complexes. *J Cell Biol*, 1997, 139(3), 773–84.

[235] Troyanovsky, SM; Troyanovsky, RB; Eshkind, LG; Krutovskikh, VA; Leube, RE; Franke, WW. Identification of the plakoglobin-binding domain indesmoglein and its

role in plaque assembly and intermediatefilament anchorage. *J Cell Biol*, 1994, 127(1), 151–60.

[236] Troyanovsky, SM; Troyanovsky, RB; Eshkind, LG; Leube, RE, Franke, WW. Identification of amino acid sequence motifs in desmocollin, a desmosomal glycoprotein, that are required for plakoglobin binding and plaque formation. *Proc Natl Acad Sci U S A*, 1994, 91(23), 10790–4.

[237] Bonne, S; van Hengel, J; van Roy, F. Chromosomal mapping of human armadillo genes belonging to thep120(ctn)/plakophilin subfamily. *Genomics*, 1998, 51(3), 452–4.

[238] Schmidt, A; Langbein, L; Pratzel, S; Rode, M; Rackwitz, HR; Franke, WW. Plakophilin 3—a novel cell-type specific desmosomal plaque protein. *Differentiation*, 1999, 64(5), 291–306.

[239] Mertens, C; Kuhn, C; Franke, WW. Plakophilins 2a and 2b: constitutive proteins of dual location in the karyoplasms and the desmosomal plaque. *J Cell Biol*, 1996, 135(4), 1009–25.

[240] Hatzfeld, M; Nachtsheim, C. Cloning andcharacterization of a new armadillo family member, p0071, associated with the junctional plaque: evidence for a subfamily of closely related proteins. *J Cell Sci*, 1996, 109(Pt 11), 2767–78.

[241] Jefferson, JJ; Ciatto, C; Shapiro, L; Liem, RK. Structuralanalysis of the plakin domain of bullous pemphigoidantigen1 (BPAG1) suggests that plakins are members of the spectrin superfamily. *J Mol Biol*, 2007, 366(1), 244–57.

[242] Armstrong, DK; McKenna, KE; Purkis, PE; et al. Haploinsufficiency of desmoplakin causes a striate subtype of palmoplantar keratoderma. *Hum Mol Genet*, 1999, 8(1), 143–8.

[243] Hatsell, S; Cowin, P. Deconstructing desmoplakin. *Nat Cell Biol*, 2001, 3(12), E270–2.

[244] Green, KJ; Parry, DA; Steinert, PM; et al. Structure ofthe human desmoplakins. Implications for function in the desmosomal plaque. *J Biol Chem*, 1990, 265(5), 2603–12.

[245] Andra, K; Lassmann, H; Bittner, R; et al. Targetedinactivation of plectin reveals essential function in maintaining the integrity of skin, muscle, and heart cytoarchitecture. *Genes Dev*, 1997, 11(23), 3143–56.

[246] Pulkkinen, L; Smith, FJ; Shimizu, H; et al. Homozygous deletion mutations in the plectin gene (PLEC1) inpatients with epidermolysis bullosa simplex associated with late-onset muscular dystrophy. *Hum Mol Genet*, 1996, 5(10), 1539–46.

[247] Vasioukhin, V; Bowers, E; Bauer, C; Degenstein, L; Fuchs, E. Desmoplakin is essential in epidermal sheet formation. *Nat Cell Biol*, 2001, 3(12), 1076–85.

[248] Hu, P; O'Keefe, EJ; Rubenstein, DS. Tyrosine phosphorylation of human keratinocyte b-catenin and plakoglobin reversibly regulates their binding to E-cadherin and a-catenin. *J Invest Dermatol*, 2001, 117, 1059e67.

[249] Yin, T; Getsios, S; Caldelari, R; Godsel, LM; Kowalczyk, AP; Muller, EJ; et al. Mechanisms of plakoglobin-dependent adhesion: desmosome-specific functions in assembly and regulation by epidermal growth factor receptor. *J Biol Chem*, 2005, 280, 40355e63.

[250] Joly, P; Litrowski, N. Pemphigus group (vulgaris, vegetans, foliaceus, herpetiformis, brasiliensis). *Clin Dermatol*, 2011, 29(4), 432–6.

[251] Diaz, LA; Giudice, GJ. End of the century overview ofskin blisters. *Arch Dermatol*, 2000, 136(1), 106–12.

[252] Ding, X; Aoki, V; Mascaro, Jr. JM; Lopez-Swiderski, A; Diaz, LA; Fairley, JA. Mucosal and mucocutaneous (generalized) pemphigus vulgaris show distinct autoantibody profiles. *J Invest Dermatol*, 1997, 109(4), 592–6.

[253] Amagai, M; Karpati, S; Prussick, R; Klaus-Kovtun, V; Stanley, JR. Autoantibodies against the aminoterminal cadherin-like binding domain of pemphigus vulgaris antigen are pathogenic. *J Clin Invest*, 1992, 90(3), 919–26.

[254] Ding, X; Diaz, LA; Fairley, JA; Giudice, GJ; Liu, Z. The anti-desmoglein 1 autoantibodies in pemphigus vulgaris sera are pathogenic. *J Invest Dermatol*, 1999, 112(5), 739–43.

[255] Amagai, M; Hashimoto, T; Shimizu, N; Nishikawa, T. Absorption of pathogenic autoantibodies by the extracellular domain of pemphigus vulgaris antigen (Dsg3) producedby baculovirus. *J Clin Invest*, 1994, 94(1), 59–67.

[256] Amagai, M; Klaus-Kovtun, V; Stanley, JR. Autoantibodies against a novel epithelial cadherin in pemphigus vulgaris, a disease of cell adhesion. *Cell*, 1991, 67(5), 869–77.

[257] Tsunoda, K; Ota, T; Saito, M; Hata, T; Shimizu, A; Ishiko, A; et al. Pathogenic relevance of IgG and IgM antibodies against desmoglein 3 in blister formation in pemphigus vulgaris. *Am J Pathol*, 2011, 179(2), 795–806.

[258] Amagai, M; Komai, A; Hashimoto, T; Shirakata, Y; Hashimoto, K; Yamada, T; et al. Usefulness of enzyme-linked immunosorbent assay using recombinant desmogleins 1 and 3 for serodiagnosis of pemphigus. *Br J Dermatol*, 1999, 140(2), 351–7.

[259] Mahoney, MG; Wang, ZH; Stanley, JR. Pemphigusvulgaris and pemphigus foliaceus antibodies arepathogenic in plasminogen activator knockout mice. *JInvest Dermatol*, 1999, 113(1), 22–5.

[260] Ota, T; Aoki-Ota, M; Tsunoda, K; Simoda, K; Nishikawa, T; Amagai, M; et al. Auto-reactive B cells againstperipheral antigen, desmoglein 3, escape from tolerancemechanism. *Int Immunol*, 2004, 16(10), 1487–95.

[261] Mouquet, H; Musette, P; Gougeon, ML; Jacquot, S; Lemercier, B; Lim, A; et al. B-cell depletion immunotherapy in pemphigus: effects on cellular and humoral immune responses. *J Invest Dermatol*, 2008, 128(12), 2859–69.

[262] Eming, R; Nagel, A; Wolff-Franke, S; Podstawa, E; Debus, D; Hertl, M. Rituximab exerts a dual effect in pemphigus vulgaris. *J Invest Dermatol*, 2008, 128(12), 2850–8.

[263] Colliou, N; Picard, D; Caillot, F; Calbo, S; Le Corre, S; Lim, A; et al. Long-term remissions of severe pemphigus after rituximab therapy are associated with prolonged failure of desmoglein B cell response. *Sci Transl Med*, 2013, 5(175), 175ra30.

[264] Wucherpfennig, KW; Yu, B; Bhol, K; Monos, DS; Argyris, E; Karr, RW; et al. Structural basis for major histocompatibility complex (MHC)-linked susceptibility to autoimmunity: charged residues of a single MHC binding pocket confer selective presentationof self-peptides in pemphigus vulgaris. *Proc Natl Acad Sci U S A*, 1995, 92(25), 11935–9.

[265] Lin, MS; Swartz, SJ; Lopez, A; Ding, X; Fernandez-Vina, MA; Stastny, P; et al. Development and characterization of desmoglein-3 specific T cells from patients with pemphigus vulgaris. *J Clin Invest*, 1997, 99(1), 31–40.

[266] Veldman, C; Stauber, A; Wassmuth, R; Uter, W; Schuler, G; Hertl, M. Dichotomy of autoreactive Th1 and Th2 cell responses to desmoglein 3 in patients with pemphigus vulgaris (PV) and healthy carriers of PV-associated HLA class II alleles. *J Immunol*, 2003, 170(1), 635–42.

[267] Riechers, R; Grotzinger, J; Hertl, M. HLA class II restriction of autoreactive T cell responses in pemphigus vulgaris: review of the literature and potential applications for the development of a specific immunotherapy. *Autoimmunity*, 1999, 30(3), 183–96.

[268] Veldman, CM; Gebhard, KL; Uter, W; et al. T cell recognition of desmoglein 3 peptides in patients with pemphigus vulgaris and healthy individuals. *J Immunol*, 2004, 172(6), 3883–92.

[269] Tony, HP; Burmester, G; Schulze-Koops, H; Grunke, M; Henes, J; Kotter, I; et al. Safety and clinical outcomesof rituximab therapy in patients with different autoimmune diseases: experience from a national registry(GRAID). *Arthritis Res Ther*, 2011, 13(3), R75.

[270] Ahmed, AR; Spigelman, Z; Cavacini, LA; Posner, MR. Treatment of pemphigus vulgaris with rituximab and intravenous immune globulin. *N Engl J Med*, 2006, 355(17), 1772–9.

[271] Joly, P; et al. A single cycle of rituximab for the treatment of severe pemphigus. *N Engl J Med*, 2007, 357(6), 545–52.

[272] Schmidt, E; Goebeler, M; Zillikens, D. Rituximab in severe pemphigus. *Ann N Y Acad Sci*, 2009, 1173, 683–91.

[273] Nagel, A; Hertl, M; Eming, R. B-cell-directed therapy for inflammatory skin diseases. *J Invest Dermatol*, 2009, 129(2), 289–301.

[274] Nagel, A; Podstawa, E; Eickmann, M; Muller, HH; Hertl, M; Eming, R. Rituximab mediates a strong elevation of B-cell-activating factor associated with increased pathogen-specific IgG but not autoantibodies in pemphigus vulgaris. *J Invest Dermatol*, 2009, 129(9), 2202–10.

[275] Hoss, DM; Shea, CR; Grant-Kels, JM. Neutrophilic spongiosis in pemphigus. *Arch Dermatol*, 1996, 132(3), 315–8.

[276] Sekiguchi, M; Futei, Y; Fujii, Y; Iwasaki, T; Nishikawa, T; Amagai, M. Dominant autoimmune epitopes recognized by pemphigus antibodies map to the N-terminal adhesive region of desmogleins. *J Immunol*, 2001, 167(9), 5439–48.

[277] Stanley, JR; Amagai, M. Pemphigus, bullous impetigo, and the staphylococcal scalded-skin syndrome. *N Engl J Med*, 2006, 355(17), 1800–10.

[278] James, KA; Culton, DA; Diaz, LA. Diagnosis and clinical features of pemphigus foliaceus. *Dermatol Clin*, 2011, 29(3), 405–12; viii.

[279] Lin, MS; Fu, CL; Aoki, V; Hans-Filho, G; Rivitti, EA; Moraes, JR; et al. Desmoglein-1-specific T lymphocytes from patients with endemic pemphigus foliaceus (fogo selvagem). *J Clin Invest*, 2000, 105(2), 207–13.

[280] Gebhard, KL; Veldman, CM; Wassmuth, R; Schultz, E; Schuler, G; Hertl, M. Ex vivo analysis of desmoglein1-responsive T-helper (Th) 1 and Th2 cells in patients with pemphigus foliaceus and healthy individuals. *Exp Dermatol*, 2005, 14(8), 586–92.

[281] Warren, SJ; Lin, MS; Giudice, GJ; et al. The prevalence of antibodies against desmoglein 1 in endemic pemphigus foliaceus in Brazil. Cooperative Group on Fogo Selvagem Research. *N Engl J Med*, 2000, 343(1), 23–30.

[282] Qaqish, BF; Prisayanh, P; Qian, Y; et al. Development of an IgG4-based predictorof endemic pemphigus foliaceus (fogo selvagem). *J Invest Dermatol*, 2009, 129(1), 110–8.

[283] Hacker-Foegen, MK; Janson, M; Amagai, M; Fairley, JA; Lin, MS. Pathogenicity and epitope characteristicsof anti-desmoglein-1 from pemphigus foliaceus patients expressing only IgG1 autoantibodies. *J Invest Dermatol*, 2003, 121(6), 1373–8.

[284] Qian, Y; Jeong, JS; Maldonado, M; et al. Cutting edge: Brazilianpemphigus foliaceus anti-desmoglein 1 autoantibodiescross-react with sand fly salivary LJM11 antigen. *J Immunol*, 2012, 189(4), 1535–9.

[285] Culton, DA; Qian, Y; Li, N; et al. Advances in pemphigus and its endemic pemphigus foliaceus (Fogo Selvagem) phenotype: a paradigm of human autoimmunity. *J Autoimmun*, 2008, 31(4), 311–24.

[286] Mimouni, D; Anhalt, GJ; Lazarova, Z; et al. Paraneoplastic pemphigusin children and adolescents. *Br J Dermatol*, 2002, 147(4), 725–32.

[287] Anhalt, GJ. Paraneoplastic pemphigus. *J Investig Dermatol Symp Proc*, 2004, 9(1), 29–33.

[288] Billet, S; Grando, S; Pittelkow, M. Paraneoplastic autoimmune multiorgan syndrome: review of the literature and support for a cytotoxic role in pathogenesis. *Autoimmunity*, 2006, 39(7), 617–30.

[289] Schepens, I; Jaunin, F; Begre, N; et al. The protease inhibitor alpha-2-macroglobulin-like-1 is the p170 antigen recognized by paraneoplastic pemphigus autoantibodiesin human. *PLoS One*, 2010, 5(8), e12250.

[290] Anhalt, GJ; Kim, SC; Stanley, JR; et al. Paraneoplasticpemphigus. An autoimmune mucocutaneous disease associated with neoplasia. *N Engl J Med*, 1990, 323(25), 1729–35.

[291] Amagai, M; Nishikawa, T; Nousari, HC; Anhalt, GJ; Hashimoto, T. Antibodies against desmoglein 3 (pemphigus vulgaris antigen) are present in sera from patients with paraneoplastic pemphigus and causeacantholysis *in vivo* in neonatal mice. *J Clin Invest*, 1998, 102(4), 775–82.

[292] Cozzani, E; Di Zenzo, G; Calabresi, V; et al. Antidesmoplakin antibodies in erythema multiforme and Stevens-Johnson syndrome sera: pathogenic or epiphenomenon? *Eur J Dermatol*, 2011, 21(1), 32–6.

[293] Fukiwake, N; Moroi, Y; Urabe, K; Ishii, N; Hashimoto, T; Furue, M. Detection of autoantibodies to desmoplakin in a patient with oral erythema multiforme. *Eur J Dermatol*, 2007, 17(3), 238–41.

[294] Hashimoto, T; Komai, A; Futei, Y; Nishikawa, T; Amagai, M. Detection of IgA autoantibodies to desmogleins by an enzyme-linked immunosorbent assay: the presence of new minor subtypes of IgA pemphigus. *Arch Dermatol*, 2001, 137(6), 735–8.

[295] Nishikawa, T; Hashimoto, T; Teraki, Y; Ebihara, T. Theclinical and histopathological spectrum of IgA pemphigus. *Clin Exp Dermatol*, 1991, 16(5), 401–2.

[296] Hashimoto, T. Immunopathology of IgA pemphigus. *Clin Dermatol*, 2001, 19(6), 683–9.

[297] Hashimoto, T; Kiyokawa, C; Mori, O; Miyasato, M; Chidgey, MA; Garrod, DR; et al. Human desmocollin1 (Dsc1) is an autoantigen for the subcorneal pustular dermatosis type of IgA pemphigus. *J Invest Dermatol*, 1997, 109(2), 127–31.

[298] Duker, I; Schaller, J; Rose, C; Zillikens, D; Hashimoto, T; Kunze, J. Subcorneal pustular dermatosis-type IgA pemphigus with autoantibodies to desmocollins 1, 2, and 3. *Arch Dermatol*, 2009, 145(10), 1159–62.

[299] Ebihara, T; Hashimoto, T; Iwatsuki, K; et al. Autoantigens for IgA antiintercellular antibodies of intercellular IgA vesiculopustulardermatosis. *J Invest Dermatol*, 1991, 97(4), 742–5.

[300] Karpati, S; Amagai, M; Liu, WL; Dmochowski, M; Hashimoto, T; Horvath, A. Identification of desmoglein1 as autoantigen in a patient with intraepidermalneutrophilic IgA dermatosis type of IgApemphigus. *Exp Dermatol*, 2000, 9(3), 224–8.

[301] Tajima, M; Mitsuhashi, Y; Irisawa, R; Amagai, M; Hashimoto, T; Tsuboi, R. IgA pemphigus reacting exclusivelyto desmoglein 3. *Eur J Dermatol*, 2010, 20(5), 626–9.

[302] Geller, S; Gat, A; Zeeli, T; et al. The expanding spectrum of IgA pemphigus: a case report and review of the literature. *Br J Dermatol*, 2014, 171(3), 650–6.

[303] Tsuruta, D; Ishii, N; Hamada, T; et al. IgA pemphigus. *Clin Dermatol*, 2011, 29(4), 437–42.

[304] Kubo, A; Amagai, M; Hashimoto, T; et al. Herpeti form pemphigus showing reactivity with pemphigus vulgaris antigen (desmoglein 3). *Br J Dermatol*, 1997, 137(1), 109–13.

[305] Kasperkiewicz, M; Kowalewski, C; Jablonska, S. Pemphigus herpetiformis: from first description until now. *J Am Acad Dermatol*, 2014, 70(4), 780–7.

[306] Ishii, K; Amagai, M; Komai, A; et al. Desmoglein 1 and desmoglein 3 are the target autoantigens in herpetiform pemphigus. *Arch Dermatol*, 1999, 135(8), 943–7.

[307] On, HR; Hashimoto, T; Kim, SC. Pemphigus herpetiformis with IgG autoantibodies to desmoglein 1 and desmocollin1. *Br J Dermatol*, 2015, 172(4), 1144-6.

[308] Rafei, D; Muller, R; Ishii, N; et al. IgG autoantibodies against desmocollin3 in pemphigus sera induces loss of keratinocyteadhesion. *Am J Pathol*, 2011, 178(2), 718–23.

[309] Nakamura, Y; Takahata, H; Teye, K; Ishii, N; Hashimoto, T; Muto, M. A case of pemphigus herpetiformis-like atypical pemphigus with IgG anti-desmocollin 3 antibodies. *Br J Dermatol*, 2014, 171(6), 1588-90.

[310] Ohyama, B; Nishifuji, K; Chan, PT; et al. Epitope spreading is rarelyfound in pemphigus vulgaris by large-scale longitudinalstudy using desmoglein 2-based swapped molecules. *J Invest Dermatol*, 2012, 132(4), 1158–68.

[311] Loiseau, P; Lecleach, L; Prost, C; et al. HLA class II polymorphism contributes to specify desmogleinderived peptides in pemphigus vulgaris and pemphigusfoliaceus. *J Autoimmun*, 2000, 15(1), 67–73.

[312] Li, N; Aoki, V; Hans-Filho, G; Rivitti, EA; Diaz, LA. Therole of intramolecular epitope spreading in the pathogenesisof endemic pemphigus foliaceus (fogo selvagem). *J Exp Med*, 2003, 197(11), 1501–10.

[313] Futei, Y; Amagai, M; Sekiguchi, M; Nishifuji, K; Fujii, Y; Nishikawa, T. Use of domain-swapped molecules forconformational epitope mapping of desmoglein 3 in pemphigus vulgaris. *J Invest Dermatol*, 2000, 115(5), 829–34.

[314] Shapiro, L; Fannon, AM; Kwong, PD; et al. Structural basis of cell-cell adhesion by cadherins. *Nature*, 1995, 374(6520), 327–37.

[315] Anhalt, GJ; Patel, HP; Labib, RS; Diaz, LA; Proud, D. Dexamethasone inhibits plasminogen activator activityin experimental pemphigus *in vivo* but does notblock acantholysis. *J Immunol*, 1986, 136(1), 113–7.

[316] Anhalt, GJ; Till, GO; Diaz, LA; Labib, RS; Patel, HP; Eaglstein, NF. Defining the role of complement inexperimental pemphigus vulgaris in mice. *J Immunol*, 1986, 137(9), 2835–40.

[317] Rock, B; Labib, RS; Diaz, LA. Monovalent Fab' immunoglobulin fragments from endemic pemphigus foliaceus autoantibodies reproduce the human disease inneonatal Balb/c mice. *J Clin Invest*, 1990, 85(1), 296–9.

[318] Tsunoda, K; Ota, T; Aoki, M; et al. Induction of pemphigus phenotypeby a mouse monoclonal antibody against the aminoterminaladhesive interface of desmoglein 3. *J Immunol*, 2003, 170(4), 2170–8.

[319] Heupel, WM; Zillikens, D; Drenckhahn, D; Waschke J. Pemphigus vulgaris IgG directly inhibit desmoglein3-mediated transinteraction. *J Immunol*, 2008, 181(3), 1825–34.

[320] Waschke, J; Menendez-Castro, C; Bruggeman, P; et al. Imaging and force spectroscopy on desmoglein 1using atomic force microscopy reveal multivalent Ca(2+)-dependent, low-affinity trans-interaction. *J Membr Biol*, 2007, 216(2–3), 83–92.

[321] Waschke, J. The desmosome and pemphigus. *Histochem Cell Biol*, 2008, 130(1), 21–54.

[322] Seishima, M; Esaki, C; Osada, K; Mori, S; Hashimoto, T; Kitajima, Y. Pemphigus IgG, but not bullous pemphigoid IgG, causes a transient increase in intracellularcalcium and inositol 1, 4, 5-triphosphate in DJM-1cells, a squamous cell carcinoma line. *J Invest Dermatol*, 1995, 104(1), 33–7.

[323] Aoyama, Y; Kitajima, Y. Pemphigus vulgaris-IgG causes a rapid depletion of desmoglein 3 (Dsg3) from the Triton X-100 soluble pools, leading to the formation of Dsg3-depleted desmosomes in a humansquamous carcinoma cell line, DJM-1 cells. *J Invest Dermatol*, 1999, 112(1), 67–71.

[324] Aoyama, Y; Owada, MK; Kitajima, Y. A pathogenic autoantibody, pemphigus vulgaris-IgG, induces phosphorylation of desmoglein 3, and its dissociation from plakoglobin in cultured keratinocytes. *Eur J Immunol*, 1999, 29(7), 2233–40.

[325] Calkins, CC; Setzer, SV; Jennings, JM; et al. Desmogleinendocytosis and desmosome disassembly are coordinated responses to pemphigus autoantibodies. *J Biol Chem*, 2006, 281(11), 7623–34.

[326] Kitajima, Y; Aoyama, Y; Seishima, M. Transmembranesignaling for adhesive regulation of desmosomes andhemidesmosomes, and for cell-cell detachment induced by pemphigus IgG in cultured keratinocytes: involvement of protein kinase C. *J Investig Dermatol Symp Proc*, 1999, 4(2), 137–44.

[327] Sato, M; Aoyama, Y; Kitajima, Y. Assembly pathway ofdesmoglein 3 to desmosomes and its perturbation by pemphigus vulgaris-IgG in cultured keratinocytes, asrevealed by time-lapsed labeling immunoelectronmicroscopy. *Lab Invest*, 2000, 80(10), 1583–92.

[328] Shu, E; Yamamoto, Y; Sato-Nagai, M; Aoyama, Y; Kitajima, Y. Pemphigus vulgaris-IgG reduces the desmoglein 3/desmocollin 3 ratio on the cell surface in cultured keratinocytes as revealed by doublestainingimmunoelectron microscopy. *J Dermatol Sci*, 2005, 40(3), 209–11.

[329] Seko, YS; Cole, W; Kasprzak, BA; et al. The role of cytokine mRNA stability in the pathogenesis of autoimmune disease. *Autoimmunity Rev*, 2006, 5(5), 299–305.

[330] Saklatvala, J. The p38 MAP kinase pathway as a therapeutic target in inflammatory disease. *Curr Opin Pharmacol*, 2004, 4(4), 372–7.

[331] Brook, MG; Sully, AR. Regulation of tumour necrosis factor α mRNA stability by the mitogenactivated protein kinase p38 signalling cascade," *FEBS Letters*, 2000, 483, 57–61.

[332] Mavropoulos, AG; Sully, AP; Clark, AR. Stabilization of IFN-γ mRNA by MAPK p38 in IL-12- and IL-18-stimulated human NK cells. *Blood*, 2005, 105, 282–8.

[333] Coulthard, LR; White, DE; Jones, DL; McDermott, MF; Burchill, SA. p38MAPK: stress responses from molecular mechanisms to therapeutics. *Trends Mol Med*, 2009, 15, 369–79.

[334] Mavropoulos, A; Orfanidou, T; Liaskos, C; et al. p38 mitogen-activated protein kinase (p38 MAPK)-mediated autoimmunity: lessons to learn from ANCA vasculitis and Pemphigus vulgaris. *Autoimmun Rev*, 2013, 12, 580–90.

[335] Johansen, C; Funding, AT; Otkjaer, K; et al. Protein expression of TNF-α in psoriatic skin is regulated at a posttranscriptional level by MAPK-activated protein kinase 2. *J Immunol*, 2006, 176, 1431–8.

[336] Mavropoulos, A; Smyk, D; Rigopoulou, EI; Bogdanos, DP. Human peripheral blood mononuclear cell culture for flow cytometric analysis of phosphorylated mitogen-activated protein kinases. *Methods Mol Biol*, 2012, 806, 275–85.

[337] Berkowitz, P; Chua, M; Liu, Z; Diaz, LA; Rubenstein, DS. Autoantibodies in the autoimmune diseasepemphigus foliaceus induce blistering via p38mitogen- activated protein kinase-dependent signalingin the skin. *Am J Pathol*, 2008, 173(6), 1628–36.

[338] Berkowitz, P; Diaz, LA; Hall, RP; Rubenstein, DS. Induction of p38MAPK and HSP27 phosphorylationin pemphigus patient skin. *J Invest Dermatol*, 2008, 128(3), 738–40.

[339] Berkowitz, P; Hu, P; Liu, Z; et al. Desmosome signaling, inhibition ofp38MAPK prevents pemphigus vulgaris IgG-induced cytoskeleton reorganization. *J Biol Chem*, 2005, 280(25), 23778–84.

[340] Cuenda, A; Rousseau, S. p38 MAP-kinases pathway regulation, function and role in human diseases. *Biochim Biophys Acta*, 2007, 1773(8), 1358–75.

[341] Schmidt, E; Gutberlet, J; Siegmund, D; Berg, D; Wajant, H; Waschke, J. Apoptosis is not required foracantholysis in pemphigus vulgaris. *Am J Physiol*, 2009, 296(1), C162–72.

[342] Lee, HE; Berkowitz, P; Jolly, PS; Diaz, LA; Chua, MP; Rubenstein, DS. Biphasic activation of p38MAPKsuggests that apoptosis is a downstream event inpemphigus acantholysis. *J Biol Chem*, 2009, 284(18), 12524–32.

[343] Nys, K; Van Laethem, A; Michiels, C; et al. Ap38(MAPK)/HIF-1 pathway initiated by UVB irradiationis required to induce Noxa and apoptosis of human keratinocytes. *J Invest Dermatol*, 2010, 130(9), 2269–76.

[344] Li, N; Zhao, M; Wang, J; Liu, Z; Diaz, LA. Involvementof the apoptotic mechanism in pemphigus foliaceusautoimmune injury of the skin. *J Immunol*, 2009, 182(1), 711–7.

[345] Gniadecki, R; Jemec, GB; Thomsen, BM; Hansen, M. Relationship between keratinocyte adhesion anddeath: anoikis in acantholytic diseases. *Arch Dermatol Res*, 1998, 290(10), 528–32.

[346] Rodrigues, DB; Pereira, SA; dos Reis, MA; et al. *In situ* detection of infl ammatory cytokines and apoptosisin pemphigus foliaceus patients. *Arch Pathol Lab Med*, 2009, 133(1), 97–100.

[347] Puviani, M; Marconi, A; Cozzani, E; Pincelli, C. Fasligand in pemphigus sera induces keratinocyte apoptosisthrough the activation of caspase-8. *J Invest Dermatol*, 2003, 120(1), 164–7.

[348] Li, J; Bu, DF; Huang, YC; Zhu, XJ. Role of autoantibodiesagainst the linker subdomains of envoplakin andperiplakin in the pathogenesis of paraneoplastic pemphigus. *Chin Med J (Engl)*, 2009, 122(5), 486–95.

[349] Schmidt, E; Waschke, J. Apoptosis in pemphigus. *Autoimmun Rev*, 2009, 8(7), 533–7.

[350] Muller, E; Caldelari, R; De Bruin, A; et al. Pathogenesis in pemphigus vulgaris: a central role for the armadilloprotein plakoglobin. *J Invest Dermatol*, 2000, 115(2), 332.

[351] Williamson, L; Hunziker, T; Suter, MM; Muller, EJ. Nuclear c-Myc: a molecular marker for early stagepemphigus vulgaris. *J Invest Dermatol*, 2007, 127(6), 1549–55.

[352] Futamura, S; Martins, C; Rivitti, EA; Labib, RS; Diaz, LA; Anhalt, GJ. Ultrastructural studies of acantholysisinduced *in vivo* by passive transfer of IgG fromendemic pemphigus foliaceus (Fogo Selvagem). *J Invest Dermatol*, 1989, 93(4), 480–5.

[353] Takahashi, Y; Patel, HP; Labib, RS; Diaz, LA; Anhalt, GJ. Experimentally induced pemphigus vulgaris in neonatal BALB/c mice: a time-course study of clinical, immunologic, ultrastructural, and cytochemicalchanges. *J Invest Dermatol*, 1985, 84(1), 41–6.

[354] Aho, S; Mahoney, MG; Uitto, J. Plectin serves as an autoantigen in paraneoplastic pemphigus. *J Invest Dermatol*, 1999, 113, 422–3.

[355] Proby, C; Fujii, Y; Owaribe, K; Nishikawa, T; Amagai, M. Human autoantibodies against HD1/plectin in paraneoplastic pemphigus. *J Invest Dermatol*, 1999, 112, 153–6.

[356] Buijsrogge, JJ. Antiplectin autoantibodies insubepidermal blistering diseases. *Br J Dermatol*, 2009, 161, 762–71.

[357] Laffitte, E. Plectin, an unusual target antigen inbullous pemphigoid. *Br J Dermatol*, 2001, 144, 136–8.

[358] Buijsrogge, JJ. Inflammatory epidermolysis bullosa acquisita with coexistent IgA antibodies to plectin. *Clin Exp Dermatol*, 2005, 30, 531–4.

[359] Tirado-Sánchez, A; León-Dorantes, G. Treatment of pemphigus vulgaris. An overview in Mexico. *Allergol Immunopathol (Madr)*, 2006, 34(1), 10-6.

[360] Beutner, EH; Jordan, RE. Demonstration of skin antibodiesin sera of pemphigus vulgaris patients bydirect immunofl uorescent staining. *Proc Soc Exp Biol Med*, 1964, 117, 505–10.

[361] Beutner, EH; Prigenzi, LS; Hale, W; Leme Cde, A; Bier, OG. Immunofluorescent studies of autoantibodies to intercellular areas of epithelia in Brazilian pemphigus foliaceus. *Proc Soc Exp Biol Med*, 1968, 127(1), 81–6.

[362] Eyre, RW; Stanley, JR. Identification of pemphigus vulgaris antigen extracted from normal human epidermis and comparison with pemphigus foliaceus antigen. *J Clin Invest*, 1988, 81(3), 807–12.

[363] Woo, TY; Hogan, VA; Patel, H; Anhalt, GJ; Labib, RS; Voorhees, JJ; et al. Specificity and inhibition of the epidermal cell detachment induced by pemphigus IgG *in vitro*. *J Invest Dermatol*, 1983, 81(1 Suppl), 115s–21.

[364] Hashimoto, K; Shafran, KM; Webber, PS; Lazarus, GS; Singer, KH. Anti-cell surface pemphigus autoantibody stimulates plasminogen activator activity of human epidermal cells. *J Exp Med*, 1983, 157, 259–72.

[365] Shimizu, A; Ishiko, A; Ota, T; Tsunoda, K; Amagai, M; Nishikawa. T. IgG binds to desmoglein 3 in desmosomesand causes a desmosomal split without keratinretraction in a pemphigus mouse model. *J Invest Dermatol*, 2004, 122(5), 1145–53.

[366] Esaki, C; Seishima, M; Yamada, T; Osada, K; Kitajima, Y. Pharmacologic evidence for involvement of phospholipase C in pemphigus IgG-induced inositol 1, 4, 5-trisphosphate generation, intracellular calcium increase, and plasminogen activator secretion in DJM-1 cells, asquamous cell carcinoma line. *J Invest Dermatol*, 1995, 105(3), 329–33.

[367] Osada, K; Seishima, M; Kitajima, Y. Pemphigus IgG activatesand translocates protein kinase C from the cytosolto the particulate/cytoskeleton fractions in human keratinocytes. *J Invest Dermatol*, 1997, 108(4), 482–7.

[368] Caldelari, R; de Bruin, A; Baumann, D; Suter, MM; Bierkamp, C; Balmer, V; et al. A central role for the armadillo protein plakoglobin in the autoimmune disease pemphigus vulgaris. *J Cell Biol*, 2001, 153(4), 823–34.

[369] Nguyen, VT; Ndoye, A; Shultz, LD; Pittelkow, MR; Grando, SA. Antibodies against keratinocyte antigensother than desmogleins 1 and 3 can induce pemphigus vulgaris-like lesions. *J Clin Invest*, 2000, 106(12), 1467–79 [comment].

[370] Nguyen, VT; Arredondo, J; Chernyavsky, AI; Kitajima, Y; Pittelkow, M; Grando, SA. Pemphigus vulgaris IgG and methylprednisolone exhibit reciprocal effects on keratinocytes. *J Biol Chem*, 2004, 279(3), 2135–46.

[371] Mascaro, Jr. JM; Espana, A; Liu, Z; et al. Mechanisms of acantholysis in pemphigus vulgaris: role of IgG valence. *Clin Immunol Immunopathol*, 1997, 85(1), 90–6.

[372] Payne, AS; Ishii, K; Kacir, S; et al. Genetic and functional characterization of human pemphigus vulgaris monoclonal autoantibodies isolated by phage display. *J Clin Invest*, 2005, 115(4), 888–99.

[373] Rogalla, T; Ehrnsperger, M; Preville, X; et al. Regulation of Hsp27 oligomerization, chaperone function, and protective activity against oxidative stress/tumor necrosis factor alpha by phosphorylation. *J Biol Chem*, 1999, 274(27), 18947–56.

[374] Lambert, H; Charette, SJ; Bernier, AF; Guimond, A; Landry, J. HSP27 multimerization mediated by phosphorylation- sensitive intermolecular interactions at the amino terminus. *J Biol Chem*, 1999, 274(14), 9378–85.

[375] Benndorf, R; Hayess, K; Ryazantsev, S; Wieske, M; Behlke, J; Lutsch, G. Phosphorylation and supramolecular organization of murine small heat shock proteinHSP25 abolish its actin polymerization-inhibitingactivity. *J Biol Chem*, 1994, 269(32), 20780–4.

[376] Geum, D; Son, GH; Kim, K. Phosphorylation-dependentcellular localization and thermoprotective role of heatshock protein 25 in hippocampal progenitor cells. *J Biol Chem*, 2002, 277(22), 19913–21.

[377] Panasenko, OO; Kim, MV; Marston, SB; Gusev, NB. Interaction of the small heat shock protein withmolecular mass 25 kDa (hsp25) with actin. *Eur JBiochem/FEBS*, 2003, 270(5), 892–901.

[378] Perng, MD; Cairns, L; van den IJssel, P; Prescott, A; Hutcheson, AM; Quinlan, RA. Intermediate filament interactions can be altered by HSP27 and alpha B crystallin. *J Cell Sci*, 1999, 112(Pt 13), 2099–112.

[379] Duverger, O; Paslaru, L; Morange, M. HSP25 is involved in two steps of the differentiation of PAM212 keratinocytes. *J Biol Chem*, 2004, 279(11), 10252–60.

[380] Lavoie, JN; Hickey, E; Weber, LA; Landry, J. Modulationof actin microfilament dynamics and fl uid phase pinocytosisby phosphorylation of heat shock protein 27. *J Biol Chem*, 1993, 268(32), 24210–4.

[381] Lavoie, JN; Lambert, H; Hickey, E; Weber, LA; Landry, J. Modulation of cellular thermoresistance and actin filament stability accompanies phosphorylationinduced changes in the oligomeric structure of heatshock protein 27. *Mol Cell Biol*, 1995, 15(1), 505–16.

[382] Guay, J; Lambert, H; Gingras-Breton, G; Lavoie, JN; Huot, J; Landry, J. Regulation of actin filament dynamics by p38 map kinase-mediated phosphorylation of heat shock protein 27. *J Cell Sci*, 1997, 110(Pt3), 357–68.

[383] Evgrafov, OV; Mersiyanova, I; Irobi, J; et al. Mutant small heat-shockprotein 27 causes axonal Charcot-Marie-Tooth disease and distal hereditary motor neuropathy. *Nat Genet*, 2004, 36(6), 602–6.

[384] Berkowitz, P; Hu, P; Warren, S; Liu, Z; Diaz, LA; Rubenstein, DS. p38MAPK inhibition prevents disease in pemphigus vulgaris mice. *Proc Natl Acad Sci U S A*, 2006, 103, 12855–60.

[385] Chernyavsky, AI; Arredondo, J; Kitajima, Y; Sato-Nagai, M; Grando, SA. Desmoglein versus non-desmoglein signaling in pemphigus acantholysis: characterization of novel signaling pathways downstream of pemphigus vulgaris antigens. *J Biol Chem*, 2007, 282(18), 13804–12.

[386] Kawasaki, Y; Aoyama, Y; Tsunoda, K; Amagai, M; Kitajima, Y. Pathogenic monoclonal antibody against desmoglein 3 augments desmoglein 3 and p38 MAPK phosphorylation in human squamous carcinoma cellline. *Autoimmunity*, 2006, 39(7), 587–90.

[387] Mao, X; Sano, Y; Park, JM; Payne, AS. p38 MAPK activation is downstream of the loss of intercellular adhesion in pemphigus vulgaris. *J Biol Chem*, 2011, 286(2), 1283–91.

[388] Waschke, J; Spindler, V; Bruggeman, P; Zillikens, D; Schmidt, G; Drenckhahn, D. Inhibition of Rho A activity causes pemphigus skin blistering. *J Cell Biol*, 2006, 175(5), 721–7.

[389] Delva, E; Jennings, JM; Calkins, CC; Kottke, MD; Faundez, V; Kowalczyk, AP. Pemphigus vulgaris IgG-induced desmoglein-3 endocytosis and desmosomal disassembly are mediated by a clathrin- and dynamin-independent mechanism. *J Biol Chem*, 2008, 283(26), 18303–13.

[390] Calkins, CC; Setzer, SV; Jennings, JM; Summers, S; Tsunoda, K; Amagai, M; et al. Desmoglein endocitosis and desmosome disassembly are coordinated responses to pemphigus autoantibodies. *J Biol Chem*, 2006, 281(11), 7623–34.

[391] Jolly, PS; Berkowitz, P; Bektas, M; Lee, HE; Chua, M; Diaz, LA; et al. p38MAPK signaling and desmoglein-3 internalization are linked events in pemphigus acantholysis. *J Biol Chem*, 2010, 285(12), 8936–41.

[392] Spindler, V; Vielmuth, F; Schmidt, E; Rubenstein, DS; Waschke, J. Protective endogenous cyclic adenosine 5′-monophosphate signaling triggered by pemphigusautoantibodies. *J Immunol*, 2010, 185(11), 6831–8.

[393] Rubenstein, DS; Werth, V; Strober, B; et al. Use of KC706 for the treatment of pemphigus vulgaris. http://clinicaltrials.gov/ct2/show/NCT00606749?term= pemphigus &rank=10.

[394] Murrell, D; Dick, S; Ahmed, A. Consensus statement on definitions of disease, end points, and therapeutic response for pemphigus. *J Am Acad Dermatol*, 2008, 58(6), 1043–6.

[395] Rosenbach, M; Murrell, DF; Bystryn, JC; Dulay, S; Dick, S; Fakharzadeh, S; et al. Reliability and convergent validity of two outcome instruments for pemphigus. *J Invest Dermatol*, 2009, 129(10), 2404–10.

[396] Muller, EJ; Hunziker, T; Suter, MM. Keratin intermediatefilament retraction is linked to plakoglobin dependent signaling in pemphigus vulgaris. *J AmAcad Dermatol*, 2007, 56(5), 890–1.

[397] Tsang, SM; Brown, L; Lin, K; Liu, L; Piper, K; O'Toole, EA; et al. Non-junctional human desmoglein 3 acts asan upstream regulator of Src in E-cadherin adhesion, a pathway possibly involved in the pathogenesis ofpemphigus vulgaris. *J Pathol*, 2012, 227(1), 81–93.

[398] Schulze, K; Galichet, A; Sayar, BS; Scothern, A; Howald, D; Zymann, H; et al. An adult passive transfer mousemodel to study desmoglein 3 signaling in pemphigus vulgaris. *J Invest Dermatol*, 2012, 132(2), 346–55.

[399] Spindler, V; Endlich, A; Hartlieb, E; Vielmuth, F; Schmidt, E; Waschke, J. The extent of desmoglein 3depletion in pemphigus vulgaris is dependent on Ca(2+)-induced differentiation: a role in suprabasalepidermal skin splitting? *Am J Pathol*, 2011, 179(4), 1905–16.

[400] Sanchez-Carpintero, I; Espana, A; Pelacho, B; LopezMoratalla, N; Rubenstein, DS; Diaz, LA; et al. *In vivo* blockade of pemphigus vulgaris acantholysis by inhibition of intracellular signal transduction cascades. *Br J Dermatol*, 2004, 151(3), 565–70.

[401] Pretel, M; Espana, A; Marquina, M; Pelacho, B; Lopez-Picazo, JM; Lopez-Zabalza, MJ. An imbalance in Akt/mTOR is involved in the apoptotic and acantholyticprocesses in a mouse model of pemphigus vulgaris. *Exp Dermatol*, 2009, 18(9), 771–80.

[402] Chernyavsky, AI; Arredondo, J; Piser, T; Karlsson, E; Grando, SA. Differential coupling of M1 muscarinic and alpha7 nicotinic receptors to inhibition of pemphigusacantholysis. *J Biol Chem*, 2008, 283(6), 3401–8.

[403] Seishima, M; Iwasaki-Bessho, Y; Itoh, Y; Nozawa, Y; Amagai, M; Kitajima, Y. Phosphatidylcholine-specificphospholipase C, but not phospholipase D, is involvedin pemphigus IgG-induced signal transduction. *Arch Dermatol Res*, 1999, 291(11), 606–13.

[404] Marconi, A; Atzei, P; Panza, C; et al. FLICE/caspase-8 activation triggers anoikis induced by beta1-integrin blockade in human keratinocytes. *J Cell Sci*, 2004, 117(Pt 24), 5815–23.

[405] Grando, SA; Bystryn, JC; Chernyavsky, AI; et al. Apoptolysis: anovel mechanism of skin blistering in pemphigus vulgarislinking the apoptotic pathways to basal cellshrinkage and suprabasal acantholysis. *Exp Dermatol*, 2009, 18(9), 764–70.

[406] Sarig, O; Bercovici, S; Zoller, L; et al. Population-specific associationbetween a polymorphic variant in ST18, encoding apro-apoptotic molecule, and pemphigus vulgaris. *J Invest Dermatol*, 2012, 132(7), 1798–805.

[407] Gazit, E; Lowenthal, R. The immunogenetics of pemphigus vulgaris. *Autoimmun Rev*, 2004, 4, 16–20.

[408] Yang, J; Siqueira, MF; Behl, Y; Alikhani, M; Graves, DT. The transcription factor ST18 regulates proapoptoticand proinflammatory gene expression in fibroblasts. *FASEB J*, 2008, 22(11), 3956–67.

[409] Pacheco-Tovar, MG; Avalos-Diaz, E; Vega-Memije, E; et al. The final destiny of acantholytic cells inpemphigus is Fas mediated. *J Eur Acad DermatolVenereol*, 2009, 23(6), 697–701.

[410] Frusic-Zlotkin, M; Raichenberg, D; Wang, X; David, M; Michel, B; Milner, Y. Apoptotic mechanism inpemphigus autoimmunoglobulins-induced acantholysis—possible involvement of the EGF receptor. *Autoimmunity*, 2006, 39(7), 563–75.

[411] Pelacho, B; Natal, C; Espana, A; Sanchez-Carpintero, I; Iraburu, MJ; Lopez-Zabalza, MJ. Pemphigus vulgarisautoantibodies induce apoptosis in HaCaT keratinocytes. *FEBS Lett*, 2004, 566(1–3), 6–10.

[412] Wang, X; Bregegere, F; Frusic-Zlotkin, M; Feinmesser, M; Michel, B; Milner, Y. Possible apoptotic mechanismin epidermal cell acantholysis induced by pemphigusvulgaris autoimmunoglobulins. *Apoptosis*, 2004, 9(2), 131–43.

[413] Wang, X; Bregegere, F; Soroka, Y; Frusic-Zlotkin, M; Milner, Y. Replicative senescence enhances apoptosis induced by pemphigus autoimmune antibodies inhuman keratinocytes. *FEBS Lett*, 2004, 567(2–3), 281–6.

[414] Pacheco-Tovar, D; Lopez-Luna, A; Herrera-Esparza, R; Avalos-Diaz, E. The caspase pathway as a posible therapeutic target in experimental pemphigus. *Autoimmun Dis*, 2011, 2011, 563091.

[415] Cirillo, N; Lanza, M; Femiano, F; et al. If pemphigus vulgaris IgG are thecause of acantholysis, new IgG-independent mechanisms are the concause. *J Cell Physiol*, 2007, 212(3), 563–7.

[416] D'Auria, L; Bonifati, C; Mussi, A; et al. Cytokines in the sera of patients with pemphigus vulgaris: interleukin-6 andtumour necrosis factor-alpha levels are significantlyincreased as compared to healthy subjects and correlate with disease activity. *Eur Cytokine Netw*, 1997, 8(4), 383–7.

[417] Siebra, MX; Santos, MA; Almeida, TL; Leite, AC; Cunha, FQ; Rocha, FA. Evidence for the participationof nitric oxide in pemphigus. *Braz J Med Biol Res*, 2006, 39(5), 671–5.

[418] Grando, SA; Glukhenky, BT; Drannik, GN; Kostromin, AP; Chernyavsky, AI. Cytotoxic proteasesin blister fluid of pemphigus and pemphigoidpatients. *Int J Tissue React*, 1989, 11(4), 195–201.

[419] Toosi, S; Habib, N; Torres, G; Reynolds, SR; Bystryn, JC. Serum levels of inhibitors of apoptotic proteins (IAPs) change with IVIg therapy in pemphigus. *J Invest Dermatol*, 2011, 131(11), 2327–9.

[420] Moravvej, H; Yousefi, M; Farrokhi, B; Mosaffa, N. Soluble Fas in pemphigus vulgaris. *Arch Iran Med*, 2011, 14(3), 200–1.

[421] Sayama, K; Yonehara, S; Watanabe, Y; Miki, Y. Expression of Fas antigen on keratinocytes *in vivo* and induction of apoptosis in cultured keratinocytes. *JInvest Dermatol*, 1994, 103(3), 330–4.

[422] Arredondo, J; Chernyavsky, AI; Karaouni, A; Grando, SA. Novel mechanisms of target cell death and survival and of therapeutic action of IVIg inpemphigus. *Am J Pathol*, 2005, 167(6), 1531–44.

[423] Orlov, MD; Chernyavsky, AI; Arredondo, J; Grando, SA. Synergistic actions of pemphigus vulgaris IgG, Fas-ligand and tumor necrosis factor-alpha duringinduction of basal cell shrinkage and acantholysis. *Autoimmunity*, 2006, 39(7), 557–62.

[424] Amagai, M; Tsunoda, K; Suzuki, H; Nishifuji, K; Koyasu, S; Nishikawa, T. Use of autoantigen- knockout mice in developing an active autoimmune disease model for pemphigus. *J Clin Invest*, 2000, 105(5), 625–31.

[425] Sinha, AA. The genetics of pemphigus. *Dermatol Clin*, 2011, 29(3), 381–91, vii.

[426] Tron, F; Gilbert, D; Joly, P; et al. Immunogenetics of pemphigus: an update. *Autoimmunity*, 2006, 39(7), 531–9.

[427] Todd, JA; Acha-Orbea, H; Bell, JI; et al. A molecularbasis for MHC class II—associated autoimmunity. *Science*, 1988, 240(4855), 1003–9.

[428] Scharf, SJ; Friedmann, A; Brautbar, C; et al. HLA classII allelic variation and susceptibility to pemphigusvulgaris. *Proc Natl Acad Sci U S A*, 1988, 85(10), 3504–8.

[429] Lee, E; Lendas, KA; Chow, S; et al. Disease relevantHLA class II alleles isolated by genotypic, haplotypic, and sequence analysis in North American Caucasianswith pemphigus vulgaris. *Hum Immunol*, 2006, 67(1–2), 125–39.

[430] Yan, L; Wang, JM; Zeng, K. Association between HLADRB1polymorphism and pemphigus vulgaris: A meta-analysis. *Br J Dermatol*, 2012, 167, 768–77.

[431] Bhanusali, D; Sachdev, A; Rahmanian, A; et al. HLAE*0103X is associated with susceptibility to pemphigus vulgaris. *Exp Dermatol*, 2013, 22(2), 108–12.

[432] Torzecka, JD; Narbutt, J; Sysa-Jedrzejowska, A; et al. Tumour necrosis factor-alpha polymorphism as one of the complex inherited factors in pemphigus. *Mediators Inflamm*, 2003, 12(5), 303–7.

[433] Martel, P; Loiseau, P; Joly, P; et al. Paraneoplastic pemphigus is associated with the DRB1* 03 allele. *J Autoimmun*, 2003, 20(1), 91–5.

[434] Liu, Q; Bu, D; Li, D; Zhu, X. Genotyping of HLA-I andHLA-II alleles in Chinese patients with paraneoplastic pemphigus. *Br J Dermatol*, 2008, 158(3), 587–91.

[435] Bordel-Gomez, MT; Sanchez-Estella, J; Yuste- Chaves, M; et al. Familial pemphigus vulgaris: immunogenetic study of HLA class II antigens. *Actas Dermosifiliogr*, 2006, 97, 509–13.

[436] Humbert, P; Dupond, JL; Vuitton, D; et al. Dermatological autoimmune diseases and the multiple autoimmunesyndromes. *Acta Derm Venereol Suppl (Stockh)*, 1989, 148, 1–8.

[437] Mohan, MP; Ramesh, TC. Multiple autoimmune syndrome. *Indian J Dermatol Venereol Leprol*, 2003, 69, 298–9.

[438] Laskaris, G; Sklavounou, A; Stavrou, A; et al. Familial pemphigus vulgaris with oral manifestationsaffecting two Greek families. *J Oral Pathol Med*, 1989, 18, 49–53.

[439] Katzenelson, V; David, M; Zamir, R; et al. Familialpemphigus vulgaris. *Dermatologica*, 1990, 181, 48–50.

[440] Feinstein, A; Yorav, S; Movshovitz, M; et al. Pemphigus in families. *Int J Dermatol*, 1991, 30, 347–51.

[441] Stavropoulos, PG; Zarafonitis, G; Petridis, A; et al. Pemphigus vulgaris in two sisters. *Acta Derm Venereol*, 2001, 81, 149.

[442] Mashiah, J; Brenner, S. Medical pearl: first step in managing pemphigus—addressing the etiology. *J Am Acad Dermatol*, 2005, 53(4), 706–7.

[443] Brenner, S. PEMPHIGUS: an acronym for a diseasewith multiple etiologies. *Skinmed*, 2003, 2(3), 163–7.

[444] Brenner, S; Tur, E; Shapiro, J; et al. Pemphigus vulgaris: environmental factors. Occupational, behavioral, medical, and qualitative food frequencyquestionnaire. *Int J Dermatol*, 2001, 40(9), 562–9.

[445] Brenner, S; Bialy-Golan, A; Ruocco, V. Drug-induced pemphigus. *Clin Dermatol*, 1998, 16(3), 393–7.

[446] Brenner, S; Wolf, R; Ruocco, V. Contact pemphigus: a subgroup of induced pemphigus. *Int J Dermatol*, 1994, 33(12), 843–5.

[447] Goldberg, I; Kashman, Y; Brenner, S. The induction of pemphigus by phenol drugs. *Int J Dermatol*, 1999, 38(12), 888–92.

[448] Tamir, A; Ophir, J; Brenner, S. Pemphigus vulgaris triggered by emotional stress. *Dermatol (Basel Switzerland)*, 1994, 189(2), 210.

[449] Jacobs, SE. Pemphigus erythematosus and ultraviolet light: a case report. *Arch Dermatol*, 1965, 91(2), 139.

[450] Brenner, S. Pemphigus and dietary factors. *Dermatology*, 1995, 190(3), 197–202.

[451] Tur, E; Brenner, S. Diet and pemphigus: in pursuit ofexogenous factors in pemphigus and fogo selvagem. *Arch Dermatol*, 1998, 134(11), 1406.

[452] Ruocco, V; Pisani, M. Induced pemphigus. *Arch Dermatol Res*, 1982, 274(1–2), 123–40.

[453] Wolf, R; Tamir, A; Brenner, S. Drug-induced versusdrug-triggered pemphigus. *Dermatologica*, 1991, 182(4), 207–10.

[454] Yamamoto, T; Takata-Michigami, M; Hisamatsu, Y; et al. A prospective analysis of anti-desmoglein antibody profiles in patients with rheumatoid arthritis treated with thiol compounds. *J Dermatol Sci*, 2010, 59(3), 170–5.

[455] Sebaratnam, DF; Martin, LK; Rubin, AI; et al. Reversible relapse of pemphigus foliaceus triggeredby topical imiquimod suggests that Toll-like receptor 7 inhibitors may be useful treatments for pemphigus. *Clin Exp Dermatol*, 2010, 36(1), 91–3.

[456] Tang, X; Zhang, X. Drug-induced pemphigus after six years of treatment with phenytoin and carbamazepine. *Int J Dermatol*, 2012, 51(4), 485–6.

[457] Valikhani, M; Kavusi, S; Chams-Davatchi, C; et al. Pemphigus and associated environmental factors: a casecontrolstudy. *Clin Exp Dermatol*, 2007, 32(3), 256–60.

[458] Valikhani, M; Kavusi, S; Chams-Davatchi, C; et al. Impact of smoking on pemphigus. *Int J Dermatol*, 2008, 47(6), 567–70.

[459] Mehta, JN; Martin, AG. A case of pemphigus vulgarisimproved by cigarette smoking. *Arch Dermatol*, 2000, 136(1), 15–7.

[460] Sullivan, TP; Elgart, GW; Kirsner, RS. Pemphigus and smoking. *Int J Dermatol.*, 2002, 41(8), 528–30.

[461] Grando, SA; Dahl, MV. Nicotine and pemphigus. *Arch Dermatol*, 2000, 136(10), 1269.

[462] Arnson, Y; Shoenfeld, Y; Amital, H. Effects of tobacco smoke on immunity, inflammation and autoimmunity. *J Autoimmun*, 2010, 34(3), J258–65.

[463] Morell-Dubois, S; Carpentier, O; Cottencin, O; et al. Stressful life events and pemphigus. *Dermatology*, 2008, 216(2), 104–8.

[464] Bastuji-Garin, S; Turki, H; Mokhtar, I; et al. Possiblerelation of Tunisian pemphigus with traditional cosmetics: a multicenter case-control study. *Am J Epidemiol*, 2002, 155(3), 249–56.

[465] Micali, G; Nasca, MR; Musumeci, ML; Innocenzi, D. Postsurgical pemphigus. *Dermatology*, 1998, 197(2), 192–3.

[466] Tur, E; Brenner, S. Contributing exogenous factors inpemphigus. *Int J Dermatol.*, 1997, 36(12), 888–93.

[467] Diaz, LA; Sampaio, SA; Rivitti, EA; et al. Endemicpemphigus foliaceus (fogo selvagem): II. Current andhistoric epidemiologic studies. *J Invest Dermatol*, 1989, 92(1), 4–12.

[468] Empinotti, JC; Aoki, V; Filgueira, A; et al. Clinical andserological follow-up studies of endemic pemphigus foliaceus (fogo selvagem) in Western Parana, Brazil (2001–2002). *Br J Dermatol*, 2006, 155(2), 446–50.

[469] Diaz, LA; Arteaga, LA; Hilario-Vargas, J; et al. Antidesmoglein-1 antibodies in onchocerciasis, leishmaniasis and Chagas disease suggest a possible etiologicallink to Fogo selvagem. *J Invest Dermatol*, 2004, 123(6), 1045–51.

[470] Qian, SX; Li, JY; Hong, M; Xu, W; Qiu HX. Nonhematological autoimmunity (glomerulosclerosis, paraneoplastic pemphigus and paraneoplasticneurological syndrome) in a patient with chronic lymphocyticleukemia: diagnosis, prognosis and management. *Leuk Res*, 2008, 33, 500–5.

[471] Moraes, ME; Fernandez-Vina, M; Lazaro, A; et al. An epitopein the third hypervariable region of the DRB1 gene is involved in the susceptibility to endemic pemphigus foliaceus (fogo selvagem) in three different Brazilian populations. *Tissue Antigens*, 1997, 49(1), 35–40.

[472] Bastuji-Garin, S; Souissi, R; Blum, L; et al. Comparativeepidemiology of pemphigus in Tunisia and France: unusual incidence of pemphigus foliaceus in young Tunisian women. *J Invest Dermatol*, 1995, 104(2), 302–5.

[473] Abida, O; Masmoudi, A; Rebai, A; et al. The familialfeature of Tunisian endemic pemphigus foliaceus. *Br J Dermatol*, 2009, 161(4), 951–3.

[474] Abida, O; Zitouni, M; Kallel-Sellami, M; et al. Tunisianendemic pemphigus foliaceus is associated with the HLA-DR3 gene: anti-desmoglein 1 antibody- positive healthy subjects bear protective alleles. *Br J Dermatol*, 2009, 161(3), 522–7.

[475] Joly, P; Mokhtar, I; Gilbert, D; et al. Immunoblot and immunoelectron microscopic analysis of endemic Tunisian pemphigus. *Br J Dermatol*, 1999, 140(1), 44–9.

[476] Kallel Sellami, M; Zitouni, M; Tombari, W; et al. Antidesmoglein-1 antibodies are prevalent in Tunisian patients with hydatidosis and leishmaniasis. *Br J Dermatol*, 2007, 156(3), 591–3.

[477] Zaraa, I; Boussoffara, T; Ben Ahmed, M; et al. Exposureto Phlebotomus papatasi and/or Leishmania major: possible etiologic link to Tunisian pemphigus. *J Invest Dermatol*, 2014, 132(2), 479–82.

[478] Lombardi, C; Borges, PC; Chaul, A; et al. Environmental risk factors in endemic pemphigus foliaceus (Fogo selvagem). 'The Cooperative Group on Fogo Selvagem Research.' *J Invest Dermatol*, 1992, 98, 847–850.

[479] Aoki, V; Sousa, JX; Jr, Diaz, LA. Pathogenesis of endemic pemphigus foliaceus. *Dermatol Clin*, 2011, 29, 413–418, viii.

[480] Wohl, Y; Brenner, S. Pemphigus in Israel _ an epidemiologic analysis of cases in search of risk factors. *Women*, 2003, 33, 60.

[481] Yazdanpanah, MJ; Ghayour-Mobarhan, M; Taji, A; et al. Serum zinc and copper status in Iranian patients with pemphigus vulgaris. *Int J Dermatol*, 2011, 50, 1343–1346.

[482] Meibodi, NT; Nahidi, Y; Mahmoudi, M; et al. Evaluation of coexistence of the human herpesvirus type 8 (HHV-8) in fection and pemphigus. *Int J Dermatol*, 2010, 49, 780–783.

[483] Fallahzadeh, MK; Lashkarizadeh, H; Kamali-Sarvestani, E; Namazi, MR. Elevation of serum prolactin levels in patients with pemphigus vulgaris: a novel finding with practical implications. *J Am Acad Dermatol*, 2010, 62, 1071–1072.

[484] Wohl, Y; Dreiher, J; Cohen, AD. Pemphigus and dyslipidaemia: a case–control study. *Br J Dermatol*, 2009, 161, 1418–1420.

[485] Da Cunha, SF; dos Santos, VM; Monteiro, JP; et al. Serum lipids of pemphigus foliaceus patients on long-term glucocorticoid therapy. *Rev Soc Bras Med Trop*, 2003, 36, 1–4.

[486] Daneshpazhooh, M; Behjati, J; Hashemi, P; et al. Thyroid autoimmunity and pemphigus vulgaris: is there a significant association? *J Am Acad Dermatol*, 2010, 62, 349–351.

[487] Kacar, N; Cevahir, N; Demirkan, N; Sanli, B. The investigation of the possible relationship between Coxsackie viruses and pemphigus. *Int J Dermatol*, 2014, 53, 312–315.

[488] Mozafari, N; Robati, RM; Younespour, S. Serum leptin levels in pemphigus: a case control study. *Biomed Res Int*, 2014, 2014, 5.

[489] Shapira, Y; Agmon-Levin, N; Shoenfeld, Y. Definingand analyzing geoepidemiology and human autoimmunity. *J Autoimmun*, 2010, 34(3), J168–77.

[490] Arbuckle, MR; McClain, MT; Rubertone, MV; et al. Development of autoantibodies before the clinicalonset of systemic lupus erythematosus. *N Engl J Med*, 2003, 349(16), 1526–33.

[491] Ortega Loayza, AG; Ramos, W; Elgart, G; et al. Antibodies against desmoglein 1 in healthy subjectsin endemic and nonendemic areas of pemphigus foliaceus(fogo selvagem) in Peru. *Int J Dermatol*, 2006, 45(5), 538–42.

[492] Amagai, M; Tsunoda, K; Zillikens, D; Nagai, T; Nishikawa, T. The clinical phenotype of pemphigus isdefined by the anti-desmoglein autoantibody profile. *J Am Acad Dermatol*, 1999, 40(2 Pt 1), 167–70.

[493] Aboobaker, J; Wojnarowska, FT; Bhogal, B; Black, MM. Chronic bullous dermatosis of childhood—clinical and immunological features seen in Africanpatients. *Clin Exp Dermatol*, 1991, 16(3), 160–4.

[494] Baican, A; Baican, C; Chiriac, G; et al. Pemphigus vulgarisis the most common autoimmune bullous diseasein northwestern Romania. *Int J Dermatol*, 2010, 49(7), 768–74.

[495] Chams-Davatchi, C; Valikhani, M; Daneshpazhooh, M; et al. Pemphigus: analysis of 1209 cases. *Int J Dermatol*, 2005, 44(6), 470–6.

[496] Hahn, K; Kippes, W; Amagai, M; Rzany, B; Brocker, EB; Zillikens, D. Clinical aspects and immunopathologyin 48 patients with pemphigus. *Hautarzt*, 2000, 51(9), 670–7.

[497] Kumar, KA. Incidence of pemphigus in Thrissur district, south India. *Indian J Dermatol Venereol Leprol*, 2008, 74(4), 349–51.

[498] Salmanpour, R; Shahkar, H; Namazi, MR; Rahman-Shenas, MR. Epidemiology of pemphigus in southwestern Iran: a 10-year retrospective study (1991–2000). *Int J Dermatol*, 2006, 45(2), 103–5.

[499] Mahe, A; Flageul, B; Cisse, I; Keita, S; Bobin, P. Pemphigus in Mali: a study of 30 cases. *Br J Dermatol*, 1996, 134(1), 114–9.

[500] Micali, G; Musumeci, ML; Nasca, MR. Epidemiologicanalysis and clinical course of 84 consecutive cases ofpemphigus in eastern Sicily. *Int J Dermatol*, 1998, 37(3), 197–200.

[501] Tallab, T; Joharji, H; Bahamdan, K; Karkashan, E; Mourad, M; Ibrahim, K. The incidence of pemphigusin the southern region of Saudi Arabia. *Int J Dermatol*, 2001, 40(9), 570–2.

[502] Uzun, S; Durdu, M; Akman, A; et al. Pemphigus in theMediterranean region of Turkey: a study of 148 cases. *Int J Dermatol*., 2006, 45(5), 523–8.

[503] V'Lckova-Laskoska, MT; Laskoski, DS; Kamberova, S; Caca-Biljanovska, N; Volckova, N. Epidemiology ofpemphigus in Macedonia: a 15-year retrospectivestudy (1990–2004). *Int J Dermatol*, 2007, 46(3), 253–8.

[504] Amin, MN; Islam, AZ. Clinical, histologic and immunologicfeatures of pemphigus in Bangladesh. *Int J Dermatol*, 2006, 45(11), 1317–8.

[505] Krain, LS. Pemphigus. Epidemiologic and survivalcharacteristics of 59 patients, 1955–1973. *Arch Dermatol*, 1974, 110(6), 862–5.

[506] Zaraa, I; Kerkeni, N; Ishak, F; et al. Spectrum of autoimmuneblistering dermatoses in Tunisia: an 11-year study and a review of the literature. *Int J Dermatol*, 2011, 50(8), 939–44.

[507] Golusin, Z; Poljacki, M; Jovanovic, M; Ethuran, V; Stojanovic, S; Rajic, N. Some epidemiological features of pemphigus chronicus in south Vojvodina: a 12-yearretrospective study. *Int J Dermatol*, 2005, 44(9), 792–3.

[508] Goncalves, GA; Brito, MM; Salathiel, AM; Ferraz, TS; Alves, D; Roselino, AM. Incidence of pemphigus vulgaris exceeds that of pemphigus foliaceus in a regionwhere pemphigus foliaceus is endemic: analysis of a21-year historical series. *An Bras Dermatol*, 2011, 86(6), 1109–12.

[509] Ahmed, AR; et al. Major histocompatibility complexhaplotype studies in Ashkenazi Jewish patientswith pemphigus vulgaris. *Proc Natl Acad Sci U S A*., 1990, 87(19), 7658–62.

[510] Hietanen, J; Salo, OP. Pemphigus: an epidemiological study of patients treated in Finnish hospitals between 1969 and 1978. *Acta Derm Venereol*, 1982, 62, 491–496.

[511] Marazza, G; Pham, HC; Scharer, L; et al. Incidence of bullous pemphigoid and pemphigus in Switzerland: a 2-year prospective study. *Br J Dermatol*, 2009, 161(4), 861–8.

[512] Michailidou, EZ; Belazi, MA; Markopoulos, AK; Tsatsos, MI; Mourellou, ON; Antoniades, DZ. Epidemiologic survey of pemphigus vulgaris with oralmanifestations in northern Greece: retrospective studyof 129 patients. *Int J Dermatol*, 2007, 46(4), 356–61.

[513] Pisanti, S; Sharav, Y; Kaufman, E; Posner, LN. Pemphigus vulgaris: incidence in Jews of differentethnic groups, according to age, sex, and initial lesion. *Oral Surg Oral Med Oral Pathol*, 1974, 38(3), 382–7.

[514] Simon, DG; Krutchkoff, D; Kaslow, RA; Zarbo, R. Pemphigus in Hartford County, Connecticut, from 1972 to 1977. *Arch Dermatol*, 1980, 116(9), 1035–7.

[515] Thomas, CW; et al. Selective inhibition of inflammatory gene expression in activated T lymphocytes: amechanism of immune suppression by thiopurines. *J Pharmacol Exp Ther*, 2005, 312, 537–45.

[516] Adam, BA. Bullous diseases in Malaysia, epidemiology and natural history. *Int J Dermatol*, 1992, 31(1), 42–5.

[517] Morini, JP; Jomaa, B; Gorgi, Y; et al. Pemphigus foliaceus in young women. An endemic focus in the Sousse area of Tunisia. *Arch Dermatol*, 1993, 129(1), 69–73.

[518] Tsankov, N; Vassileva, S; Kamarashev, J; Kazandjieva, J; Kuzeva, V. Epidemiology of pemphigus in Sofia, Bulgaria. A 16-year retrospective study (1980–1995). *Int J Dermatol*, 2000, 39(2), 104–8.

[519] Bertram, F; Brocker, EB; Zillikens, D; Schmidt, E. Prospective analysis of the incidence of autoimmunebullous disorders in Lower Franconia, Germany. *J Dtsch Dermatol Ges*, 2009, 7(5), 434–40.

[520] Hahn-Ristic, K; Rzany, B; Amagai, M; Brocker, EB; Zillikens, D. Increased incidence of pemphigus vulgaris in southern Europeans living in Germany comparedwith native Germans. *J Eur Acad Dermatol Venereol*, 2002, 16(1), 68–71.

[521] Bozdag, K; Bilgin, I. Epidemiology of pemphigus inthe western region of Turkey: retrospective analysis of 87 patients. *Cutan Ocul Toxicol*, 2012, 31, 280–5.

[522] Langan, SM; Smeeth, L; Hubbard, R; Fleming, KM; Smith, CJ; West, J. Bullous pemphigoid and pemphigusvulgaris—incidence and mortality in the UK: population based cohort study. *BMJ*, 2008, 337(7662), 160.

[523] Huang, YH; Kuo, CF; Chen, YH; Yang, YW. Incidence, mortality, and causes of death of patients with pemphigusin Taiwan: a nationwide population-basedstudy. *J Invest Dermatol*, 2012, 132(1), 92–7.

[524] Marinovic, B; Lipozencic, J; Jukic, IL. Autoimmuneblistering diseases: incidence and treatment in Croatia. *Dermatol Clin*, 2011, 29(4), 677–9.

[525] Groves, RW; Bhogal, B; Taghipour, K; Caposciutti, P; Saha, M. Bullous pemphigoid: is the incidence ofpemphigoid really increasing? *BMJ*, 2008, 337, a1138.

[526] Wilson, C. Pemphigus in Oxford, UK, and NewDelhi, India; a comparative study of disease characteristics and HLA antigens. *Dermatology*, 1994, 189(1), 108–10.

[527] Bickle, KM; Roark, TR; Hsu, S. Autoimmune bullous dermatoses: a review. *Am Fam Physician*, 2002, 65(9), 1861–82.

[528] Mutasim, DF. Immunobullous diseases. *J Am Acad Dermatol*, 2005, 52(6), 1029–43.

[529] Chmurova, N; Svecova, D. Pemphigus vulgaris: a 11-year review. *Bratisl Lek Listy*, 2009, 110(8), 500–3.

[530] Gorsky, M; Raviv, M; Raviv, E. Pemphigus vulgaris in adolescence: a case presentation and review of the literature. *Oral Surg Oral Med Oral Pathol*, 1994, 77(6), 620–2.

[531] Baican, A; Chiorean, R; Leucuta, DC; Baican, C; Danescu, S; Ciuce, D; Sitaru, C. Prediction of survival for patients with pemphigus vulgaris and pemphigus foliaceus: a retrospective cohort study. *Orphanet J Rare Dis*, 2015, 10, 48.

[532] Saha, M; Bhogal, B; Black, MM; Cooper, D; Vaughan, RW; Groves, RW. Prognostic factors in pemphigus vulgaris and pemphigus foliaceus. *Br J Dermatol*, 2014, 170(1), 116-22.

[533] Risser, J; Lewis, K; Weinstock, MA. Mortality of bullous skin disorders from 1979 through 2002 in theUnited States. *Arch Dermatol*, 2009, 145(9), 1005–8.

[534] Ahmed, AR; Moy, R. Death in pemphigus. *J Am Acad Dermatol*, 1982, 7(2), 221–8.

[535] Leshem, YA; Katzenelson, V; Yosipovitch, G; David, M; Mimouni, D. Autoimmune diseases in patients with pemphigus and their first-degree relatives. *Int JDermatol*, 2011, 50(7), 827–31.

[536] Wohl, Y; Dreiher, J; Cohen, AD. Pemphigus and osteoporosis: a case-control study. *Arch Dermatol*, 2010, 146(10), 1126–31.

[537] Tee, SI; Yosipovitch, G; Chan, YC; et al. Prevention of glucocorticoid-induced osteoporosis in immunobullous diseases with alendronate: a randomized, double blind, placebo-controlled study. *Arch Dermatol*, 2012, 148(3), 307–14.

[538] Diaz, LA; Sampaio, SA; Rivitti, EA; et al. Endemicpemphigus foliaceus (fogo selvagem). I. Clinical featuresand immunopathology. *J Am Acad Dermatol*, 1989, 20(4), 657–69.

[539] Robledo, MA; Prada, S; Jaramillo, D; Leon, W. South American pemphigus foliaceus: study of an epidemicin El Bagre and Nechi, Colombia 1982 to 1986. *Br J Dermatol*, 1988, 118(6), 737–44.

[540] Abreu-Velez, AM; Hashimoto, T; Bollag, WB; et al. Aunique form of endemic pemphigus in northern Colombia. *J Am Acad Dermatol*, 2003, 49(4), 599–608.

[541] Abreu-Velez, AM; Howard, MS; Jiao, Z; et al. Cardiac autoantibodies from patients affected by a new variant of endemic pemphigus foliaceus in Colombia, SouthAmerica. *J Clin Immunol*, 2011, 31(6), 985–97.

[542] Abreu-Velez, AM; Howard, MS; Yi, H; Gao, W; Hashimoto, T; Grossniklaus, HE. Neural system antigensare recognized by autoantibodies from patients affected by a new variant of endemic pemphigus foliaceusin Colombia. *J Clin Immunol*, 2011, 31(3), 356–68.

[543] Zimmermann, J; Bahmer, F; Rose, C; Zillikens, D; Schmidt, E. Clinical and immunopathological spectrumof paraneoplastic pemphigus. *J Dtsch Dermatol Ges*, 2010, 8(8), 598–605.

[544] Leger, S; Picard, D; Ingen-Housz-Oro, S; et al. Prognostic factors of paraneoplastic pemphigus. *Arch Dermatol*, 2012, 16, 1–8.

[545] Joly, P; Richard, C; Gilbert, D; et al. Sensitivity and specificity of clinical, histologic, and immunologic features in the diagnosis of paraneoplastic pemphigus. *J Am Acad Dermatol*, 2000, 43(4), 619–26.

[546] Ohyama, M; Amagai, M; Hashimoto, T; Nousari, HC;Anhalt, GJ; Nishikawa, T. Clinical phenotype and antidesmoglein autoantibody profile in paraneoplastic pemphigus. *J Am Acad Dermatol*, 2001, 44(4), 593–8.

[547] Huilgol, SC; Black, MM. Management of the immunobullous disorders. II. Pemphigus. *Clin Exp Dermatol*, 1995, 20(4), 283–93.

[548] Bédane, C; Prost, C; Thomine, E; et al. Binding of autoantibodiesis not restricted to desmosomes in pemphigus vulgaris, comparison of 14 cases of pemphigus vulgaris and 10 cases of pemphigus foliaceus studied by western immunoblot and immunoelectron microscopy. *Arch Dermatol Res*, 1996, 288(7), 343–52.

[549] Meurer, M. Oral pemphigus vulgaris: a report often cases. *Arch Dermatol*, 1977, 113(11), 1520.

[550] Sirois, DA. Diagnostic patterns and delays inpemphigus vulgaris: experience with 99 patients. *Arch Dermatol*, 2000, 136(12), 1569.

[551] Goldberg, NS; Weiss, SS. Pemphigus vulgaris of the esophagus in women. *J Am Acad Dermatol*, 1989, 21(5), 1115–8.

[552] Baykal, H. Severe eye involvement in pemphigus vulgaris. *Ophthalmologe*, 1995, 92(6), 854.

[553] Hodak, E. Conjunctival involvement in pemphigus vulgaris: a clinical, histopathological and immunofluorescence study. *Br J Dermatol*, 1990, 123(5), 615–20.

[554] Batta, K; Munday, P; Tatnall, F. Pemphigus vulgaris localized to the vagina presenting as chronic vaginal discharge. *Br J Dermatol*, 1999, 140(5), 945–7.

[555] Chan, E. Pemphigus vulgaris of the cervix andupper vaginal vault: a cause of atypical Papanicolaou smears. *Arch Dermatol*, 1998, 134(11), 1485.

[556] Malik, M; Ahmed, AR. Involvement of the femalegenital tract in pemphigus vulgaris. *Obstet Gynecol*, 2005, 106(5, Part 1), 1005.

[557] Malik, M; El Tal, AE; Ahmed, AR. Anal involvementin pemphigus vulgaris. *Dis Colon Rectum*, 2006, 49(4), 500–6.

[558] Hale, EK; Bystryn, JC. Laryngeal and nasal involvement in pemphigus vulgaris. *J Am Acad Dermatol*, 2001, 44(4), 609–11.

[559] Sami, N; Ahmed, AR. Penile pemphigus. *Arch Dermatol*, 2001, 137(6), 756.

[560] Korman, N. Pemphigus. *J Am Acad Dermatol*, 1988, 18(6), 1219–38.

[561] Udey, MC; Stanley, JR. Pemphigus—diseases of antidesmosomal autoimmunity. *JAMA*, 1999, 282(6), 572–6.

[562] Yesudian, PD. Postpemphigus acanthomata: a sign of clinical activity? *Int J Dermatol*, 1997, 36(3), 194–6.

[563] Yoshida, K. Cutaneous type pemphigus vulgaris: a rare clinical phenotype of pemphigus. *J Am Acad Dermatol*, 2005, 52(5), 839–45.

[564] Kolivras, A; Gheeraert, P; Andre, J. Nail destructionin pemphigus vulgaris. *Dermatology*, 2003, 206(4), 351–2.

[565] Berker, D. Pemphigus associated with naildystrophy. *Br J Dermatol.*, 1993, 129(4), 461–4.

[566] Robinson, ND; Hashimoto, T; Amagai, M; Chan, LS. The new pemphigus variants. *J Am Acad Dermatol*, 1999, 40, 649–71.

[567] Santi, CG; Maruta, CW; Aoki, V; et al. Pemphigus herpetiformisis a rare clinical expression of non-endemicpemphigus foliaceus: fogo selvagem and pemphigusvulgaris. *J Am Acad Dermatol*, 1996, 34(1), 40–6.

[568] Yamamoto, S; Kanekura, T; Gushi, A; et al. A case oflocalized pemphigus foliaceus. *J Dermatol*, 1996, 23, 893–5.

[569] Nousari, HC; Moresi, M; Klapper, M; Anhalt GJ. Nonendemic pemphigus foliaceus presenting as fatal bullous exfoliative erythroderma. *Cutis*, 2001, 67, 251–2.

[570] Auad, A; Castro, RM; Fraga, S; et al. The treatment of Brazilian pemphigus foliaceus (fogo selvagem). *Int J Dermatol*, 1970, 9(2), 130–6.

[571] Meyer, N; Misery, L. Geoepidemiologic considerations of auto-immune pemphigus. *Autoimmun Rev*, 2010, 9, A379–82.

[572] Penas, PF; Buezo, GF; Carvajal, I; et al. D-Penicillamine-induced pemphigus foliaceus with autoantibodies todesmoglein-1 in a patient with mixed connective tissue disease. *J Am Acad Dermatol*, 1997, 37, 121–3.

[573] Ong, CS; Cook, N; Lee, S. Drug-related pemphigus andangiotensin converting enzyme inhibitors. *Australas J Dermatol*, 2000, 41, 242–6.

[574] Lee, CW; Lim, JH; Kang, HJ. Pemphigus foliaceus induced by rifampicin. *Br J Dermatol*, 1984, 111, 619–22.

[575] Lin, R; Ladd, Jr. DJ; Powell, DJ; Way, BV. Localizedpemphigus foliaceus induced by topical imiquimodtreatment. *Arch Dermatol*, 2004, 140(7), 889–90.

[576] Cram, DL; Winkelmann, RK. Ultraviolet-induced acantholysis in pemphigus. *Arch Dermatol*, 1965, 92, 7–13.

[577] Low, GJ; Keeling, JH. Ionizing radiation-induced pemphigus: case presentations and literature review. *Arch Dermatol*, 1990, 126, 1319–23.

[578] Korman, NJ; Stanley, JR; Woodley, DT. Coexistence ofpemphigus foliaceus and bullous pemphigoid. *Arch Dermatol*, 1991, 127, 387–90.

[579] Ishiko, A; Hashimoto, T; Shimizu, H; et al. Combined features of pemphigus foliaceus and bullous pemphigoid: immunoblot and immunoelectron microscopic studies. *Arch Dermatol*, 1995, 131, 732–4.

[580] Imamura, S; Takigawa, M; Ikai, K; et al. Pemphigusfoliaceus, myasthenia gravis, thymoma and red cellaplasia. *Clin Exp Dermatol*, 1978, 3, 285–91.

[581] Ng, PP; Ng, SK; Chng, HH. Pemphigus foliaceus andoral lichen planus in a patient with systemic lupus erythematosus and thymoma. *Clin Exp Dermatol*, 1998, 23, 181–4.

[582] Kwon, HH; Kwon, IH; Chung, JH; Youn, JI. Pemphigus foliaceus associated with psoriasis during the course of narrow-band UVB therapy: a simple coincidence? *Ann Dermatol*, 2011, 23(3), S281–4.

[583] Cowley, NC; Neill, SM; Staughton, RCD. Pemphigus foliaceus and non-Hodgkin's lymphoma. *Int J Dermatol*, 1994, 33, 510–1.

[584] Rybojad, M; Leblanc, T; Flageul, B; et al. Paraneoplasticpemphigus in a child with a T-cell lymphoblastic lymphoma. *Br J Dermatol*, 1993, 128, 418–22.

[585] Ota, M; Sato-Matsumura, KC; Matsumura, T; et al. Pemphigus foliaceus and figurate erythema in a patient with prostate cancer. *Br J Dermatol*, 2000, 142, 816–8.

[586] Inaoki, M; Kodera, M; Fujimoto, A; Nousari, H; Anhalt, G; Takehara, K. Paraneoplastic pemphigus withoutantidesmoglein 3 or antidesmoglein 1 autoantibodies. *Br J Dermatol.*, 2001, 144(3), 610–3.

[587] Kawana, S; Hashimoto, T; Nishikawa, T; et al. Changesin clinical features, histologic findings, and antigen profiles with development of pemphigus foliaceus from pemphigus vulgaris. *Arch Dermatol*, 1994, 130, 1534–8.

[588] Tsuji, Y; Kawashima, T; Yokota, K; et al. Clinical andserological transition from pemphigus vulgaris topemphigus foliaceus demonstrated by desmoglein ELISA system. *Arch Dermatol*, 2002, 138, 95–6.

[589] Ishii, K; Amagai, M; Ohata, Y; et al. Development of pemphigus vulgaris in a patient with pemphigus foliaceus: antidesmoglein antibody profile shift confirmedby enzyme-linked immunosorbent assay. *J Am Acad Dermatol*, 2000, 42, 859–61.

[590] Maeda, JY; Moura, AK; Maruta, CW; et al. Changes inthe autoimmune blistering response: a clinical andimmunopathological shift from pemphigus foliaceusto bullous pemphigoid. *Clin Exp Dermatol*, 2006, 31(5), 653–5.

[591] Amerian, ML; Ahmed, AR. Pemphigus erythematosus: presentation of four cases and review of literature. *J Am Acad Derm*, 1984, 10(2), 215–22.

[592] Bruckner, N; Katz, RA; Hood, AF. Pemphigus foliaceus resembling eruptive seborrheic keratoses. *Arch Dermatol*, 1980, 116, 815–6.

[593] Kahana, M; Trau, H; Schewach-Millet, M; et al. Pemphigusfoliaceus presenting as multiple giant seborrheic keratoses. *J Am Acad Dermatol*, 1984, 11, 299–300.

[594] Metry, DW; Hebert, AA; Jordon, RE. Nonendemic pemphigus foliaceus in children. *J Am Acad Dermatol*, 2002, 46, 419–22.

[595] Ohata, C; Akamatsu, K; Imai, N; Sumimura, Y. Localized pemphigus foliaceus exclusively involving the follicular infundibulum: a novel peau d'orangeappearance. *Eur J Dermatol*, 2011, 21, 392–5.

[596] Nagao, K; Tanikawa, A; Yamamoto, N; Amagai, M. Declineof anti-desmoglein 1 IgG ELISA scores by withdrawal of D-penicillamine in drug-induced pemphigus foliaceus. *Clin Exp Dermatol*, 2005, 30(1), 43–5.

[597] Camisa, C; Helm, TN. Paraneoplastic pemphigus is adistinct neoplasia-induced autoimmune disease. *Arch Dermatol*, 1993, 129(7), 883.

[598] Nguyen, V; Ndoye, A; Bassler, K; Shultz, L; Shields, M; Ruben, B; et al. Classification, clinical manifestations, and immunopathological mechanisms of the epithelialvariant of paraneoplastic autoimmune multiorgan syndrome: a reappraisal of paraneoplastic pemphigus. *Arch Dermatol*, 2001, 137(2), 193.

[599] Kaplan, I; Hodak, E; Ackerman, L; Mimouni, D; Anhalt, GJ; Calderon, S. Neoplasms associated with paraneoplasticpemphigus, a review with emphasis on nonhematologicmalignancy and oral mucosalmanifestations. *Oral Oncol*, 2004, 40(6), 553–62.

[600] Wang, J; Zhu, X; Li, R; Tu, P; Wang, R; Zhang, L; et al. Paraneoplastic pemphigus associated with Castlemantumor: a commonly reported subtype of paraneoplasticpemphigus in China. *Arch Dermatol*, 2005, 141(10), 1285.

[601] Lemon, M; Weston, W; Huff, J. Childhood paraneoplasticpemphigus associated with Castleman's tumour. *Br J Dermatol*, 1997, 136(1), 115–7.

[602] Zhang, J; Qiao Q; Chen, X; et al. Improved outcomes after complete resection ofunderlying tumors for patients with paraneoplasticpemphigus: a single-center experience of 22 cases. *J Cancer Res Clin Oncol*, 2011, 137(2), 229–34.

[603] Lee, IJ; Kim, SC; Kim, HS; et al. Paraneoplastic pemphigus associated with follicular dendritic cell sarcoma arising from Castleman's tumor. *J Am Acad Dermatol*, 1999, 40(2), 294–7.

[604] Wang, J; Bu, D; Li, T; Zheng, R; Zhang, B; Chen, X; et al. Autoantibody production from a thymoma and a folliculardendritic cell sarcoma associated with paraneoplastic pemphigus. *Br J Dermatol*, 2005, 153(3), 558–64.

[605] Choi, PCL; To, K; Lai, FMM; Lee, TW; Yim, APC; Chan, JKC. Follicular dendritic cell sarcoma of the neck. *Cancer*, 2000, 89(3), 664–72.

[606] Kim, WY; Kim, H; Jeon, YK; Kim, CW. Follicular dendriticcell sarcoma with immature T-cell proliferation. *Hum Pathol*, 2010, 41(1), 129–33.

[607] Haeryfar, S; Hickman, HD; Irvine, KR; Tscharke, DC; Bennink, JR; Yewdell, JW. Terminal deoxynucleotidyltransferase establishes and broadens antiviral CD8+ Tcell immunodominance hierarchies. *J Immunol*, 2008, 181(1), 649.

[608] Kedzierska, K; Thomas, PG; Venturi, V; Davenport, MP; Doherty, PC; Turner, SJ; et al. Terminal deoxynucleotidyltransferase is required for the establishment of privatevirus-specific CD8+ T-cell receptor repertoires andfacilitates optimal CTL responses. *J Immunol*, 2008, 181(4), 2556.

[609] Rosen, D; Lee, JH; Cuttitta, F; Rafiqi, F; Degan, S; Sunday, ME. Accelerated thymic maturation and autoreactiveT cells in bronchopulmonary dysplasia. *Am JRespir Crit Care Med*, 2006, 174(1), 75.

[610] Wang, L; Bu, D; Yang, Y; Chen, X; Zhu, X. Castleman'stumours and production of autoantibody in paraneoplasticpemphigus. *Lancet*, 2004, 363(9408), 525–31.
[611] Sklavounou, A; Laskaris, G. Paraneoplastic pemphigus: a review. *Oral Oncol*, 1998, 34(6), 437–40.
[612] Fullerton, S; Woodley, DT; Smoller, BR; Anhalt, GJ. Paraneoplastic pemphigus with autoantibody depositionin bronchial epithelium after autologous bonemarrow transplantation. *JAMA*, 1992, 267(11), 1500.
[613] Fried, R; Lynfield, Y; Vitale, P; Anhalt, G. Paraneoplasticpemphigus appearing as bullous pemphigoid-like eruption after palliative radiation therapy. *J Am Acad Dermatol*, 1993, 29(5), 815–7.
[614] Hashimoto, T; Maciejewskab, B; Amagaid, M; Anhalte, GJ; Jablonskaa S. Paraneoplastic pemphigus associated with Castleman tumor, myasthenia gravis and bronchiolitis obliterans. *J Am Acad Dermatol*, 1999, 41(3), 393–400.
[615] Powell, A; Albert, S; Oyama, N; Sakuma-Oyama, Y; Bhogal, B; Black M. Paraneoplastic pemphigus secondaryto fludarabine evolving into unusual oral pemphigus vegetans. *J Eur Acad Dermatol Venereol*, 2004, 18(3), 360–4.
[616] Sapadin, A; Anhalt, G. Paraneoplastic pemphigus with a pemphigus vegetans-like plaque as the only cutaneous manifestation. *J Am Acad Dermatol.*, 1998, 39(5), 867–71.
[617] Camisa, C; Helm, TN; Liu, YC; et al. Paraneoplastic pemphigus: a report of three cases including one long-term survivor. *J Am Acad Dermatol*, 1992, 27(4), 547–53.
[618] Wadhera, A; Maverakis, E; Mitsiades, N; Lara, PN; Fung, MA; Lynch, PJ. Thymoma-associated multiorgan autoimmunity: a graft-versus-host–like disease. *J Am Acad Dermatol*, 2007, 57(4), 683–9.
[619] Cummins, DL; Mimouni, D; Tzu, J; Owens, N; Anhalt, GJ; Meyerle, JH. Lichenoid paraneoplastic pemphigusin the absence of detectable antibodies. *J Am Acad Dermatol*, 2007, 56(1), 153–9.
[620] Preisz, K; Horvath, A; Sardy, M; et al. Exacerbation of paraneoplastic pemphigus by cyclophosphamide treatment: detection of novel autoantigens and bronchial autoantibodies. *Br J Dermatol*, 2004, 150(5), 1018–24.
[621] Czernik, A; Camilleri, M; Pittelkow, MR; Grando, SA. Paraneoplastic autoimmune multiorgan syndrome: 20 years after. *Int J Dermatol*, 2011, 50(8), 905–14.
[622] Wakahara, M; Kiyohara, T; Kumakiri, M; et al. Paraneoplastic pemphigus with wide spread mucosal involvement. *Acta DermVenereol*, 2005, 85(6), 530.
[623] Miida, H; Kazama, T; Inomata, N; et al. Severe gastrointestinal involvement inparaneoplastic pemphigus. *Eur J Dermatol*, 2006, 16, 420–2.
[624] Nousari, HC; Brodsky, RA; Jones, RJ; Grever, MR; Anhalt, GJ. Immunablative high-dose cyclophosphamide without stem cell rescue in paraneoplastic pemphigus: report of a case and review of this new therapyfor severe autoimmune disease. *J Am Acad Dermatol*, 1999, 40, 750–4.
[625] Qian, SX; Li, JY; Hong, M; Xu, W; Qiu, H. Non hematological autoimmunity (glomerulosclerosis; paraneoplastic pemphigus and paraneoplastic neurological syndrome) in a patient with chronic lymphocyticleukemia: diagnosis, prognosis and management. *Leuk Res*, 2009, 33(3), 500.
[626] Hayanga, AJ; Lee, TM; Pannucci, CJ; et al. Paraneoplastic pemphigus in aburn intensive care unit: case report and review of the literature. *J Burn Care Res*, 2010, 31(5), 826.

[627] Woodrow, JP; Shlobin, OA; Barnett, SD; Burton, N; Nathan, SD. Comparison of bronchiolitis obliterans syndrome to other forms of chronic lung allograftdys function after lung transplantation. *J Heart Lung Transplant*, 2010, 29(10), 1159–64.

[628] Maldonado, F; Pittelkow, MR; Ryu, JH. Constrictivebronchiolitis associated with paraneoplastic autoimmunemulti-organ syndrome. *Respirology*, 2009, 14(1), 129–33.

[629] Wang, J; Bu, D; Zhu, X. Immunoglobulin variable region gene analysis to the autoantibody-secreting Bcells from tumors in association with paraneoplasticautoimmune multiorgan syndrome. *Int J Dermatol*, 2007, 46(11), 1146–54.

[630] Helou, J; Allbritton, J; Anhalt, GJ. Accuracy of indirect immunofluorescence testing in the diagnosis of paraneoplastic pemphigus. *J Am Acad Dermatol*, 1995, 32(3), 441–7.

[631] Probst, C; Schlumberger, W; Stocker, W; et al. Development of ELISA for the specific determination of autoantibodies against envoplakin and periplakin in paraneoplastic pemphigus. *Clin Chim Acta*, 2009, 410(1–2), 13–8.

[632] Ishii, N; Hamada, T; Koga, H; Sogame, R; Ohyama, B; Fukuda, S; et al. Decline of disease activity and autoantibodiesto desmoglein 3 and envoplakin by oralprednisolone in paraneoplastic pemphigus withbenign thymoma. *Eur J Dermatol*, 2012, 22(4), 547–9.

[633] Bennett, DD; Busick, TL. Delayed detection of autoantibodies in paraneoplastic pemphigus. *J Am Acad Dermatol*, 2007, 57(6), 1094–5.

[634] Barnadas, MA; Curell, R; Alomar, A; Gelpí, C. Paraneoplastic pemphigus with negative direct immunofluorescence in epidermis or mucosa but positive findings in adnexal structures. *J Cutan Pathol*, 2009, 36(1), 34–8.

[635] Inaoki, M; Kaji, K; Furuse, S; et al. Pemphigus foliaceusdeveloping after metastasis of cutaneous squamouscell carcinoma to regional lymph nodes. *J AmAcad Dermatol*, 2001, 45, 767–70.

[636] Brandt, O; Rafei, D; Podstawa, E; et al. Differential IgG recognition of desmoglein 3 by paraneoplastic pemphigus and pemphigus vulgaris sera. *J Invest Dermatol*, 2012, 132(6), 1738–41.

[637] Reich, K; Brinck, U; Letschert, M; et al. Graft-versus-host disease-like immunophenotypeand apoptotic keratinocyte death in paraneoplasticpemphigus. *Br J Dermatol*, 1999, 141, 739–46.

[638] Lim, YJ; Chang, SE; Choi, JH; et al. Expression of inducible nitric oxide synthasein skin lesions of acute herpes zoster. *J Dermatol Sci*, 2002, 29(3), 201–5.

[639] Iranzo, P; Xaubet, A; Carrera, C; et al. Bronchiolitis obliterans associated withparaneoplastic pemphigus: a paraneoplastic autoimmune multiorgan syndrome. *Arch Bronconeumol*, 2004, 40(5), 240–3.

[640] Horn, TD; Anhalt, GJ. Histologic features of paraneoplastic pemphigus. *Arch Dermatol*, 1992, 128(8), 1091-5.

[641] Yong, AA; Tey, HL. Paraneoplastic pemphigus. *Austral J Dermatol*, 2015, 54, 241-250.

[642] Zhang, J; Qiao, QL; Chen, XX; et al. Improved outcomes after complete resection of underlying tumors for patients with paraneoplastic pemphigus: a single-center experience of 22 cases. *J Cancer Res Clin Oncol*, 2010, 14.

[643] Anhalt, GJ. Paraneoplastic pemphigus. *Adv Dermatol*, 1997, 12, 77–96, discussion 7.

[644] Hohwy, T; Bang, K; Steiniche, T; Peterslund, NA; d'Amore, F. Alemtuzumab-induced remission of both severe paraneoplastic pemphigus and leukaemic bone marrow infiltration in a case of treatment-resistantB-cell chronic lymphocytic leukaemia. *Eur J Haematol*, 2004, 73(3), 206–9.

[645] Borradori, L; Lombardi, T; Samson, J; Girardet, C; Saurat, JH; Hugli, A. Anti-CD20 monoclonal antibody (rituximab) for refractory erosive stomatitis secondary toCD20+ follicular lymphoma-associated paraneoplasticpemphigus. *Arch Dermatol*, 2001, 137(3), 269.

[646] Heizmann, M; Itin, P; Wernli, M; Borradori, L; Bargetzi, M. Successful treatment of paraneoplastic pemphigusin follicular NHL with rituximab: report of a case andreview of treatment for paraneoplastic pemphigus inNHL and CLL. *Am J Hematol*, 2001, 66(2), 142–4.

[647] Barnadas, M; Roe, E; Brunet, S; et al. Therapy of paraneoplastic pemphiguswith Rituximab, a case report and review of literature. *J Eur Acad Dermatol Venereol*, 2006, 20(1), 69–74.

[648] Grando, S. New approaches to the treatment of pemphigus. *J Invest Dermatol Symp Proc*, 2004, 9, 84–91.

[649] Ekbäck, M; Uggla, B. Paraneoplastic pemphigus associated with chronic lymphocytic leukaemia: treatment with alemtuzumab. *Leuk Res*, 2012, 36, e190–1.

[650] Kimyai-Asadi, A; Jih, MH. Paraneoplastic pemphigus. *Int J Dermatol*, 2001, 40(6), 367–72.

[651] Nousari, HC; Deterding, R; Wojtczack, H; et al. The mechanism of respiratory failure in paraneoplastic pemphigus. *N Engl J Med*, 1999, 340(18), 1406–10.

[652] Hashimoto, T; Ebihara, T; Dmochowski, M; et al. IgA antikeratinocyte surface autoantibodies from two types of intercellular IgA vesiculopustular dermatosis recognize distinct isoforms of desmocollin. *Arch Dermatol Res*, 1996, 288(8), 447–52.

[653] Hashimoto, T; Ebihara, T; Nishikawa, T. Studies of autoantigens recognized by IgA anti-keratinocyte cellsurface antibodies. *J Dermatol Sci*, 1996, 12(1), 10–7.

[654] Hashimoto, T; Yasumoto, S; Nagata, Y; Okamoto, T; Fujita, S. Clinical, histopathological and immunological distinction in two cases of IgA pemphigus. *Clin Exp Dermatol*, 2002, 27(8), 636–40.

[655] Wallach, D. Intraepidermal IgA pustulosis. *J Am Acad Dermatol*, 1992, 27(6 Pt 1), 993–1000.

[656] Gengoux, P; Tennstedt, D; Lachapelle, JM. Intraepidermalneutrophilic IgA dermatosis: pemphigus-like IgA deposits. *Dermatology*, 1992, 185(4), 311–3.

[657] Teraki, Y; Amagai, N; Hashimoto, T; Kusunoki, T; Nishikawa. T. Intercellular IgA dermatosis of childhood. Selective deposition of monomer IgA1 in the intercellular space of the epidermis. *Arch Dermatol*, 1991, 127(2), 221–4.

[658] Chorzelski, TP; Beutner, EH; Kowalewski, C; et al. IgA pemphigus foliaceus with a clinical presentation of pemphigus herpetiformis. *J Am Acad Dermatol*, 1991, 24(5 Pt 2), 839–44.

[659] Erdag, G; Qureshi, HS; Greer, KE; Patterson, JW. Immunoglobulin A pemphigus involving the perianal skin and oral mucosa: an unusual presentation. *Cutis*, 2007, 80(3), 218–20.

[660] Zaraa, I; Kerkeni, N; Sellami, M; Chelly, I; Zitouna, M; Makni, S; et al. IgG/IgA pemphigus with IgG and IgAantidesmoglein 3 antibodies and IgA antidesmoglein

1antibodies detected by enzyme-linked immunosorbent assay: a case report and review of the literature. *Int J Dermatol*, 2010, 49(3), 298–302.

[661] Kopp, T; Sitaru, C; Pieczkowski F; Schneeberger A; Fodinger D; Zillikens D; et al. (2006). IgA pemphigus—occurrence of anti-desmocollin 1 and anti-desmoglein1 antibody reactivity in an individual patient. *J Dtsch Dermatol Ges*, *4*(12), 1045–50.

[662] Kim SC; Won JH; Chung, J; Bang, DS. IgA pemphigus: report of a case with immunoelectron localizationof bound IgA in the skin. *J Am Acad Dermatol*, 1996, 34(5 Pt 1), 852–4.

[663] Carayannopoulos, L; Hexham, JM; Capra, JD. Localization of the binding site for the monocyteimmunoglobulin (Ig) A-Fc receptor (CD89) to the domain boundary between C alpha2 and C alpha3 in human IgA1. *J Exp Med*, 1996, 183(4), 1579–86.

[664] Petropoulou, H; Politis, G; Panagakis, P; Hatziolou, E; Aroni, K; Kontochristopoulos, G. Immunoglobulin apemphigus associated with immunoglobulin A gammopathy and lung cancer. *J Dermatol*, 2008, 35(6), 341–5.

[665] Hodak, E; David, M; Ingber, A; Rotem, A; Hazaz, B; Shamai-Lubovitz, O; et al. The clinical and histopathological spectrum of IgA-pemphigus—report of twocases. *Clin Exp Dermatol*, 1990, 15(6), 433–7.

[666] Ishii, N; Ishida-Yamamoto, A; Hashimoto, T. Immunolocalization of target autoantigens in IgA pemphigus. *Clin Exp Dermatol*, 2004, 29(1), 62–6.

[667] Yasuda, H; Kobayashi, H; Hashimoto, T; Itoh, K; Yamane, M; Nakamura, J. Subcorneal pustular dermatosistype of IgA pemphigus, demonstration of autoantibodies to desmocollin-1 and clinical review. *Br J Dermatol*, 2000, 143(1), 144–8.

[668] Endo, Y; Tsujioka, K; Tanioka, M; et al. Bullous dermatosis associated with IgG antibodies specific for desmocollins. *Eur J Dermatol*, 2010, 20(5), 620–5.

[669] Camisa C; Warner M. Treatment of pemphigus. *Dermatol Nurs*, 1998, 10(2), 115–8, 23–31.

[670] McLeish, KR; Miller, FN; Stelzer, GT; Wellhausen, SR. Mechanism by which methylprednisolone inhibitsacute immune complex-induced changes in vascularperme ability. *Inflammation*, 1986, 10(3), 321–32.

[671] Williams, RN; Paterson, CA. The influence of topicalcorticosteroid therapy upon polymorphonuclear leukocytedistribution, vascular integrity and ascorbate levels in endotoxin-induced inflammation of the rabbit eye. *Exp Eye Res*, 1987, 44(2), 191–8.

[672] Zurier, RB; Weissman, G. Anti-immunologic and antiinflammatory effects of steroid therapy. *Med Clin N Am*, 1973, 57(5), 1295–307.

[673] Gruss, C; Zillikens, D; Hashimoto, T; et al. Rapid response of IgA pemphigus of subcorneal pustular dermatosis type to treatment with isotretinoin. *J Am Acad Dermatol*, 2000, 43(5 Pt2), 923–6.

[674] Ruiz-Genao, DP; Hernandez-Nunez, A; Hashimoto, T; Amagai, M; Fernandez-Herrera J; Garcia-Diez, A. A case of IgA pemphigus successfully treated withacitretin. *Br J Dermatol*, 2002, 147(5), 1040–2.

[675] Howell, SM; Bessinger, GT; Altman, CE; Belnap, CM. Rapid response of IgA pemphigus of the subcornealpustular dermatosis subtype to treatment with adalimumab and mycophenolate mofetil. *J Am Acad Dermatol*, 2005, 53(3), 541–3.

[676] Mahalingam, M. Follicular acantholysis: a subtle clue to the early diagnosis of pemphigus vulgaris. *Am J Dermatopathol*, 2005, 27, 237–9.

[677] Emmerson, RW; Wilson, JE. Eosinophilic spongiosis in pemphigus. *Arch Dermatol*, 1968, 97, 252–7.

[678] Ahmed, AR; Blose, DA. Pemphigus vegetans. Neumann type and Hallopeau type. *Int J Dermatol*, 1984, 23, 135–41.

[679] Sladden, C; Kirchhof, MG; Crawford, RI. Biopsylocation for direct immunofluorescence in patients with suspected bullous pemphigoid impacts probability of a positive test result. *J Cutan Med Surg*, 2014, 18, 392–6.

[680] Jablonska, S; Chorzelski, T; Beutner, EH; et al. Herpetiform pemphigus: a variable pattern of pemphigus. *Int J Dermatol*, 1975, 14, 353–9.

[681] Kanitakis, J; Wang, YZ; Roche, P; et al. Immuno histopathological study of autoimmune pemphigus. Lack of strictly specific histological and indirect immunofluorescence criteria for paraneoplastic pemphigus. *Dermatology*, 1994, 188, 282–5.

[682] Wang, J; Kwon, J; Ding, X; Fairley, JA; Woodley, DT; Chan, LS. Nonsecretory IgA1 autoantibodies targeting desmosomal component desmoglein 3 inintraepidermal neutrophilic IgA dermatosis. *Am J Pathol*, 1997, 150, 1901–7.

[683] Borradori, L; Saada, V; Rybojad, M; et al. Oral intraepidermalIgA pustulosis and Crohn's disease. *Br J Dermatol*, 1992, 126, 383–6.

[684] Storch, WB. Ed. Immunofluorescence in Clinical Immunology. *Germany*, 2000, Pp. 231. ISBN. 978-3-7643-6182-2.

[685] Ullman, S. Immunofluorescence and diseases of the skin. *Acta Derm Venereol Suppl* (Stockh), 1988, 140, 1–31.

[686] Michel, B; Milner, Y; David, K. Preservation of tissue-fixed immunoglobulins in skin biopsies of patients with lupus erythematosus and bullous diseases-preliminary report. *J Invest Dermatol*, 1973, 59, 449–52.

[687] Vaughan Jones, SA; Salas, J; McGrath, JA; Palmer, I; Bhogal, GS; Black, MM. A retrospective analysis of tissue-fixed immunoreactants from skin biopsiesmaintained in Michel's medium. *Dermatology*, 1994, 189 Suppl 1, 131–2.

[688] Vodegel, RM; de Jong, MC; Meijer, HJ; Weytingh, MB; Pas, HH; Jonkman, MF. Enhanced diagnostic immunofluorescence using biopsies transported insaline. *BMC Dermatol*, 2004, 4, 10.

[689] Arbesman, J; Grover, R; Helm, TN; Beutner, EH. Can direct immunofluorescence testing still be accurate if performed on biopsy specimens after brief in advertent immersion in formalin? *J Am Acad Dermatol*, 2011, 65, 106–11.

[690] Beutner, EH; Lever, WF; Witebsky, E; Jordon, R; Chertock, B. Autoantibodies in pemphigus vulgaris, response to an intercellular substance of epidermis. *JAMA*, 1965, 192, 682–8.

[691] Ratnam, KV; Pang, BK. Pemphigus in remission: value of negative direct immunofluorescence in management. *J Am Acad Dermatol*, 1994, 30, 547–50.

[692] de Messias, IT; von Kuster, LC; Santamaria, J; Kajdacsy-Balla, A. Complement and antibody depositionin Brazilian pemphigus foliaceus and correlationof disease activity with circulating antibodies. *Arch Dermatol*, 1988, 124, 1664–8.

[693] Nikolskaia, OV; Nousari, CH; Anhalt, GJ. Paraneoplasticpemphigus in association with Castleman's disease. *Br J Dermatol*, 2003, 149, 1143–51.

[694] Zhou, S; Wakelin, SH; Allen, J; Wojnarowska, F. Blister fluid for the diagnosis of subepidermal immunobullousdiseases: a comparative study of basement membrane

zone autoantibodies detected in blister fluid and serum. *Br J Dermatol*, 1998, 139, 27–32.

[695] Allen, J; Shears, E; Powell, J; Wojnarowska, F. Assessment of skin basement membrane zone antibodiesin the urine of patients with acquired subepidermalimmunobullous diseases. *Br J Dermatol*, 2001, 144, 540–5.

[696] Judd, KP; Lever, WF. Correlation of antibodies in skin and serum with disease severity in pemphigus. *ArchDermatol*, 1979, 115, 428–32.

[697] Ahmed, AR; Workman, S. Presence in serum samples of 14 patients without pemphigus. *Arch Dermatol*, 1983, 119, 17–21.

[698] Creswell, SN; Black, MM; Bhogal, B; Skeete, MV. Correlation of circulating intercellular antibodytitres in pemphigus with disease activity. *Clin ExpDermatol*, 1981, 6, 477–83.

[699] Feibelman, C; Stolzner, G; Provost, TT. Pemphigusvulgaris. Superior sensitivity of monkey esophagusin the determination of pemphigus antibody. *Arch Dermatol*, 1981, 117, 561–2.

[700] Matis, WL; Anhalt, GJ; Diaz, LA; Rivitti, EA; Martins, CR; Berger, RS. Calcium enhances the sensitivity of immunofluorescence for pemphigus antibodies. *J Invest Dermatol*, 1987, 89, 302–4.

[701] Squiquera, HL; Diaz, LA; Sampaio, SA; et al. Serologic abnormalitiesin patients with endemic pemphigus foliaceus (Fogoselvagem), their relatives, and normal donors fromendemic and non-endemic areas of Brazil. *J Invest Dermatol*, 1988, 91, 189–91.

[702] Rowilson-Cunha, P; Bystryn, JC. Sensitivity of indirect immunofluorescence and immunoblotting for the detection of intercellular antibodies inendemic pemphigus foliaceus (fogo selvagem). *Int J Dermatol*, 1999, 38, 41–5.

[703] Jiao, D; Bystryn, JC. Sensitivity of indirect immunofluorescence, substrate specificity, and immunoblottingin the diagnosis of pemphigus. *J Am Acad Dermatol*, 1997, 37, 211–6.

[704] Su, WP; Oursler, JR; Muller, SA. Paraneoplastic pemphigus: a case with high titer of circulating antibasement membrane zone autoantibodies. *J Am Acad Dermatol*, 1994, 30, 841–4.

[705] Liu, AY; Valenzuela, R; Helm, TN; Camisa, C; Melton, AL; Bergfeld, WF. Indirect immunofluorescence onrat bladder transitional epithelium: a test with highspecificity for paraneoplastic pemphigus. *J Am Acad Dermatol*, 1993, 28, 696–9.

[706] Foedinger, D; Sterniczky, B; Elbe, A; Anhalt, G; Wolff, K; Rappersberger, K. Autoantibodies against desmoplakin I and II define a subset of patients witherythema multiforme major. *J Invest Dermatol*, 1996, 106, 1012–6.

[707] Mimouni, D; Foedinger, D; Kouba, DJ; Orlow, SJ; Rappersberger, K; Sciubba, JJ; et al. Mucosal dominant pemphigus vulgaris with anti-desmoplakinautoantibodies. *J Am Acad Dermatol*, 2004, 51, 62–7.

[708] Lleo, A; Invernizzi, P; Gao, B; Podda, M; Gershwin, ME. Definition of human autoimmunity—autoantibodies versus autoimmune disease. *Autoimmun Rev*, 2010, 9(5), A259–66.

[709] Cunha, PR; Barraviera, SR. Autoimmune bullous dermatoses. *An Bras Dermatol*, 2009, 84(2), 111–24.

[710] Vaughan, FL; Bernstein, IA. Molecular aspects ofcontrol in epidermal differentiation. *Mol Cell Biochem*, 1976, 12(3), 171–9.

[711] Brooke, MA; Nitoiu, D; Kelsell, DP. Cell-cell connectivity: desmosomes and disease. *J Pathol*, 2012, 226(2), 158–71.
[712] Green, KJ; Simpson, CL. Desmosomes: new perspectiveson a classic. *J Invest Dermatol*, 2007, 127(11), 2499–515.
[713] Sterk, LM; Geuijen, CA; Oomen, LC; Calafat, J; Janssen, H; Sonnenberg, A. The tetraspan molecule CD151, a novel constituent of hemidesmosomes, associates with the integr in alpha6 beta4 and may regulate the spatial organization of hemidesmosomes. *J Cell Biol*, 2000, 149(4), 969–82.
[714] Tsuruta, D; Kobayashi, H; Imanishi, H; Sugawara, K; Ishii, M; Jones, JC. Laminin-332-integrin interaction, atarget for cancer therapy? *Curr Med Chem*, 2008, 15(20), 1968–75.
[715] Koster, J; Geerts, D; Favre, B; Borradori, L; Sonnenberg, A. Analysis of the interactions between BP180, BP230, plectin and the integrin alpha6beta4 importantfor hemidesmosome assembly. *J Cell Sci*, 2003, 116(Pt2), 387–99.
[716] Koster, J; van Wilpe, S; Kuikman, I; Litjens, SH; Sonnenberg, A. Role of binding of plectin to the integrinbeta4 subunit in the assembly of hemidesmosomes. *Mol Biol Cell*, 2004, 15(3), 1211–23.
[717] Schmidt, E; Brocker, EB; Zillikens, D. Pemphigus. Loss of desmosomal cell-cell contact. *Hautarzt*, 2000, 51(5), 309–18.
[718] Fontao, L; Favre, B; Riou, S; et al. Interaction of the bullous pemphigoid antigen 1 (BP230) and desmoplakin with intermediate filaments is mediated by distinct sequences within their COOH terminus. *Mol Biol Cell*, 2003, 14(5), 1978–92.
[719] Karashima, T; Tsuruta, D; Hamada, T; et al. Interaction of plectin andintermediate filaments. *J Dermatol Sci*, 2012, 66(1), 44–50.
[720] Monshi, B; Marker, M; Feichtinger, H; et al. Pemphigus vegetans—immunopathological findings in a rare variant of pemphigus vulgaris. *J Dtsch Dermatol Ges*, 2010, 8(3), 179–83.
[721] Tsuruta, D; Kobayashi H. Recent patents in pemphigus research, prophylaxis, diagnosis and treatment in USA (1988–2006). *Recent Pat Inflamm Allergy Drug Discov*, 2007, 1(1), 77–81.
[722] Tateishi, C; Tsuruta, D; Nakanishi, T; et al. Antidesmocollin-1 antibody- positive, antidesmoglein antibody-negativepemphigus herpetiformis. *J Am Acad Dermatol*, 2010, 63(1), e8–10.
[723] Harman, KE. New laboratory techniques for theassessment of acquired immunobullous disorders. *Clin Exp Dermatol*, 2002, 27(1), 40–6.
[724] Ishii, K; Amagai, M; Hall, RP; et al. Characterization of autoantibodies in pemphigus using antigen-specific enzyme-linkedimmunosorbent assays with baculovirus-expressed recombinant desmogleins. *J Immunol*, 1997, 159(4), 2010–7.
[725] Miida, H; Fujiwara, H; Ito, M. Association betweeneffective dose of prednisolone, alone or in conjunctionwith other immunosuppressants, and titre ofanti-bullous pemphigoid 180 antibody: a retrospectivestudy of 42 cases. *Clin Exp Dermatol*, 2011, 36(5), 485–8.
[726] Lee, JB; Fumimori, T; Kurose, K; Mori, O; Hashimoto, T. A case of bullous pemphigoid successfully treated byplasmapheresis: assessment of the change in titers ofcirculating antibodies by immunoblotting and enzyme-linked immunosorbent assay. *J Dermatol*, 2003, 30(4), 326–31.

[727] Natsuga, K; Nishie, W; Shinkuma, S; et al. Circulating IgA and IgE autoantibodies in antilaminin-332 mucous membrane pemphigoid. *Br J Dermatol*, 2010, 162(3), 513–7.

[728] Dmochowski, M; Hashimoto, T; Bhogal, BS; Black, MM; Zone, JJ; Nishikawa, T. Immunoblotting studiesof linear IgA disease. *J Dermatol Sci*, 1993, 6(3), 194–200.

[729] Ohata, Y; Hashimoto, T; Nishikawa, T. Comparativestudy of autoantigens for various bullous skin diseasesby immunoblotting using different dermo-epidermal separation techniques. *Clin Exp Dermatol*, 1995, 20(6), 454–8.

[730] Kowalczyk, AP; Anderson, JE; Borgwardt, JE; Hashimoto, T; Stanley, JR; Green, KJ. Pemphigus sera recognize conformationally sensitive epitopes in theamino-terminal region of desmoglein-1. *J Invest Dermatol*, 1995, 105(2), 147–52.

[731] Nagata, Y; Karashima, T; Watt, FM; Salmhofer, W; Kanzaki, T; Hashimoto, T. Paraneoplastic pemphigussera react strongly with multiple epitopes on the various regions of envoplakin and periplakin, except for the c-terminal homologous domain of periplakin. *J Invest Dermatol*, 2001, 116(4), 556–63.

[732] Prost, C; Dubertret, L; Fosse, M; Wechsler, J; Touraine, R. A routine immuno-electron microscopic technique for localizing an auto-antibody on epidermal basementmembrane. *Br J Dermatol*, 1984, 110(1), 1–7.

[733] Prost, C; Labeille, B; Chaussade, V; Guillaume, JC; Martin, N; Dubertret, L. Immunoelectron microscopyin subepidermal autoimmune bullous diseases: a prospectivestudy of IgG and C3 bound *in vivo* in 32 patients. *J Invest Dermatol*, 1987, 89(6), 567–73.

[734] Bédane, C; Prost, C; Bernard, P; Catanzano, G; Bonnetblanc, JM; Dubertret, L. Cicatricial pemphigoidantigen differs from bullous pemphigoid antigen byits exclusive extracellular localization: a study byindirect immunoelectronmicroscopy. *J Invest Dermatol*, 1991, 97(1), 3–9.

[735] Bédane, C; McMillan, JR; Balding, SD; et al. Bullous pemphigoid and cicatricial pemphigoidautoantibodies react with ultrastructurally separable epitopes on the BP180 ectodomain: evidence that BP180 spans the lamina lucida. *J Invest Dermatol*, 1997, 108(6), 901–7.

[736] Tanaka, H; Ishida-Yamamoto, A; Hashimoto, T; et al. A novel variant ofacquired epidermolysis bullosa with autoantibodies against the central triple-helical domain of type VII collagen. *Lab Invest*, 1997, 77(6), 623–32.

[737] Ishiko, A; Shimizu, H; Masunaga, T; et al. 97-kDa linear IgA bullous dermatosis(LAD)antigen localizes to the lamina lucida ofthe epidermal basement membrane. *J Invest Dermatol*, 1996, 106(4), 739–43.

[738] Tidman, MJ; Eady, RA. Ultrastructural morphometry of normal human dermal-epidermal junction. The influence of age, sex, and body region on laminar and nonlaminar components. *J Invest Dermatol*, 1984, 83(6), 448–53.

[739] Liu, Z; Li, N; Diaz, LA. Immunopathological mechanismsof acantholysis in pemphigus vulgaris: an explanation by ultrastructural observations. *J Invest Dermatol*, 2004, 122(5), XIII–XIV.

[740] Shimizu, H; Masunaga, T; Ishiko, A; Kikuchi, A; Hashimoto, T; Nishikawa, T. Pemphigus vulgaris and pemphigus foliaceus sera show an inversely graded binding pattern to extracellular regions of desmosomesin different layers of human epidermis. *J Invest Dermatol*, 1995, 105(2), 153–9.

[741] Zhou, S; Ferguson, DJ; Allen, J; Wojnarowska, F. The location of binding sites of pemphigus vulgaris and pemphigus foliaceus autoantibodies: a postembedding immunoelectron microscopic study. *Br J Dermatol*, 1997, 136(6), 878–83.

[742] Akiyama, M; Hashimoto, T; Sugiura, M; Nishikawa, T. Ultrastructural localization of pemphigus vulgarisand pemphigus foliaceus antigens in cultured humans quamous carcinoma cells. *Br J Dermatol*, 1991, 125(3), 233–7.

[743] Kárpáti, S; Amagai, M; Prussick, R; Cehrs, K; Stanley, JR. Pemphigus vulgaris antigen, a desmoglein type of cadherin, is localized within keratinocyte desmosomes. *J Cell Biol*, 1993, 122(2), 409–15.

[744] Chorzelski, T; Biczysko, W; Dabrowski, J; Jarzabek, M. Ultrastructural localization of pemphigus autoantibodies. *J Invest Dermatol*, 1968, 50(1), 36–40.

[745] Wolff, K; Schreiner, E. Ultrastructural localization of pemphigus autoantibodies within the epidermis. *Nature*, 1971, 229(5279), 59–61.

[746] Hönigsmann, H; Holubar, K; Wolff, K; Beutner, EH. Immunochemical localization of *in vivo* boundimmunoglobulins in pemphigus vulgaris epidermis. Employment of a peroxidase-antiperoxidase multisteptechnique for light and electron microscopy. *Arch Dermatol Res*, 1975, 254(2), 113–20.

[747] Patel, HP; Diaz, LA; Anhalt, GJ; Labib, RS; Takahashi, Y. Demonstration of pemphigus antibodies on the cell surface of murine epidermal cell monolayersand their internalization. *J Invest Dermatol*, 1984, 83(6), 409–15.

[748] Wang, W; Amagai, M; Ishiko, A. Desmosome splitting is a primary ultrastructural change in the acantholysis of pemphigus. *J Dermatol Sci*, 2009, 54(1), 59–61.

[749] Diercks, GF; Pas, HH; Jonkman, MF. The ultrastructure of acantholysis in pemphigus vulgaris. *Br JDermatol*, 2009, 160(2), 460–1.

[750] Wilgram, G; Caulfield, J; Lever, W. An electronmicroscopic study of acantholysis in pemphigus vulgaris. *J Invest Dermatol*, 1961, 36(5), 373–82.

[751] Wilgram, GF; Caulfield, JB; Madgic, EB. An electronmicroscopic study of acantholysis and dyskeratos is in pemphigus foliaceus: with a special note on peculiarintracytoplasmic bodies. *J Invest Dermatol*, 1964, 43, 287–99.

[752] Hashimoto, K; Lever, WF. An electron microscopicstudy on pemphigus vulgaris of the mouth and the skin with special reference to the intercellularcement. *J Invest Dermatol*, 1967, 48(6), 540–52.

[753] Sotto, MN; Shimizu, SH; Costa, JM; De Brito, T. South American pemphigus foliaceus: electron microscopy and immunoelectron localization of boundimmunoglobulin in the skin and oral mucosa. *Br J Dermatol*, 1980, 102(5), 521–7.

[754] Hu, CH; Michel, B; Schiltz, JR. Epidermal acantholysisinduced *in vitro* by pemphigus autoantibody. An ultrastructural study. *Am J Pathol*, 1978, 90(2), 345–62.

[755] Barnett, ML; Beutner, EH; Chorzelski, TP. Organculture studies of pemphigus antibodies. II. Ultrastructural comparison between acantholytic changes *in vitro* and human pemphigus lesions. *J Invest Dermatol*, 1977, 68(5), 265–71.

[756] Lanza, A; De Rosa, A; Femiano, F; et al. Internalization of non-clustered desmoglein 1 withoutdepletion of desmoglein 1 from adhesion complexesin an experimental model of the autoimmunedisease pemphigus foliaceus. *Int J Immunopathol Pharmacol*, 2007, 20(2), 355–61.

[757] Oktarina, DA; van der Wier, G; Diercks, GF; Jonkman, MF; Pas, HH. IgG-induced clustering ofdesmogleins 1 and 3 in skin of patients withpemphigus fits with the desmoglein nonassemblydepletion hypothesis. *Br J Dermatol*, 2011, 165(3), 552–62.

[758] Costello, MJ; Jaimovich, L; Dannenberg, M. Treatment of pemphigus with corticosteroids; study of fifty-two patients. *J Am Med Assoc*, 1957, 165(10), 1249–55.

[759] Almugairen, N. Assessment of the rate of long term complete remission off therapy in patients with pemphigus treated with different regimens including medium- and high-dose corticosteroids. *J Am Acad Dermatol*, 2013, 069(4), 583–8.

[760] Dick, SE; Werth, VP. Pemphigus: a treatment update. *Autoimmunity*, 2006, 39(7), 591–9.

[761] Mimouni, D; Nousari, CH; Cummins, DL; et al. Differences and similarities among expert opinions on the diagnosis and treatment of pemphigus vulgaris. *J Am Acad Dermatol*, 2003, 49, 1059–1062.

[762] Sagi, L. The role of the rapeutic plasma exchangein pemphigus vulgaris. *J Eur Acad Dermatol Venereol*, 2011, 25(1), 82–6.

[763] Fernandes, NC; Perez, M. Treatment of pemphigusvulgaris and pemphigus foliaceus: experience with 71 patients over a 20 year period. *Rev Inst Med Trop Sao Paulo*, 2001, 43(1), 33–6.

[764] Ratnam, KV; Phay, KL; Tan, CK. Pemphigus therapy with oral prednisolone regimens. A 5-year study. *Int J Dermatol*, 1990, 29(5), 363–7.

[765] Hofmann, SC. Results of a survey of Germandermatologists on the therapeutic approaches to pemphigusand bullous pemphigoid. *J Dtsch Dermatol Ges*, 2009, 7(3), 227–33.

[766] Schmidt, E. Rituximab in autoimmune bullousdiseases: mixed responses and adverse effects. *Br J Dermatol*, 2007, 156(2), 352–6.

[767] Kasperkiewicz, M; Schmidt, E; Zillikens, D. Current therapy of the pemphigus group. *Clin Dermatol.*, 2012, 30(1), 84–94.

[768] Dehen, L. Comparative study of the developmentand prognosis of pemphigus vulgaris and seborrheicpemphigus. *Ann Dermatol Venereol*, 1993, 120(12), 874–8.

[769] Lever, WF; Schaumburg-Lever, G. Treatment of pemphigus vulgaris. Results obtained in 84 patients between 1961 and 1982. *Arch Dermatol*, 1984, 120(1), 44–7.

[770] Lapidoth, M. The efficacy of combined treatment with prednisone and cyclosporine in patients with pemphigus: preliminary study. *J Am Acad Dermatol*, 1994, 30(5 Pt 1), 752–7.

[771] Lever, WF; White, H. Treatment of pemphigus with corticosteroids. Results obtained in 46 patients over aperiod of 11 years. *Arch Dermatol*, 1963, 87, 12–26.

[772] Hashimoto, T. Treatment strategies for pemphigus vulgaris in Japan. *Expert Opin Pharmacother*, 2008, 9(9), 1519–30.

[773] Toth, GG; van de Meer, JB; Jonkman, MF. Dexamethasone pulse therapy in pemphigus. *J Eur Acad Dermatol Venereol*, 2002, 16(6), 607–11.

[774] Mentink, LF; Mackenzie, MW; Toth, GG; et al. Randomized controlled trial of adjuvant oral dexamethasone pulse therapy in pemphigus vulgaris: PEMPULS trial. *Arch Dermatol*, 2006, 142, 570–576.

[775] Aberer, W. Azathioprine in the treatment of pemphigusvulgaris. A long-term follow-up. *J Am Acad Dermatol*, 1987, 16(3 Pt 1), 527–33.

[776] Benoit Corven C. Treatment of pemphigus vulgarisby azathioprine and low doses of prednisone (Lever scheme). *Ann Dermatol Venereol*, 2003, 130(1Pt 1), 13–5.
[777] Mourellou, O. The treatment of pemphigusvulgaris. Experience with 48 patients seen over an11-year period. *Br J Dermatol*, 1995, 133(1), 83–7.
[778] Akhtar, SJ; Hasan, MU. Treatment of pemphigus: a local experience. *J Pak Med Assoc*, 1998, 48(10), 300–4.
[779] Chaidemenos, G. High dose oral prednisonevs. prednisone plus azathioprine for the treatment of oral pemphigus: a retrospective, bi-centre, comparativestudy. *J Eur Acad Dermatol Venereol*, 2011, 25(2), 206–10.
[780] Sebaratnam, D; Murrell, DF. Treatment of pemphigusvulgaris and pemphigus foliaceus. *Expert Rev Dermatol*, 2009, 4(5), 469–81.
[781] Martin, LK; Werth, VP; Villaneuva, EV; Murrell, DF. Asystematic review of randomized controlled trials forpemphigus vulgaris and pemphigus foliaceus. *J Am Acad Dermatol*, 2011, 64(5), 903–8.
[782] Anstey, A; Wakelin, S; Reynolds, N. Guidelines for prescribingazathioprine in dermatology. *Br J Dermatol*, 2004, 151(6), 1123–32.
[783] Pasricha, J; Sood, V; Minocha, Y. Treatment of pemphiguswith cyclophosphamide. *Br J Dermatol*, 1975, 93(5), 573–6.
[784] Chams-Davatchi, C; Esmaili, N; Daneshpazhooh, M; et al. Randomized controlled open-label trial of four treatment regimens for pemphigus vulgaris. *J Am Acad Dermatol*, 2007, 57, 622–8.
[785] Rose, E; Wever, S; Zilliken, D; et al. Intravenousdexamethasone- cyclophosphamide pulse therapy in comparison with oral methylprednisolone- azathioprinetherapy in patients with pemphigus vulgaris: results of amulticenter prospectively randomized study. *J Dermatol Ges*, 2005, 3 (3), 200–6.
[786] Powell, AM; Albert, S; Al Fares, S; Harman, KE; Setterfield, J; Bhogal, B; Black MM. An evaluation of the usefulness of mycophenolate mofetil in pemphigus. *Br J Dermatol*, 2003, 149, 138–45.
[787] Qin, Y; Zhang, F; Shen, B; Liu, Y; Qiu, J; Guo, Y; Fan, Y. Efficacy and safety of enteric-coated mycophenolate sodium in patients with de novo and maintenance renal transplantation. *Int J Clin Pract Suppl*, 2014, 181, 17-22.
[788] Zwerner, J; Fiorentino, D. Mycophenolate mofetil. *Dermatol Ther*, 2007, 20(4), 229–38.
[789] Nousari, H; Anhalt, G. Pemphigus and bullous pemphigoid. *Lancet*, 1999, 354, 667–72.
[790] Orvis, AK; Wesson, SK; Breza, Jr TS; Church, AA; Mitchell, CL; Watkins, SW. Mycophenolate mofetil indermatology. *J Am Acad Dermatol*, 2009, 60, 183–99, quiz 200–182.
[791] Mimouni, D. Treatment of pemphigus vulgaris and pemphigus foliaceus with mycophenolatemofetil. *Arch Dermatol*, 2003, 139(6), 739.
[792] Scheinfeld, N. Red blood cell anemia in a patient withpemphigus vulgaris induced by the use of mycophenolatemofetil and prednisone. *J Dermatol Treat*, 2007, 18(4), 243–5.
[793] Sterneck, M. Mycophenolate mofetil for preventionof liver allograft rejection: initial results of a controlled clinical trial. *Ann Transplant*, 2000, 5(1), 43–6.

[794] Lever, WF; Schaumburg-Lever, G. Immunosuppressantsand prednisone in pemphigus vulgaris: the rapeutic results obtained in 63 patients between 1961 and 1975. *Arch Dermatol*, 1977, 113(9), 1236–41.

[795] Lever, WF. Methotrexate and prednisone in pemphigusvulgaris: the rapeutic results obtained in 36 patients between 1961 and 1970. *Arch Dermatol*, 1972, 106(4), 491.

[796] Mashkilleyson, N; Mashkilleyson, A. Mucous membranemanifestations of pemphigus vulgaris. A25-year survey of 185 patients treated with corticosteroidsor with combination of corticosteroids with methotrexate or heparin. *Acta Derm Venereol*, 1988, 68(5), 413.

[797] Smith, TJ; Bystryn, JC. Methotrexate as an adjuvanttreatment for pemphigus vulgaris. *Arch Dermatol*, 1999, 135(10), 1275.

[798] Gürcan, H; Razzaque Ahmed, A. Analysis of currentdata on the use of methotrexate in the treatment of pemphigus and pemphigoid. *Br J Dermatol*, 2009, 161(4), 723–31.

[799] Chrysomallis, F. Treatment of oral pemphigusvulgaris. *Int J Dermatol*, 1994, 33(11), 803–7.

[800] Ioannides, D; Chrysomallis, F; Bystryn, JC. Ineffectiveness of cyclosporine as an adjuvant to corticosteroids in the treatment of pemphigus. *Arch Dermatol*, 2000, 136(7), 868.

[801] Bystryn, JC; Steinman, NM. The adjuvant therapy of pemphigus. An update. *Arch Dermatol*, 1996, 132(2), 203–12.

[802] Werth, VP; Fivenson, D; Pandya, AG; et al. Multicenter randomized, double blind, placebo-controlled, clinical trial of dapsone as a glucocorticoid-sparing agent in the maintenance-phase pemphigus vulgaris. *ArchDermatol*, 2008, 144(1), 25–32.

[803] Gurcan, HM; Ahmed, AR. Efficacy of dapsone in thetreatment of pemphigus and pemphigoid: analysis of current data. *Am J Clin Dermatol*, 2009, 10(6), 383–96.

[804] Calebotta, A. Pemphigus vulgaris: benefits of tetracycline as adjuvant therapy in a series of thirteen patients. *Int J Dermatol*, 1999, 38(3), 217–21.

[805] Alpsoy, E. Is the combination of tetracycline and nicotinamide therapy alone effective in pemphigus? *Arch Dermatol*, 1995, 131(11), 1339.

[806] Chaffins, ML; Collison, D; Fivenson, DP. Treatment of pemphigus and linear IgA dermatosis with nicotinamideand tetracycline: a review of 13 cases. *J Am Acad Dermatol*, 1993, 28(6), 998.

[807] Turner, MS; Sutton, D; Sauder, DN. The use of plasmapheresis and immunosuppression in the treatment of pemphigus vulgaris. *J Am Acad Dermatol*, 2000, 43(6), 1058–64.

[808] Roujeau, JC. Plasma exchange in pemphigus. Uncontrolled study of ten patients. *Arch Dermatol*, 1983, 119(3), 215–21.

[809] Tan-Lim, R; Bystryn, JC. Effect of plasmapheresis therapy on circulating levels of pemphigus antibodies. *J Am Acad Dermatol*, 1990, 22(1), 35–40.

[810] Guillaume, JC. Controlled study of plasma exchange in pemphigus. *Arch Dermatol*, 1988, 124(11), 1659–63.

[811] Braun, N; Kadar, JG; Risler, T. Therapeutic immunoadsorption—its role in clinical practice. *Transfus Sci*, 1998, 19(Suppl), 65–9.

[812] Eming, R; Hertl, M. Immunoadsorption in pemphigus. *Autoimmunity*, 2006, 39(7), 609–16.

[813] Schoen, H. Immunoapheresis in paraneoplasticpemphigus. *Arch Dermatol*, 1998, 134(6), 706–10.

[814] Luftl, M. Successful removal of pathogenic autoantibodiesin pemphigus by immunoadsorption with a tryptophan-linked polyvinylalcohol adsorber. *Br J Dermatol*, 2003, 149(3), 598–605.

[815] Frost, N. Treatment of pemphigus vulgaris with protein A immunoadsorption, case report of long- termhistory showing favorable outcome. *Ann N Y Acad Sci*, 2005, 1051, 591–6.

[816] Schneider, KM. Plasmapheresis and immunoadsorption: different techniques and their current role inmedical therapy. *Kidney Int Suppl*, 1998, 64, S61–5.

[817] Amagai, M; Ikeda, S; Shimizu, H; et al. A randomized double-blind trial of intravenousimmunoglobulin for pemphigus. *J Am Acad Dermatol*, 2009, 60(4), 595–603.

[818] Prins, C; Gelfand, EW; French, LE. Intravenousimmunoglobulin: properties, mode of action andpractical use in dermatology. *Acta Derm Venereol*, 2007, 87(3), 206–18.

[819] Zhu, KY. Intravenous immunoglobulin suppresses experimental myasthenia gravis: immunological mechanisms. *J Neuroimmunol*, 2006, 176(1–2), 187–97.

[820] Aoyama, Y. What's new in i.v. immunoglobulin therapyand pemphigus: high-dose i.v. immunoglobulintherapy and its mode of action for treatment of pemphigus. *J Dermatol*, 2010, 37(3), 239–45.

[821] Green, MG; Bystryn, JC. Effect of intravenousimmunoglobulin therapy on serum levels of IgG1and IgG4 antidesmoglein 1 and antidesmoglein 3 antibodies in pemphigus vulgaris. *Arch Dermatol*, 2008, 144(12), 1621–4.

[822] Mimouni, D. Protective effect of intravenous immunoglobulin (IVIG) in an experimental model of pemphigusvulgaris. *Clin Exp Immunol*, 2005, 142(3), 426–32.

[823] Bystryn, J; Jiao, D; Natow, S. Treatment of pemphiguswith intravenous immunoglobulin. *J Am Acad Dermatol*, 2002, 47(3), 358–63.

[824] Arnold, D; Burton, J; Shine, B; Wojnarowska, F; Misbah, S. An 'n-of-1' placebo-controlled crossover trial ofintravenous immunoglobulin as adjuvant therapy. *Br J Dermatol*, 2009, 160(5), 1098-102.

[825] Di Gaetano, N. Complement activation determines the therapeutic activity of rituximab *in vivo*. *J Immunol*, 2003, 171(3), 1581–7.

[826] Looney, RJ. B cells as a therapeutic target in autoimmune diseases other than rheumatoid arthritis. *Rheumatology (Oxford)*, 2005, 44 Suppl 2, ii13–7.

[827] Zambruno, G; Borradori, L. Rituximab immunotherapy in pemphigus: therapeutic effects beyond B-cell depletion. *J Invest Dermatol*, 2008, 128(12), 2745–7.

[828] Herrmann, G; Hunzelmann, N; Engert, A. Treatment ofpemphigus vulgaris with anti-CD20 monoclonal antibody (rituximab). *Br J Dermatol*, 2003, 148(3), 602–3.

[829] Faurschou, A; Gniadecki, R. Two courses of rituximab (anti-CD20 monoclonal antibody) for recalcitrant pemphigus vulgaris. *Int J Dermatol*, 2008, 47(3), 292–4.

[830] Hertl, M. Recommendations for the use of rituximab (anti-CD20 antibody) in the treatment of autoimmunebullous skin diseases. *J Dtsch Dermatol Ges*, 2008, 6(5), 366–73.

[831] Dupuy, A. Treatment of refractory pemphigus vulgaris with rituximab (anti-CD20 monoclonal antibody). *Arch Dermatol*, 2004, 140(1), 91–6.

[832] Morrison, LH. Therapy of refractory pemphigus vulgaris with monoclonal anti-CD20 antibody (rituximab). *J Am Acad Dermatol*, 2004, 51(5), 817–9.

[833] Bikowski, J; Pillai, R. The position not the presence of the halogen in corticosteroids infl uences potency andside effects. *Drugs Dermatol*, 2006, 5(2), 125–30.

[834] Williams, LC; Nesbitt, Jr LT. Update on systemic glucocorticosteroids in dermatology. *Dermatol Clin*, 2001, 19(1), 63–77.

[835] McClain, R; Yentzer, B; Fledman, S. Comparison of skin concentration following topical versus oral corticosteroid treatment: reconsidering the treatment of common inflammatory dermatoses. *Drugs Dermatol*, 2009, 8(12), 1076–9.

[836] Murrell, D; Daniel, B; Joly, P; et al. Definitions and outcome measures for bullous pemphigoid: recommendations by an international panel of experts. *J Am Acad Dermatol*, 2012, 66(3), 479–85.

[837] Martin, L; Agero, AL; Werth, V; et al. Interventions for Pemphigus Vulgaris and Pemphigus Foliaceus (Review). *Cochrane Database Syst Rev*, 2009, (1), CD006263.

[838] Harman, KE; Albert, S; Black, MM. Guidelines for the management of pemphigus vulgaris. *Br J Dermatol*, 2003, 149, 926–37.

[839] Lapiere, K; Caers, S; Lambert, J. A case of long standing pemphigus vulgaris on the scalp. *Dermatology*, 2004, 209, 162–3.

[840] Baykal, C; Azizlerli, G; Thoma-Uszynski, S; et al. Pemphigus vulgaris localized to the nose and cheeks. *J Am Acad Dermatol*, 2002, 47, 875–8.

[841] Dagistan, S; Goregen, M; Miloglu, O; et al. Oral pemphigus vulgaris: a case report with review of the literature. *J Oral Sci*, 2008, 50(3), 359–62.

[842] Hanna, A; Sebaratnam, D; Chee, S; et al. The development of a disease-specific quality of lifeinstrument for autoimmune bullous dermatoses: the ABQOL. *J Invest Dermatol*, 2011, 131 Suppl 2, S33.

[843] Gulko, PS; Mulloy, AL. Glucocorticoid-induced osteoporosis: pathogenesis, prevention and treatment. *Clin Exp Rheumatol*, 1996, 14, 199–206.

[844] Compston, J. Management of glucocorticoid-induced osteoporosis. *Nat Rev Rheumatol*, 2010, 6, 82–8.

[845] Stoch, SA; Saag, KG; Greenwald, M; et al. Onceweeklyoral alendronate 70mg in patients with glucocorticoidinduced bone loss: a 12 month randomizes, placebo controlled clinical trial. *J Rheumatol*, 2009, 36(8), 1705–14.

[846] Cohen, S; Levy, R; Keller, M; et al. Risendronate therapyprevents corticosteroid induced bone loss: atwelve month, multicenter, randomized, double blindplacebo controlled parallel group study. *Arthritis Rheumatol*, 1999, 42(11), 2309–18.

[847] Minden, S; Orav, J; Schildkraut, J. Hypomanic reactionsto ACTH and prednisone in treatment for multiplesclerosis. *Neurology*, 1988, 38(10), 1631–4.

[848] Patten, SB; Neutel, CI. Corticosteroid-induced adverse psychiatric effects. *Drug Saf*, 2000, 22(2), 111–22.

[849] Chau, SY; Mok, CC. Factors predictive of corticosteroidpsychosis in patients with systemic lupus erythematosus. *Neurology*, 2003, 61(1), 104–7.

[850] Keenan, P; Jacobson, M; Soleymani, R; et al. The effect onmemory of chronic prednisone treatment in patients withsystemic disease. *Neurology*, 1996, 47((6), 1396–402.

[851] Trikudanathan, S; McMahon, GT. Optimum managementof glucocorticoid treated patients. *Nat Rev Endocrinol*, 2008, 4, 62–271.

[852] Souverein, P; Berars, A; Van Staa, T. Use of oral glucocorticoids and risk of cardiovascular and cerebrovasculardisease in a population based case-control study. *Heart*, 2004, 90(8), 859–65.

[853] Lehman, JS; Murrell, DF; Camilleri, MJ; Kalaaji, AN. Infection and infection prevention in patients treated with immunosuppressive medications for autoimmune bullous disorders. *Dermatol Clin*, 2011, 29, 591–8.

[854] LoCascio, V; Bonucci, E; Imbimbo, B; et al. Boneloss in response to long-term glucocorticoid therapy. *Bone Miner*, 1990, 8(1), 39–51.

[855] Canalis, E; Mazziotti, G; Giustina, A; Bilezikian, JP. Glucocorticoid-induced osteoporosis: pathophysiology and therapy. *Osteoporos Int*, 2007, 18, 1319–28.

[856] Weinstein, RS; Nicholas, RW; Manolagas, SC. Apoptosis of osteocytes in glucocorticoid- induced osteonecrosis of the hip. *J Clin Endocrinol Metab*, 2000, 85(8), 2907.

[857] Jia, D; O'Brien, CA; Stewart, SA; Manolagas, SC; Weinstein, RS. Glucocorticoids act directly on osteoclasts to increase their life span and reduce bonedensity. *Endocrinology*, 2006, 147(12), 5592–9.

[858] Hahn, TJ; Halstead, LR; Baran, DT. Effects off short term glucocorticoid administration on intestinal calcium absorption and circulating vitamin D metabolite concentrations in man. *J Clin Endocrinol Metab*, 1981, 52(1), 111–5.

[859] Suzuki, Y; Ichikawa, Y; Saito, E; Homma, M. Importance of increased urinary calcium excretion in the development of secondary hyperparathyroidism of patients under glucocorticoid therapy. *Metabolism*, 1983, 32(2), 151–6.

[860] Bonadonna, S; Burattin, A; Nuzzo, M; et al. Chronicglucocorticoid treatment alters spontaneous pulsatileparathyroid hormone secretory dynamics in humansubjects. *Eur J Endocrinol*, 2005, 152, 199–205.

[861] Lombardi, G; Colarusso, S; Di Somma, C; Guerra, E; Tauchmanova, L; Colao, A. The role of growthhormone in glucocorticoid-induced osteoporosis. *J Endocrinol Invest*, 2008, 31(7 Suppl), 38–42.

[862] Pearce, G; Tabensky, DA; Delmas, PD; Baker, HW; Seeman, E. Corticosteroid-induced bone loss in men. *J Clin Endocrinol Metab*, 1998, 83(3), 801.

[863] Van Staa, TP; Laan, RF; Barton, IP; Cohen, S; Reid, DM; Cooper, C. Bone density threshold and other predictors of vertebral fracture in patients receiving oral glucocorticoid therapy. *Arthritis Rheum*, 2003, 48(11), 3224–9.

[864] van Staa, TP; Leufkens, HGM; Cooper, C. The epidemiology of corticosteroid-induced osteoporosis: a metaanalysis. *Osteoporos Int*, 2002, 13, 777–87.

[865] Van Staa, TP; Leufkens, HG; Abenhaim, L; Zhang, B; Cooper, C. Use of oral corticosteroids and risk of fractures. *J Bone Miner Res*, 2000, 15(6), 993–1000.

[866] Scully, C; Paes de Almedia, O; Porter, SR; et al. Pemphigus vulgaris: the manifestations and long-term management of 55 patients with oral lesions. *Br J Dermatol*, 1999, 140, 84–9.

[867] Grossman, JM; Gordon, R; Ranganath, VK; et al. American College of Rheumatology 2010 recommendations for the prevention and treatment of glucocorticoid- induced osteoporosis. *Arthritis Care Res (Hoboken)*, 2010, 62(11), 1515–26.

[868] Cruse, LM; Valeriano, J; Vasey, FB; et al. Prevalence of evaluation and treatment of glucocorticoid-induced osteoporosis in men. *J Clin Rheumatol*, 2006, 12(5), 221–5.

[869] Feldstein, AC; Elmer, PJ; Nichols, GA; Herson, M. Practice patterns in patients at risk for glucocorticoidinducedosteoporosis. *Osteoporos Int*, 2005, 16(12), 2168–74.

[870] Homik, J; Suarez-Almazor, ME; Shea, B; et al. Calcium and vitamin D for corticosteroid-induced osteoporosis. *Cochrane Database Syst Rev*, 2000, 2, CD000952.

[871] Wang, L; Manson, JE; Sesso, HD. Calcium intake andrisk of cardiovascular disease: a review of prospective studies and randomized clinical trials. *Am J Cardiovasc Drugs*, 2012, 12(2), 105–16.

[872] Richy, F; Ethgen, O; Bruyere, O; et al. Efficacy of alphacalcidol and calcitriol in primary andcorticosteroid- induced osteoporosis: a meta-analysisof their effects on bone mineral density and fracturerate. *Osteoporos Int*, 2004, 15(4), 301–10.

[873] Sambrook, PN; Kotowicz, M; Nash, P; et al. Prevention and treatment of glucocorticoid-induced osteoporosis: a comparison of calcitriol, vitamin D plus calcium, and alendronate plus calcium. *J Bone Miner Res*, 2003, 18(5), 919–24.

[874] de Nijs, RN; Jacobs, JW; Lems, WF; et al. Alendronate or alfacalcidol in glucocorticoid-induced osteoporosis. *N Engl J Med*, 2006, 355(7), 675–84.

[875] Kanis, JA; Borgstrom, F; De Laet, C; et al. Assessment of fracture risk. *Osteoporos Int*, 2005, 16, 581–9.

[876] Siris, ES; Chen, YT; Abbott, TA; et al. Bone mineraldensity thresholds for pharmacological interventionto prevent fractures. *Arch Intern Med*, 2004, 164(10), 1108–12.

[877] The International Society for Clinical Densitometry, International Osteoporosis Foundation. 2010 official positions on FRAX. (http://www.iscd.org/Visitors/pdfs/Official%20Positions%20ISCD-IOF%20FRAX.pdf).

[878] Tosteson, AN; Melton 3rd, LJ; Dawson-Hughes, B; et al. Cost-effective osteoporosis treatment thresholds: the United States perspective. *Osteoporos Int*, 2008, 19(4), 437–47.

[879] Kanis, JA; Borgstrom, F; Zethraeus, N; et al. Interventionthresholds for osteoporosis in the UK. *Bone*, 2005, 36(1), 22–32.

[880] Kanis, JA; Borgstrom, F; Johnell, O; et al. Costeffectiveness of risedronate for the treatment of osteoporosisand prevention of fractures in postmenopausalwomen. *Osteoporos Int*, 2004, 15(11), 862–71.

[881] Borgstrom, F; Johnell, O; Kanis, JA; et al. Cost effectivenessof raloxifene in the treatment of osteoporosisin Sweden: an economic evaluation based on theMORE study. *Pharmacoeconomics*, 2004, 22(17), 1153–65.

[882] Saag, KG; Emkey, R; Schnitzer, TJ; et al. Alendronate for the prevention and treatment of glucocorticoid induced osteoporosis. Glucocorticoid-Induced Osteoporosis Intervention Study Group. *N Engl J Med*, 1998, 339(5), 292–9.

[883] Homik, J; Cranney, A; Shea, B; et al. Bisphosphonates for steroid induced osteoporosis. *Cochrane Database Syst Rev*, 2000, (2), CD001347.

[884] Plotkin, LI; Weinstein, RS; Parfitt, AM; et al. Preventionof osteocyte and osteoblast apoptosis by bisphosphonates and calcitonin. *J Clin Invest*, 1999, 104, 1363–74.

[885] Weinstein, RS; Chen, JR; Powers, CC; et al. Promotion of osteoclast survival and antagonism of bisphosphonate- induced osteoclast apoptosis by glucocorticoids. *J Clin Invest*, 2002, 109, 1041–8.

[886] Wang, J; Stern, PH. Dose-dependent differential effects of risedronate on gene expression in osteoblasts. *Biochem Pharmacol*, 2011, 81(8), 1036–42.

[887] Brown, JP; Kendler, DL; McClung, MR; et al. The efficacy and tolerability of risedronate once a week forthe treatment of postmenopausal osteoporosis. *Calcif Tissue Int*, 2002, 71(2), 103–11.

[888] Reid, DM; Hughes, RA; Laan, RF; et al. Efficacy andsafety of daily risedronate in the treatment ofcorticosteroid- induced osteoporosis in men andwomen: a randomized trial. European Corticosteroid-Induced Osteoporosis Treatment Study. *J Bone MinerRes*, 2000, 15, 1006–113.

[889] Reid, DM; Devogelaer, JP; Saag, K; et al. Zoledronicacid and risedronate in the prevention and treatmentof glucocorticoid-induced osteoporosis (HORIZON): a multicenter, double-blind, double-dummy, randomizedcontrolled trial. *Lancet*, 2009, 373, 1253–63.

[890] Agrawal, Krueger DC; Engelke, JA; et al. Between mealrisedronate does not alter bone turnover in nursinghome residents. *J Am Geriatr Soc*, 2006, 54(5), 790–5.

[891] Bauer, DC; Black, D; Ensrud, K; et al. Upper gastrointestinaltract safety profile of alendronate: the fractureintervention trial. *Arch Intern Med*, 2000, 160(4), 517–25.

[892] Cardwell, CR; Abnet, CC; Cantwell, MM; et al. Exposure to oral bisphosphonates and risk of esophagealcancer. *JAMA*, 2010, 304, 657–63.

[893] Khosla, S; Burr, D; Cauley, J; et al. Bisphosphonate associated osteonecrosis of the jaw: report of a taskforce of the American Society for Bone and MineralResearch. *J Bone Miner Res*, 2007, 22(10), 1479–91.

[894] Odvina, CV; Zerwekh, JE; Rao, DS; et al. Severely suppressed bone turnover: a potential complication of alendronate therapy. *J Clin Endocrinol Metab*, 2005, 90(3), 1294–301.

[895] Park-Wyllie, LY; Mamdani, MM; Juurlink, DN; et al. Bisphosphonate use and the risk of subtrochanteric or femoral shaft fractures in older women. *JAMA*, 2011, 305(8), 783–9.

[896] Bone, HG; Hosking, D; Gevogelaer, JP; et al. Ten years' experience with alendronate for osteoporosis in postmenopausalwomen. *N Engl J Med*, 2004, 350, 1189–99.

[897] Whitaker, M; Guo, J; Kehoe, T; et al. Bisphosphonatesfor osteoporosis—where do we go from here? *N Engl J Med*, 2012, 366, 2048–51.

[898] Khosla, S; Bilezikian, JP; Dempster, DW; et al. Benefitsand risks of bisphosphonate therapy for osteoporosis. *J Clin Endocrinol Metab*, 2012, 97(7), 2272–82.

[899] Lane, NE; Sanchez, S; Modin, GW; et al. Parathyroid hormone treatment can reverse corticosteroid-induced osteoporosis. Results of a randomized controlledclinical trial. *J Clin Invest*, 1998, 102, 1627–33.

[900] Compston, JE. Skeletal actions of intermittent parathyroidhormone: effects on bone remodeling andstructure. *Bone*, 2007, 40, 1447–52.

[901] Saag, KG; Shane, E; Boonen, S; et al. Teriparatide oralendronate in glucocorticoid-induced osteoporosis. *N Engl J Med*, 2007, 357, 2028–39.

[902] Saag. KG; Zanchetta. JR; Devogelaer. JP; et al. Effects of teriparatide versus alendronate for treating glucocorticoid-induced osteoporosis: thirty-six month results of a randomized, double-blind, controlled trial. *Arthritis Rheum*, 2009, 60, 3346–55.

[903] Murad, MH; Drake, MT; Mullan, RJ; et al. Comparative effectiveness of drug treatments to prevent fragility fractures: a systematic review and network metaanalysis. *J Clin Endocrinol Metab*, 2012, 97(6), 1871–90.

[904] Sambrook, PN; Birmingham, J; Kelly, P; et al. Prevention of corticosteroid osteoporosis: a comparison of calcium, calcitriol, and calcitonin. *N Engl JMed*, 1993, 328, 1747–52.

[905] Luengo, M; Pons, F; Martinez de Osaba, JM; et al. Prevention of further bone mass loss by nasal calcitoninin patients on long term glucocorticoid therapy forasthma: a two year follow up study. *Thorax*, 1994, 49, 1099–102.

[906] Cranney, A; Welch, V; Adachi, JD; et al. Calcitonin for the treatment and prevention of corticosteroid-induced osteoporosis Cochrane review. In: The Cochrane library. Issue 2. Oxford: Update Software, 2000.

[907] Bolognese, MA; Teglbjaerg, CD; Zanchetta, JR; et al. Denosumab significantly increases DXA BMD atboth trabecular and cortical sites: results from the FREEDOM study. *J Clin Densitom*, 2013, 16(2), 147–53.

[908] Dore, RK; Cohen, SB; Lane, NE; et al. Effects of denosumab on bone mineral density and bone turnover in patients with rheumatoid arthritis receiving concurrent glucocorticoids or bisphosphonates. *Ann Rheum Dis*, 2010, 69, 872–5.

[909] Cummings, SR; Karpf, DB; Harris, F; et al. Improvement in spine bone density and reduction in risk of vertebral fractures during treatment with antiresorptive drugs. *Am J Med*, 2002, 112(4), 281–9.

[910] Lenchik, L; Keibzak, GM; Blunt, BA; et al. What is the role of serial bone mineral density measurements inpatient management? *J Clin Densitom*, 2002, 5, S29–38.

[911] Binkley, N; Bilezikian, JP; Kendler, DL; et al. Official positions of the International Society for Clinical Densitometry and Executive Summary of the 2005 position development conference. *J Clin Densitom*, 2006, 9, 4–14.

[912] Clore, JN; Thurby-Hay, L. Glucocorticoid-induced hyperglycemia. *Endocr Pract*, 2009, 15(5), 469–74.

[913] Gurwitz, JH. Glucocorticoids and the risk for initiation of hypoglycemic therapy. *Arch Intern Med*, 1994, 154(1), 97–101.

[914] Lansang, MC; Hustak, LK. Glucocorticoid-induced diabetesand adrenal suppression: how to detect and managethem. *Cleve Clin J Med*, 2011, 78(11), 748–56.

[915] Hoogwerf, B; Danese, RD. Drug selection and themanagement of corticosteroid-related diabetes mellitus. *Rheumatol Dis Clin N Am*, 1999, 25(3), 489–505.

[916] Hoogwerf, BJ; Goetz, FC. Urinary C-peptide: a simplemeasure of integrated insulin production with emphasison the effects of body size, diet, and corticosteroids. *J Clin Endocrinol Metab*, 1983, 56(1), 60–7.

[917] Ceriello, A. Oscillating glucose is more deleteriousto endothelial function and oxidative stress thanmean glucose in normal and type 2 diabetic patients. *Diabetes*, 2008, 57(5), 1349–54.

[918] Campbell, IW. Epidemiology and clinical presentation of type 2 diabetes. *Value Health*, 2000, 3 Suppl 1, 3–6.

[919] American Diabetes Association. Standards of medicalcare in diabetes—2012. *Diabetes Care*, 2012, 35 Suppl1, S11–63.

[920] Moleiro, S. Atypical response to treatment in linearIgA bullous dermatosis of childhood: revision of literature. *Dermatol Online J*, 2011, 17(6), 5.

[921] Trence, DL; Hirsch, IB. Hyperglycemic crises in diabetesmellitus type 2. *Endocrinol Metab Clin North Am*, 2001, 30(4), 817–31.

[922] Davidson, J. New-onset diabetes after transplantation: 2003 International consensus guidelines. Proceedings of an international expert panel meeting. Barcelona, Spain, 19 February 2003. *Transplantation*, 2003, 75(10), SS3–24.

[923] Attaway, A; Mersfelder, TL; Vaishnav, S; Baker, JK. Bullous pemphigoid associated with dipeptidyl peptidase IV inhibitors. A case report and review of literature. *J Dermatol Case Rep*, 2014, 8(1), 24-8.

[924] Gerstein, HC. Effects of intensive glucose loweringin type 2 diabetes. *N Engl J Med*, 2008, 358(24), 2545–59.

[925] Wysocki, AB. Evaluating and managing open skin wounds: colonization versus infection. *AACN Clin Issues*, 2002, 13(3), 382–97.

[926] Clay, T; Pandya, AG. Minimizing complications in autoimmune blistering diseases. *Dermatol Clin*, 2011, 29, 577–83.

[927] Altemus, M; Rao, B; Dhabhar, FS; Ding, W; Granstein RD. Stress-induced changes in skin barrier function in healthy women. *J Invest Dermatol*, 2001, 117(2), 309–17.

[928] Belgnaoui, FZ; Senouci, K; Chraibi, H; et al. Predisposition to infection in patients with pemphigus. Retrospective study of 141 cases. *Presse Med*, 2007, 36(11 Pt 1), 1563–9.

[929] Langan, SM; Hubbard, R; Fleming, K; et al. A population-based study of acute medical conditions associated with bullous pemphigoid. *Br J Dermatol*, 2009, 161(5), 1149–52.

[930] Savin, JA; Noble, WC. Immunosuppression and skin infection. *Br J Dermatol*, 1975, 93(1), 115–20.

[931] Robson, MC. Wound infection: a failure of wound healing caused by an imbalance of bacteria. *Surg Clin N Am*, 1997, 77(3), 637–50.

[932] Boughrara, Z; Ingen-Housz-Oro, S; Legrand, P; et al. Cutaneous infections in bullous pemphigoid patients treated with topical corticosteroids. *Ann Dermatol Venereol*, 2010, 137(5), 345–51.

[933] Tirado-Sánchez, A; Bonifaz, A; Ponce-Olivera, RM. Increasing prevalence of antimicrobial resistance among gram-negative isolates in patients with pemphigus vulgaris. *J Am Acad Dermatol*, 2014, 66, e16-8.

[934] Feldmeyer, L; Trüeb, RM; French, LE; et al. Pitfall: pemphigus herpeticatus should not be confounded with resistant pemphigus vulgaris. *J Dermatol Treat*, 2010, 21(5), 311–3.

[935] Nikkels, AF; Delvenne, P; Herfs, M; et al. Occult herpessimplex virus colonization of bullous dermatitides. *Am J Clin Dermatol*, 2008, 9(3), 163–8.

[936] Avalos-Peralta, P; Herrera, A; Rios-Martin, JJ; et al. Localized Kaposi's sarcoma in a patient with pemphigusvulgaris. *J Eur Acad Dermatol Venereol*, 2006, 20(1), 79–83.

[937] Adachi, M; Tsuruta, D; Imanishi, H; et al. Necrotizing fasciitis caused by Cryptococcus neoformans in apatient with pemphigus vegetans. *Clin Exp Dermatol*, 2009, 34(8), e751–3.

[938] Yoo, SS; Tran, M; Anhalt, G; et al. Disseminatedcellulitic cryptococcosis in the setting of prednisone monotherapy for pemphigus vulgaris. *J Dermatol*, 2003, 30(5), 405–10.

[939] Uslan, DZ; Kowalski, TJ; Wengenack, NL; et al. Skin and soft tissue infections due to rapidly growing mycobacteria: comparison of clinical features, treatment, and susceptibility. *Arch Dermatol*, 2006, 142(10), 287–92.

[940] Kawabata, E; Morita, K; Matsuyoshi, N; et al. Bilateral inguinal scrofuloderma during steroid therapy in a patient with bullous pemphigoid. *J Dermatol*, 1995, 22(8), 582–6.

[941] Steele, RW. Should immunocompromised patients have pets? *Ochsner J*, 2008, 8(3), 134–9.

[942] Fiore, AE; Uyeki, TM; Broder, K; et al. General recommendationson immunization—recommendations ofthe Advisory Committee on Immunization Practices (ACIP). National Center for Immunization and Respiratory Diseases. *MMWR Recomm Rep*, 2011, 60(2), 1–64.

[943] Harpaz, R; Ortega-Sanchez, IR; Seward, JF. Advisory Committee on Immunization Practices (ACIP), Centers for Disease Control and Prevention (CDC). Prevention of herpes zoster: recommendations of the Advisory Committee on Immunization Practices (ACIP). *MMWR Recomm Rep*, 2008, 57(RR-5), 1–30.

[944] Huang, JT; Rademaker, A; Paller, AS. Dilute bleachbaths for Staphylococcus aureus colonization inatopic dermatitis to decrease disease severity. *Arch Dermatol*, 2011, 147(2), 246–7.

[945] Craig, FE; Smith, EV; Williams, HC. Bleach baths to reduce severity of atopic dermatitis colonized by Staphylococcus. *Arch Dermatol*, 2010, 146(5), 541–3.

[946] Gerhart, JL; Kalaaji, AN. Development of Pneumocystiscarinii pneumonia in patients with immunobullous and connective tissue disease receiving immune suppressive medications. *J Am Acad Dermatol*, 2010, 62(6), 957–61.

[947] Lehman, JS; Kalaaji, AN. Role of primary prophylaxisfor pneumocystis pneumonia in patients treated withsystemic corticosteroids or other immune suppressive agents for immune-mediated dermatologic conditions. *J Am Acad Dermatol*, 2010, 63(5), 815–23.

[948] Calne, RY. The rejection of renal homografts. Inhibitionin dogs by 6-mercaptopurine. *Lancet*, 1960, 1, 417–8.

[949] Elion, GB. The purine path to chemotherapy. *Science*, 1989, 244, 41–7.

[950] Calne, RY. Renal transplantation in man: a report of five cases, using cadaveric donors. *Br Med J*, 1963, 2, 645–51.

[951] Karran, P; Attard, N. Thiopurines in current medical practice: molecular mechanisms and contributions totherapy-related cancer. *Nat Rev Cancer*, 2008, 8, 24–36.

[952] Szawlowski, PW. Azathioprine suppresses themixed lymphocyte reaction of patients with Lesch-Nyhan syndrome. *Br J Clin Pharmacol*, 1985, 20, 489–91.

[953] Uchiyama, K. Thiopurine S-methyltransferase and inosine triphosphate pyrophosphohydrolasegenes in Japanese patients with infl ammatory boweldisease in whom adverse drug reactions were induced by azathioprine/6-mercaptopurine treatment. *J Gastroenterol*, 2009, 44, 197–203.

[954] Aarbakke, J. Thiopurine biology and pharmacology. *Trends Pharmacol Sci*, 1997, 18, 3–7.

[955] Tiede, I. CD28-dependent Rac1 activation is themolecular target of azathioprine in primary human CD4+T lymphocytes. *J Clin Invest*, 2003, 111, 1133–45.

[956] Marinkovic, G. Inhibition of GTPase Rac1 in endothelium by 6-mercaptopurine results in immunosuppression in nonimmune cells: new target for an olddrug. *J Immunol*, 2014, 192, 4370–8.

[957] Yamamoto, H. NF-kappaB activation in CD27 signaling: involvement of TNF receptor-associatedfactors in its signaling and identification of functionalregion of CD27. *J Immunol*, 1998, 161, 4753–9.

[958] Aldinucci, A. Modulating dendritic cells (DC) from immunogenic to tolerogenic responses: a novelmechanism of AZA/6-MP. *J Neuroimmunol*, 2010, 218, 28–35.

[959] Krakowski, A. Pemphigus vulgaris. *Arch Dermatol*, 1969, 100, 117.

[960] Wolff, K; Schreiner, E. Immunosuppressive therapy of pemphigus vulgaris. Preliminary results of azathioprine (Imuran) treatment). *Arch Klin Exp Dermatol*, 1969, 235, 63–77.

[961] Beissert, S; Mimouni, D; Kanwar, AJ; Solomons, N; Kalia, V; Anhalt, GJ. Treating pemphigus vulgaris with prednisone and mycophenolate mofetil: a multicenter, randomized, placebo-controlled trial. *J Invest Dermatol*, 2010, 130, 2041–8.

[962] Beissert, S; Werfel, T; Frieling, U; et al. A comparison of oral methylprednisolone plusazathioprine or mycophenolate mofetil for the treatmentof pemphigus. *Arch Dermatol*, 2006, 142, 1447–54.

[963] Chams-Davatchi, C. Randomized double blindtrial of prednisolone and azathioprine, vs. prednisoloneand placebo, in the treatment of pemphigus vulgaris. *J Eur Acad Dermatol Venereol*, 2013, 27, 1285–92.

[964] Zillikens, D. IgA pemphigus foliaceus: a case report. *Dermatologica*, 1990, 181, 304–7.

[965] Frew, JW; Murrell, DF. Current management strategies in paraneoplastic pemphigus (paraneoplastic autoimmunemultiorgan syndrome). *Dermatol Clin*, 2011, 29, 607–12.

[966] Lam, S. Paraneoplastic pemphigus, cicatricial conjunctivitis, and acanthosis nigricans with pachydermatoglyphyin a patient with bronchogenic squamous cellcarcinoma. *Ophthalmology*, 1992, 99, 108–13.

[967] Verrinim A. A patient with immunological featuresof paraneoplastic pemphigus in the absence of a detectablemalignancy. *Acta Derm Venereol*, 2002, 82, 382–4.

[968] Behzad, M; Möbs, C; Kneisel, A; et al. Combined treatmentwith immunoadsorption and rituximab leads tofast and prolonged clinical remission in difficult-to-treat pemphigus vulgaris. *Br J Dermatol*, 2012, 166, 844–52.

[969] Ostensen, M. Treatment with immunosuppressive anddisease modifying drugs during pregnancy and lactation. *Am J Reprod Immunol*, 1992, 28, 148–52.

[970] Janssen, NM; Genta, MS. The effects of immunosuppressiveand anti-infl ammatory medications on fertility, pregnancy, and lactation. *Arch Intern Med*, 2000, 160, 610–9.

[971] Tendron, A. In utero exposure to immunosuppressive drugs: experimental and clinical studies. *Pediatr Nephrol*, 2002, 17, 121–30.

[972] Marder, W. In utero azathioprine exposure andincreased utilization of special educational services in children born to mothers with systemic lupus erythematosus. *Arthr Care Res (Hoboken)*, 2013, 65, 759–66.

[973] Tichy M. Life-threatening course of pemphigusvulgaris complicated by sepsis caused by azathioprine induced bone marrow suppression: successfully managedwith combination therapy. Dermatol Ther 2014, 27,183–6.

[974] Anstey, A. Pancytopenia related to azathioprine—an enzyme deficiency caused by a commongenetic polymorphism: a review. *J R Soc Med*, 1992, 85, 752–6.

[975] Otterness, D. Human thiopurine methyltransferaseharmacogenetics: gene sequence polymorphisms. *Clin Pharmacol Ther*, 1997, 62, 60–73.

[976] Kumagai, K. Allelotype frequency of the thiopurine methyltransferase (TPMT) gene in Japanese. *Pharmacogenetics*, 2001, 11, 275–8.

[977] Lennard, L. Pharmacogenetics of acute azathioprine toxicity: relationship to thiopurine methyltransferase genetic polymorphism. *Clin Pharmacol Ther*, 1989, 46, 149–54.

[978] Sumi, S. Genetic basis of inosine triphosphatepyrophosphohydrolase deficiency. *Hum Genet*, 2002, 111, 360–7.

[979] Carney, DM. Massive azathioprine overdose. Case report and review of the literature. *Am J Med*, 1974, 56, 133–6.

[980] Mahmood, K. Intentional overdose of azathioprinein a patient with systemic lupus erythematosus. *Scott Med J*, 2013, 58, e3–4.

[981] Silman, AJ. Lymphoproliferative cancer and other malignancy in patients with rheumatoid arthritistreated with azathioprine: a 20 year follow up study. *Ann Rheum Dis*, 1988, 47, 988–92.

[982] Pasternak, B. Use of azathioprine and the risk of cancer in inflammatory bowel disease. *Am J Epidemiol*, 2013, 177, 1296–305.

[983] Khan, N. Risk of lymphoma in patients with ulcerativecolitis treated with thiopurines: a nationwide retrospective cohort study. *Gastroenterology*, 2013, 145, 1007–15.

[984] Pedersen, EG. Risk of non-melanoma skin cancerin myasthenia patients treated with azathioprine. *Eur J Neurol*, 2014, 21, 454–8.

[985] Pedersen, EG. Use of azathioprine for nonthymomamyasthenia and risk of cancer: a nationwide case-control study in Denmark. *Eur J Neurol*, 2013, 20, 942–8.

[986] van den Reek, JM. Increased incidence of squamous cell carcinoma of the skin after long-term treatment with azathioprine in patients with auto-immune inflammatory rheumatic diseases. *J Eur Acad Dermatol Venereol*, 2014, 28, 27–33.

[987] Ramsay, HM. Non-melanoma skin cancer risk in the Queensland Renal transplant population. *Br J Dermatol*, 2002, 147, 950–6.

[988] O'Donovan, P. Azathioprine and UVA light generate mutagenic oxidative DNA damage. *Science*, 2005, 309, 1871–4.

[989] Hemmens, VJ; Moore, DE. Photochemical sensitizationby azathioprine and its metabolites—I.6- Mercaptopurine. *Photochem Photobiol*, 1986, 43, 247–55.

[990] Reeve, VE. Effect of immunosuppressive agents and sunscreens on UV carcinogenesis in the hairless mouse. *Aust J Exp Biol Med Sci*, 1985, 63(Pt 6), 655–65.

[991] Allison, AC. Mechanisms of action of mycophenolate mofetil. *Lupus*, 2005, 14 Suppl 1, s2–8.

[992] Allison, AC; Eugui, EM. Immunosuppressive and other effects of mycophenolic acid and an ester prodrug, mycophenolate mofetil. *Immunol Rev*, 1993, 136, 5–28.

[993] Carr, SF; Papp, E; Wu, JC; Natsumeda, Y. Characterization of human type I and type II IMP dehydrogenases. *J Biol Chem*, 1993, 268, 27286–90.

[994] Allison, AC; Eugui, EM. Mycophenolate mofetil andits mechanisms of action. *Immunopharmacology*, 2000, 47, 85–118.

[995] Cohn, RG; Mirkovich, A; Dunlap, B; Burton, P; Chiu, SH; Eugui, E; Caulfield, JP. Mycophenolic acid increases apoptosis, lysosomes and lipid droplets in human lymphoid and monocytic cell lines. *Transplantation*, 1999, 68, 411–8.

[996] Allison, AC; Almquist, SJ; Muller, CD; Eugui, EM. *In vitro* immunosuppressive effects of mycophenolic acid and an ester pro-drug, RS-61443. *Transplant Proc*, 1991, 23, 10–4.

[997] Blaheta, RA; Leckel, K; Wittig, B; et al. Mycophenolate mofetil impairs transendothelialmigration of allogeneic CD4 and CD8T-cells. *Transplant Proc*, 1999, 31, 1250–2.

[998] Morath, C; Schwenger, V; Beimler, J; Mehrabi, A; Schmidt, J; Zeier, M; Muranyi, W. Antifibrotic actions of mycophenolic acid. *Clin Transplant*, 2006, 20 Suppl 17, 25–9.

[999] Colic, M; Stojic-Vukanic, Z; Pavlovic, B; Jandric, D; Stefanoska, I. Mycophenolate mofetil inhibits differentiation, maturation and allostimulatory function ofhuman monocyte-derived dendritic cells. *Clin Exp Immunol*, 2003, 134, 63–9.

[1000] Lagaraine, C; Lebranchu, Y. Effects of immunosuppressivedrugs on dendritic cells and tolerance induction. *Transplantation*, 2003, 75, 37S–42.

[1001] Senda, M; DeLustro, B; Eugui, E; Natsumeda, Y. Mycophenolic acid, an inhibitor of IMP dehydrogenase that is also an immunosuppressive agent, suppressesthe cytokine-induced nitric oxide production in mouseand rat vascular endothelial cells. *Transplantation*, 1995, 60, 1143–8.

[1002] Bullingham, R; Monroe, S; Nicholls, A; Hale, M. Pharmacokinetics and bioavailability of mycophenolatemofetil in healthy subjects after single-doseoral and intravenous administration. *J Clin Pharmacol*, 1996, 36, 315–24.

[1003] Sweeney, MJ. Mycophenolic acid and its mechanismof action in cancer and psoriasis. *Jpn J Antibiot*, 1977, 30(Suppl), 85–92.

[1004] Bullingham, RE; Nicholls, AJ; Kamm, BR. Clinical pharmacokinetics of mycophenolate mofetil. *Clin Pharmacokinet*, 1998, 34, 429–55.

[1005] Behrend, M. Adverse gastrointestinal effects of mycophenolatemofetil: aetiology, incidence and management. *Drug Saf*, 2001, 24, 645–63.

[1006] Goldblum, R. Therapy of rheumatoid arthritis with mycophenolate mofetil. *Clin Exp Rheumatol.*, 1993, 11Suppl 8, S117–9.

[1007] Mimouni, D; Anhalt, GJ; Cummins, DL; Kouba, DJ;Thorne, JE; Nousari, HC. Treatment of pemphigus vulgaris and pemphigus foliaceus with mycophenolatemofetil. *Arch Dermatol*, 2003, 139, 739–42.

[1008] Bjarnason, I. Enteric coating of mycophenolatesodium: a rational approach to limit topical gastrointestinallesions and extend the therapeutic index ofmycophenolate. *Transplant Proc*, 2001, 33, 3238–40.

[1009] Salvadori, M; Holzer, H; de Mattos, A; Sollinger, H; Arns, W; Oppenheimer, F; Maca, J; Hall, M. Enteric coated mycophenolate sodium is therapeuticallyequivalent to mycophenolate mofetil in de novo renaltransplant patients. *Am J Transplant*, 2004, 4, 231–6.

[1010] Budde, K; Curtis, J; Knoll, G; Chan, L; Neumayer, HH; Seifu, Y; Hall, M. Enteric-coated mycophenolatesodium can be safely administered in maintenance renal transplant patients: results of a 1-year study. *Am J Transplant*, 2004, 4, 237–43.

[1011] Kobashigawa, JA; Renlund, DG; Gerosa, G; et al. Similar efficacy and safety of entericcoatedmycophenolate sodium (EC-MPS, myfortic)compared with mycophenolate mofetil (MMF) in denovo heart transplant recipients: results of a 12-month, single-blind, randomized, parallel-group, multicenter study. *J Heart Lung Transplant*, 2006, 25, 935–41.

[1012] Chan, L; Mulgaonkar, S; Walker, R; Arns, W; Ambuhl, P; Schiavelli R. Patient-reported gastrointestinal symptomburden and health-related quality of life following conversionfrom mycophenolate mofetil to enteric-coatedmycophenolate sodium. *Transplantation*, 2006, 81, 1290–7.

[1013] Sabbatini, M; Capone, D; Gallo, R; et al. EC-MPS permits lower gastrointestinal symptom burden despite higher MPA exposure in patients with severe MMF-related gastrointestinal side-effects. *Fundam Clin Pharmacol*, 2009, 23, 617–24.

[1014] Engelen, W; Verpooten, GA; Van der Planken, M; Helbert, MF; Bosmans, JL; De Broe, ME. Four cases ofred blood cell aplasia in association with the use ofmycophenolate mofetil in renal transplant patients. *Clin Nephrol*, 2003, 60, 119–24.

[1015] Arbeiter, K; Greenbaum, L; Balzar, E; Muller, T; Hofmeister, F; Bidmon, B; Aufricht, C. Reproducible erythroid aplasia caused by mycophenolate mofetil. *Pediatr Nephrol*, 2000, 14, 195–7.

[1016] Mydlarski, PR. Mycophenolate mofetil: a dermatologicperspective. *Skin Therapy Lett*, 2005, 10, 1–6.

[1017] Epinette, WW; Parker, CM; Jones, EL; Greist, MC. Mycophenolic acid for psoriasis. A review of pharmacology, long-term efficacy, and safety. *J Am Acad Dermatol*, 1987, 17, 962–71.

[1018] Simmons, WD; Rayhill, SC; Sollinger, HW. Preliminary risk-benefit assessment of mycophenolate mofetil in transplant rejection. *Drug Saf*, 1997, 17, 75–92.

[1019] Hambach, L; Stadler, M; Dammann, E; Ganser, A; Hertenstein, B. Increased risk of complicated CMV infection with the use of mycophenolate mofetil inallogeneic stem cell transplantation. *Bone Marrow Transplant*, 2002, 29, 903–6.

[1020] Sarmiento, JM; Dockrell, DH; Schwab, TR; Munn, SR; Paya, CV. Mycophenolate mofetil increases cytomegalovirusinvasive organ disease in renal transplantpatients. *Clin Transplant*, 2000, 14, 136–8.

[1021] ter Meulen, CG; Wetzels, JF; Hilbrands, LB. The influence of mycophenolate mofetil on the incidence andseverity of primary cytomegalovirus infections anddisease after renal transplantation. *Nephrol DialTransplant*, 2000, 15, 711–4.

[1022] Weber, SC; Uhlenberg, B; Raile, K; Querfeld, U; Muller, D. Polyoma virus-associated progressive multifocal leukoencephalopathy after renal transplantation: regression following withdrawal of mycophenolate mofetil. *Pediatr Transplant*, 2011, 15, E19–24.

[1023] Manfro, RC; Vedolin, L; Cantarelli, M; Oppitz, P; Antunes, AC; Rieder, CR. Progressive multifocal leukoencephalopathyin a kidney transplant recipientafter conversion to mycophenolic acid therapy. *Transpl Infect Dis*, 2009, 11, 189–90.

[1024] Lefevre, G; Queyrel, V; Maurage, CA; et al. Effective immune restoration after immunosuppressant discontinuation in a lupus patient presenting progressive multifocal leukoencephalopathy. *J Neurol Sci*, 2009, 287, 246–9.

[1025] Kitchin, JE; Pomeranz, MK; Pak, G; Washenik, K; Shupack, JL. Rediscovering mycophenolic acid: a review of its mechanism, side effects, and potential uses. *J Am Acad Dermatol*, 1997, 37, 445–9.

[1026] Mathew, TH. A blinded, long-term, randomized multicenterstudy of mycophenolate mofetil in cadaveric renaltransplantation: results at three years. Tricontinental Mycophenolate Mofetil Renal Transplantation Study Group. *Transplantation*, 1998, 65, 1450–4.

[1027] Robson, R; Cecka, JM; Opelz, G; Budde, M; Sacks, S. Prospective registry-based observational cohort study of the long-term risk of malignancies in renaltransplant patients treated with mycophenolate mofetil. *Am J Transplant*, 2005, 5, 2954–60.

[1028] O'Neill, JO; Edwards, LB; Taylor, DO. Mycophenolate mofetil and risk of developing malignancy after orthotopic heart transplantation: analysis of the transplant registry of the International Society for Heart and Lung Transplantation. *J Heart Lung Transplant*, 2006, 25, 1186–91.

[1029] Lynch, WS; Roenigk, Jr HH. Mycophenolic acid for psoriasis. *Arch Dermatol*, 1977, 113, 1203–8.

[1030] Sifontis, NM; Coscia, LA; Constantinescu, S; Lavelanet, AF; Moritz, MJ; Armenti, VT. Pregnancy outcomes insolid organ transplant recipients with exposure tomycophenolate mofetil or sirolimus. *Transplantation*, 2006, 82, 1698–702.

[1031] Le Ray, C; Coulomb, A; Elefant, E; Frydman, R; Audibert, F. Mycophenolate mofetil in pregnancy afterrenal transplantation: a case of major fetal malformations. *Obstet Gynecol*, 2004, 103, 1091–4.

[1032] Tjeertes, IF; Bastiaans, DE; van Ganzewinkel, CJ; Zegers, SH. Neonatal anemia and hydrops fetalis aftermaternal mycophenolate mofetil use. *J Perinatol*, 2007, 27, 62–4.

[1033] Anderka, MT; Lin, AE; Abuelo, DN; Mitchell, AA; Rasmussen, SA. Reviewing the evidence for mycophenolatemofetil as a new teratogen: case report andreview of the literature. *Am J Med Genet A*, 2009, 149A, 1241–8.

[1034] Gimenez, F; Foeillet, E; Bourdon, O; Weller, S; Garret, C; Bidault, R; Singlas, E. Evaluation of pharmacokinetic interactions after oral administration of mycophenolate mofetil and valaciclovir or aciclovir to healthy subjects. *Clin Pharmacokinet*, 2004, 43, 685–92.

[1035] Jones, EL; Epinette, WW; Hackney, VC; Menendez, L; Frost, P. Treatment of psoriasis with oral mycophenolic acid. *J Invest Dermatol*, 1975, 65, 537–42.

[1036] Gomez, EC; Menendez, L; Frost, P. Efficacy of mycophenolicacid for the treatment of psoriasis. *J AmAcad Dermatol*, 1979, 1, 531–7.

[1037] Enk, AH; Knop, J. Mycophenolate is effective in the treatment of pemphigus vulgaris. *Arch Dermatol*, 1999, 135, 54–6.

[1038] Chams-Davatchi, C; Nonahal Azar, R; Daneshpazooh, M; et al. Open trial of mycophenolate mofetil in thetreatment of resistant pemphigus vulgaris. *Ann Dermatol Venereol*, 2002, 129, 23–5.

[1039] Esmaili, N; Chams-Davatchi, C; Valikhani, M; Farshidfar, F; Parvaneh, N; Tamizifar, B. Treatment of pemphigus vulgaris with mycophenolate mofetil as a steroid-sparing agent. *Eur J Dermatol*, 2008, 18, 159–64.

[1040] Grundmann-Kollmann, M; Korting, HC; Behrens, S; et al. Mycophenolate mofetil: a new therapeutic option inthe treatment of blistering autoimmune diseases. *J Am Acad Dermatol*, 1999, 40, 957–60.

[1041] Baskan, EB; Yilmaz, M; Tunali, S; Saricaoglu, H. Efficacy and safety of long-term mycophenolatesodium therapy in pemphigus vulgaris. *J Eur Acad Dermatol Venereol*, 2009, 23, 1432–4.

[1042] Williams, JV; Marks, Jr JG; Billingsley, EM. Use of mycophenolate mofetil in the treatment of paraneoplastic pemphigus. *Br J Dermatol*, 2000, 142, 506–8.

[1043] Zuidema, J; Hilbers-Modderman, ESM; Merkus, FWHM. Clinical pharmokinetics of dapsone. *Clin Pharmacokinet*, 1986, 11, 299–315.

[1044] May, DG; Arns, PA; Richards, WO; et al. The disposition of dapsone in cirrhosis. *Clin Pharmacol Ther*, 1992, 51, 689–700.

[1045] Caproni, M; Antiga, E; Melani, L; et al. Guidelines for the diagnosis and treatment of dermatitis herpetiformis. *J Eur Acad Dermatol Venereol*, 2009, 23, 633–8.

[1046] Zhu, YI; Stiller, MJ. Dapsone and sulfones in dermatology: overview and update. *J Am Acad Dermatol*, 2001, 45(3), 420–34.

[1047] Mentink, LF; de Jong, MC; Kloosterhuis, GJ; et al. Coexistence of IgA antibodies to desmogleins 1 and 3 inpemphigus vulgaris, pemphigus foliaceus and paraneoplastic pemphigus. *Br J Dermatol*, 2007, 156(4), 635–41.

[1048] Winkelmann, RK; Roth, HL. Dermatitis herpetiformis with acantholysis or pemphigus with response to sulfonamides: report of two cases. *Arch Dermatol*, 1960, 82, 385–90.

[1049] Basset, N; Guillot, B; Michel, B; et al. Dapsone as initialtreatment in superficial pemphigus. Report of nine cases. *Arch Dermatol*, 1987, 123(6), 783–5.

[1050] Beutner, EH; Chorzelski, TP; Wilson, RM; et al. IgA pemphigus foliaceus. *J Am Acad Dermatol*, 1989, 20, 89–97.

[1051] Niimi, Y; Kawana, S; Kusunoki, T. IgA pemphigus: acase report and its characteristic clinical features comparedto subcorneal pustular dermatosis. *J Am Acad Dermatol*, 2000, 43(3), 546–9.

[1052] Suzuki, M; Karaube, S; Kobori, Y; et al. IgA pemphigusoccurring in a 1-month-old infant. *J Am Acad Dermatol*, 2003, 48(2 Suppl), S22–4.

[1053] Hirata, Y; Abe, R; Kikuchi, K; et al. Intraepidermal neutrophilic IgA pemphigus successfully treated with dapsone. *Eur J Dermatol*, 2011, 22(2), 282–3.

[1054] Kishimoto, K; Iwatsuki, K; Akiba, H; et al. Subcorneal pustular dermatosis-type IgA pemphigus induced by thiol drugs. *Eur J Dermatol*, 2001, 11(1), 41–4.

[1055] Gniadecki, R; Bygum, A; Clemeensen, O; et al. IgA pemphigus: the first two Scandinavian cases. *Acta Dermatol*, 2002, 82(6), 441–5.

[1056] Monshi, B; Ritcher, L; Hashimoto, T; et al. IgA pemphigus of the subcorneal pustular dermatosis type: successful therapy with a combination of dapsone andacitretin. *Hautartz*, 2012, 63(6), 482–6. Only Abstract.

[1057] Jing, Z; Quan, T; Shu-Feng, Z. Clinical pharmacology of cyclophosphamide and ifosfamide. *Curr Drug Ther*, 2006, 1, 55–84.

[1058] Sethy, P; Khandpur, S; Sharma, V. Randomized open comparative trial of dexamethasone-cyclophosphamidepulse and daily oral cyclophosphamide versus cyclophosphamide pulse and daily oral prednisolone in pemphigus vulgaris. *Indian J Dermatol Venereol Leprol*, 2009, 75(5), 476–82.

[1059] Herzberg, MS; Schiffer, M; Sullivan, J; Stapleton, K. Paraneoplastic pemphigus in two patients with B-cell non-Hodgkin's lymphoma: significant responses to cyclophosphamide and prednisolone. *Am J Hematol*, 2000, 63, 105–6.

[1060] Becker, LR; Bastian, BC; Wesselmann, U; Karls, A; Hamm, H; Bröker, EB. Paraneoplastic pemphigus treated with dexamethasone/cyclophosphamide pulse therapy. *Eur J Derm*, 1998, 8, 551–3.

[1061] Meurer, M. Immunosuppressive therapy for autoimmune bullous diseases. *Clin Dermatol*, 2012, 30, 78–83.

[1062] Monach, PA; Arnold, LM; Merkel, PA. Incidence and prevention of bladder toxicity from cyclophosphamide in the treatment of rheumatic diseases. *Arthritis Rheum*, 2010, 62(1), 9–21.

[1063] Schuchter, LM; Hensley, ML; Meropol, NJ; Winer, EP. 2002 update of recommendations for the use of chemotherapyand radiotherapy protectants: clinical practice guidelines of the American Society of Clinical Oncology. *J Clin Oncol*, 2002, 20(12), 2895–903.

[1064] Sneddon, IB. A clinical trial of tetracycline in rosacea. *Br J Dermatol*, 1966, 78(12), 649–52.

[1065] Monk, E; Shalita, A; Siegel, DM. Clinical applications of non-antimicrobial tetracyclines in dermatology. *Pharmacol Res*, 2011, 63(2), 130–45.

[1066] Viera, MH; Perez, OA; Berman, B. Incyclinide. *Drugs Fut.*, 2007, 32(3), 209.

[1067] Bastos, FFS. Tetracyclines and Pain. *Naunyn-Schmiedeberg's Arch Pharmacol*, 2012, 385(3), 225–41.

[1068] Dezube, BJ. Randomized phase II trial of matrix metalloproteinase inhibitor COL-3 in AIDS-relatedKaposi's sarcoma: an AIDS malignancy consortium study. *J Clin Oncol*, 2006, 24(9), 1389–94.

[1069] Sapadin, AN; Fleischmajer, R. Tetracyclines: nonantibiotic properties and their clinical implications. *J Am Acad Dermatol*, 2006, 54(2), 258–65.

[1070] Fivenson, DP. Nicotinamide and tetracycline therapy of bullous pemphigoid. *Arch Dermatol*, 1994, 130(6), 753.

[1071] Ozog, DM. Minocycline-induced hyperpigmentationin patients with pemphigus and pemphigoid. *Arch Dermatol*, 2000, 136(9), 1133.

[1072] Fine, JD. Management of acquired bullous skin diseases. *N Engl J Med*, 1995, 333(22), 1475–84.

[1073] Wojnarowska, F. Guidelines for the managementof bullous pemphigoid. *Br J Dermatol*, 2002, 147(2), 214–21.

[1074] Kasperkiewicz, M; Schmidt, E. Current treatment of autoimmune blistering diseases. *Curr Drug Discov Technol*, 2009, 6(4), 270.

[1075] Bhatia, N. Use of antibiotics for noninfectious dermatologicdisorders. *Dermatol Clin*, 2009, 27(1), 85–9.

[1076] Gelfand, E. Differences between IGIV products: impact on clinical outcome. *Int Immunopharmacol*, 2006, 6, 592–9.

[1077] Frauger, E; Grassi, J; Pradel, V; et al. Use of intravenous immunoglobulins in clinical practice: data from three French university hospitals. *Fund Clin Pharmacol*, 2011, 25, 753–61.

[1078] Robinson, P; Anderson, D; Brouwers, M; Feasby, T; Hume, H. Evidence-based guidelines on the use of intravenous immune globulin for hematologic and neurologic conditions. *Trans Med Rev*, 2007, 21(2), S3–8.

[1079] Smith, S; Dennington, P; Cooper, A. Use of intravenous immunoglobulin for treatment of dermatological conditions in Australia: a review. *Australas J Dermatol.*, 2010, 51, 227–37.

[1080] Sami, N; Bhol, K; Ahmed, A. Influence of IVIg therapy on autoantibody titers to desmoglein 1 in patients with pemphigus foliaceus. *Clin Immunol*, 2002, 105, 192–8.

[1081] Nousari, HC. Mycophenolate mofetil in autoimmuneand inflammatory skin disorders. *J Am Acad Dermatol*, 1999, 40(2), 265–8.

[1082] Lolis, M; Toosi, S; Czernick, A; Bystryn, J. Effect ofintravenous immunoglobulin with or without cytotoxicdrugs on pemphigus intercellular antibodies. *J Am Acad Dermatol*, 2011, 64(3), 484–9.

[1083] Feldmeyer, L; Benden, C; Haile, S; et al. Not all intravenous immunoglobulin preparations are equally well tolerated. *Acta Derm Venereol*, 2010, 90(5), 494–7.

[1084] Ballow, M. Immunoglobulin therapy: methods of delivery. *J Allergy Clin Immunol*, 2008, 122(5), 1038–9.

[1085] Carr, DR; Heffernan, MP. Innovative uses of rituximab in dermatology. *Dermatol Clin*, 2010, 28(3), 547–57.

[1086] Joly, P; Mouquet, H; Roujeau, JC; et al. A single cycle of rituximab for the treatment of severe pemphigus. *N Engl J Med*, 2007, 357(6), 545–52.

[1087] Sanz, I. Indications of rituximab in autoimmune diseases. *Drug Discov Today Ther Strateg*, 2009, 6(1), 13–9.

[1088] Maloney, DG. Phase I clinical trial using escalating single-dose infusion of chimeric anti-CD20 monoclonal antibody (IDEC-C2B8) in patients with recurrent B-cell lymphoma. *Blood*, 1994, 84(8), 2457–66.

[1089] Edwards, JC; Cambridge, G. B-cell targeting in rheumatoid arthritis and other autoimmune diseases. *Nat Rev Immunol*, 2006, 6(5), 394–403.

[1090] Schmidt, E. Rituximab in refractory autoimmune bullous diseases. *Clin Exp Dermatol*, 2006, 31(4), 503–8.

[1091] McDonald, V; Leandro, M. Rituximab in non haematological disorders of adults and its mode of action. *Br J Haematol*, 2009, 146(3), 233–46.

[1092] Onrust, SV; Lamb, HM; Balfour, JA. Rituximab. *Drugs*, 1999, 58(1), 79–88, discussion 89–90.

[1093] Horvath, B. Low-dose rituximab is effective in pemphigus. *Br J Dermatol*, 2012, 166(2), 405–12.

[1094] Winkler, U; Jensen, M; Manzke, O; Schulz, H; Diehl, V; Engert, A. Cytokine-release syndrome in patients with B-cell chronic lymphocytic leukemia and high lymphocyte counts after treatment with an anti-CD20 monoclonal antibody (rituximab, IDEC-C2B8). *Blood*, 1999, 94, 2217-24.

[1095] Arin, MJ; Hunzelmann, N. Anti-B-cell-directed immunotherapy (rituximab) in the treatment of refractory pemphigus-an update. *Eur J Dermatol*, 2005, 15, 224-30.

[1096] Lowndes, S; Darby, A; Mead, G; Lister, A. Stevens-Johnson syndrome after treatment with rituximab. *Ann Oncol*, 2002, 13, 1948-50.

[1097] Yang, H; Rosove, MH; Figlin, RA. Tumor lysis syndrome occurring after the administration of rituximab in lymphoproliferative disorders: high-grade non-Hodgkins lymphoma and chronic lymphocytic leukaemia. *Ann J Haematol*, 1999, 62, 247-50.

[1098] Bermudez, A; Marco, F; Conde, E; Mazo, E; Recio, M; Zubizaretta, A. Fatal varicella-zoster infection following rituximab and chemotherapy treatment in a patient with follicular lymphoma. *Haematologica*, 2000, 85, 894-5.

[1099] Quartier, P; Tournilhac, O; Archimbaud, C; et al. Enteroviral meningoencephalitis after anti-CD20 (rituximab) treatment. *Clin Infect Dis*, 2003, 36, 47-9.

[1100] Jourdan, E; Topart, D; Richard, B; Jourdan, J; Sotto, A. Severe autoimmune hemolytic anemia following rituximab therapy in a patient with a lymphoproliferative disorder. *Leuk Lymphoma*, 2003, 44, 889-90.

[1101] Qazilbash, MH; Qu, Z; Hosing, C; et al. Rituximab-induced acute liver failure after an allogeneic transplantation for chronic myeloid leukemia. *Am J Hematol*, 2005, 80, 43-5.

[1102] Clifford, KS; Demierre, MF. Progression of classic Kaposi's sarcoma with rituximab. *J Am Acad Dermatol*, 2005, 53, 155-7.

[1103] Dunleavy, K; Hakim, F; Kim, HK; Janik, JE; Grant, N; Nakayama, T; et al. B-cell recovery following rituximab-based therapy is associated with perturbations in stromal derived factor-1 and granulocyte homeostasis. *Blood*, 2005, 106, 795-802.

[1104] Le Roux-Villet, C; et al. Rituximab for patients withrefractory mucous membrane pemphigoid. *ArchDermatol.*, 2011, 147, 843–9.

[1105] Mercader, P. Fatal Pseudomona pneumonia followingrituximab therapy in a patient with epidermolysisbullosa acquisita. *J Eur Acad Dermatol Venereol*, 2007, 21(8), 1141–2.

[1106] Rios-Fernandez, R. Late-onset neutropenia following rituximab treatment in patients with autoimmune diseases. *Br J Dermatol*, 2007, 157(6), 1271–3.

[1107] Li, WW. Haemolytic anaemia following rituximab treatment in a patient with pemphigus vulgaris. *Br J Dermatol*, 2009, 161(1), 205–6.

[1108] Smith, MR. Rituximab (monoclonal anti-CD20 antibody): mechanism of action and resistance. *Oncogene*, 2003, 22, 7359-68.

[1109] Maloney, DG; Smith, B; Rose, A. Rituximab: mechanism of actionand resistance. *Semin Oncol*, 2002, 29(Suppl 2), 2-9.

[1110] Matsukura, S. Effect of a single-cycle alternative dosing regimen for rituximab for recalcitrant pemphigus: a case series of 9 patients. *Arch Dermatol*, 2012, 148(6), 734–9.

[1111] Diab, M. Treatment of refractory pemphigus erythematosus with rituximab. *Int J Dermatol*, 2008, 47(12), 1317–8.

[1112] Fernando, SL; O'Connor, KS. Treatment of severe pemphigus foliaceus with rituximab. *Med J Aust*, 2008, 189(5), 289–90.

[1113] Serrao, VV. Successful treatment of recalcitrant pemphigus foliaceus with rituximab. *J Eur Acad Dermatol Venereol*, 2008, 22(6), 768–70.

[1114] Sorce, M; Arico, M; Bongiorno, MR. Rituximab in refractory pemphigus vulgaris. *Dermatol Ther*, 2008, 21 Suppl 1, S6–9.

[1115] Goh, MS. Rituximab in the adjuvant treatment of pemphigus vulgaris: a prospective open-label pilot study in five patients. *Br J Dermatol*, 2007, 156(5), 990–6.

[1116] Marzano, AV. Treatment of refractory pemphigus with the anti-CD20 monoclonal antibody (rituximab). *Dermatology*, 2007, 214(4), 310–8.

[1117] Arin, MJ. Anti-CD20 monoclonal antibody (rituximab) in the treatment of pemphigus. *Br J Dermatol*, 2005, 153(3), 620–5.

[1118] Cooper, HL. Treatment of resistant pemphigus vulgaris with an anti-CD20 monoclonal antibody (Rituximab). *Clin Exp Dermatol*, 2003, 28(4), 366–8.

[1119] Virgolini, L; Marzocchi, V. Anti-CD20 monoclonal antibody (rituximab) in the treatment of autoimmune diseases. Successful result in refractory Pemphigus vulgaris: report of a case. *Haematologica*, 2003, 88(7), ELT24.

[1120] Fuertes, I. Rituximab in childhood pemphigus vulgaris: a long-term follow-up case and review of the literature. *Dermatology*, 2010, 221(1), 13–6.

[1121] Connelly, EA. Generalized erythrodermic pemphigus foliaceus in a child and its successful response to rituximab treatment. *Pediatr Dermatol*, 2007, 24(2), 172–6.

[1122] Kong, HH. Successful treatment of refractory childhood pemphigus vulgaris with anti-CD20 monoclonal antibody (rituximab). *Pediatr Dermatol*, 2005, 22(5), 461–4.

[1123] Schmidt, E. Long-standing remission of recalcitrantjuvenile pemphigus vulgaris after adjuvant therapywith rituximab. *Br J Dermatol*, 2005, 153(2), 449–51.

[1124] Ahmed, A. Use of intravenous immunoglobulin therapy in autoimmune blistering diseases. *IntImmunopharmacol*, 2006, 6, 557–78.

[1125] Cianchini, G. Treatment of severe pemphiguswith rituximab: report of 12 cases and a review of theliterature. *Arch Dermatol*, 2007, 143(8), 1033–8.

[1126] Cianchini, G. Therapy with rituximab for autoimmunepemphigus: results from a single-centerobservational study on 42 cases with long-term follow-up. *J Am Acad Dermatol*, 2012, 67(4), 617–22.

[1127] Kim, JH. Clinical efficacy of different doses of rituximab in the treatment of pemphigus: a retrospective study of 27 patients. *Br J Dermatol*, 2011, 165(3), 646–51.

[1128] Lunardon, L. Adjuvant rituximab therapy of pemphigus: a single-center experience with 31 patients. *Arch Dermatol*, 2012, 148(9), 1031–6.

[1129] Weger, W; Aberer, E. Treatment failure with rituximab in a patient with pemphigus vulgaris. *J Eur Acad Dermatol Venereol*, 2008, 22(3), 387–9.

[1130] Karampetsou, MP; Liossis, SNC; Sfikakis, PP. TNFα antagonists beyond approved indications: stories of success and prospects for the future. *Q J Med*, 2010, 103, 917-28.

[1131] Bachmann, F; Nast, A; Sterry, W; Phillips, S. Safety and efficacy of the tumor necrosis factor antagonists. *Semin Cutan Med Surg*, 2010, 29, 35-47.

[1132] Guhl, G; Diaz-Ley, B; Fernandez-Herrera, J. Off-label use of biologic agents in the treatment of dermatosis, Part 2: Etanercept, Efalizumab, Alefacept, Rituximab, Daclizumab, Basiliximab, Omalizumab y Cetuximab. *Actas Dermosifiliogr*, 2008, 99, 5-33.

[1133] Fiorentino, DF; García, MS; Rehmus, W; BoerKimball, AB. A pilot study of etanercept treatment for pemphigus vulgaris. *Arch Dermatol*, 2011, 147 (1), 117-8.

[1134] Lin, MH; Hsu, CK; Lee, JY. Successful treatment of recalcitrant pemphigus vulgaris and pemphigus vegetans with etanercept and carbon dioxide laser. *Arch Dermatol*, 2005, 141, 680-2.

[1135] Ikumi, N; Matsukawa, Y; Kuwana, Y; et al. Staphylococcus aureus sepsis after etanercept induction in a hemodialysis patient. *Hemodial Int*, 2013, 17(1), 133-5.

[1136] Díaz-Lagares, C; Pérez-Alvarez, R; García-Hernández, FJ; et al. Rates of, and risk factors for, severe infections in patients with systemic autoinmune diseases receiving biological agents off-label. *Arthritis Res Ther*, 2011, 13, R1-12.

[1137] Daulat, S; Detweiler, JG; Pandya, AG. Development of pemphigus vulgaris in a patient with psoriasis treated with etanercept. *JEADV*, 2009, 23, 441-6.

[1138] Tirado-Sánchez, A; Bonifaz, A; Montes de Oca-Sánchez, G; Ponce-Olivera, RM. Etanercept plus methotrexate: An effective combination therapy for recalcitrant pemphigus. *J Res Med Sci*, 2015, 20, 317.

[1139] Hall, R; Fairley, J; Woodley, D; Werth, V. Treatment of pemphigus vulgaris patients with infliximab and prednisone is associated with decreased autoantibodies and an increase in immature B cells. *J Investig Dermatol*, 2012, 132, S89.

[1140] Hall, RP; 3rd; Fairley, J; Woodley, D; et al. A multicentre randomized trial of the treatment of patients with pemphigus vulgaris with infliximab and prednisone compared with prednisone alone. *Br J Dermatol*, 2015, 172(3), 760-8.

[1141] Anolik, JH; Ravikumar, R; Barnard, J et al. Cutting edge: anti-tumor necrosis factor therapy in rheumatoid arthritis inhibits memory B lymphocytes via effects on lymphoid germinal centers and follicular dendritic cell networks. *J Immunol*, 2008, 180, 688–92.

[1142] El-Darouti, M; Marzouk, S; Abdel Hay, R; et al. The use of sulfasalazine and pentoxifylline (low cost antitumour necrosis factor drugs) as adjuvant therapy for thetreatment of pemphigus vulgaris: a comparative study. *Br JDermatol*, 2009, 161(2), 313–9.

[1143] Rashid, RM; Ibrahim, S; Patel, V. Painful pemphigus vulgaris. *Anesth Analg*, 2007, 104, 233.

[1144] Iraji, F; Yoosefi, A. Healing effect of pilocarpine gel 4% on skin lesions of pemphigus vulgaris. *Int J Dermatol*, 2006, 45, 743–746.

[1145] Bystryn, JC; Rudolph, JL. Pemphigus. *Lancet*, 2005, 366, 61–73.

[1146] Vun, YY; Lun, K; Strutton, G. Use of biosynthetic dressings in paraneoplastic pemphigus. *Australas J Dermatol*, 2004, 45, 133–135.

[1147] Epstein, JB; Gorsky, M; Epstein, MS; et al. Topical azathioprine in the treatment of immune-mediated chronic oral inflammatory conditions: a series of cases. *Oral Surg Oral Med Oral Pathol Oral Radiol Endod*, 2001, 91, 56–61.

[1148] Lozada-Nur, F; Miranda, C; Maliksi, R. Double-blind clinical trial of 0.05% clobetasol propionate (corrected from propionate) ointment in Orabase and 0.05% fluocinonide ointment in Orabase in the treatment of patients with oral vesiculoerosive diseases. *Oral Surg Oral Med Oral Pathol*, 1994, 77, 598–604.

[1149] Gach, JE; Ilchyshyn, A. Beneficial effects of topical tacrolimus on recalcitrant erosions of pemphigus vulgaris. *Clin Exp Dermatol*, 2004, 29, 271–272.

[1150] Martin, L; Murrell, D. Measuring the immeasurable: a systematic review of outcome measures in pemphigus. *Australas J Dermatol*, 2006, 47(Suppl1), A32–3.

[1151] Sebaratnam, D; Murrell, D. Objective scoring systemsfor disease activity in autoimmune bullous disease. *Dermatol Clin*, 2011, 29(3), 515–20.

[1152] Pfutze, M; Niedermeier, A; Hertl, M; et al. Introducinga novel Autoimmune Bullous Skin Disorder IntensityScore (ABSIS) in pemphigus. *Eur J Dermatol*, 2007, 17(1), 4–11.

[1153] Saraswat, A; Kumar, B. A new grading system for oralpemphigus. *Int J Dermatol*, 2003, 42(5), 413–4.

[1154] Pfütze, M; Eming, R; Kneisel, A; et al. Clinical andimmunological follow-up of pemphigus patients onadjuvant treatment with immunoadsorption or rituximab. *Dermatology*, 2009, 218, 237–45.

[1155] Zhong, S; Qiu, YF; Han, BB; et al. Detection of serumdesmoglein antibody level using enzyme-linkedimmunosorbent assay (ELISA) for monitoring diseaseactivity in patients with pemphigus vulgaris. *Beijing Da Xue Xue Bao*, 2011, 43, 414–5.

[1156] Souza, SR; Azulay-Abulafia, L; Nascimento, LV. Validation of the commitment index of skin andmucous membranes in pemphigus vulgaris for the clinical evaluation of patients with pemphigus vulgaris. *An Bras Dermatol*, 2011, 86(2), 284–91.

[1157] Agarwal, M; Walia, R; Kochhar, AM; et al. Pemphigus Area and Activity Score (PAAS)—a novel clinical scoring method for monitoring of pemphigus vulgaris patient. *Int J Dermatol*, 1998, 37(2), 158–9.

[1158] Herbst, A; Bystryn, JC. Patterns of remission in pemphigus vulgaris. *J Am Acad Dermatol*, 2000, 42(3), 422–7.

[1159] Mahanjan, VK; Sharma, NL; Sharma, RC; et al. Twelveyearclinico-therapeutic experience in pemphigus, aretrospective study of 54 cases. *Int J Dermatol*, 2005, 44(10), 821–7.

[1160] Harman, KE; Seed, PT; Gratian, MJ; et al. The severity of cutaneous and oral pemphigus is related to desmoglein1 and 3 antibody levels. *Br J Dermatol*, 2001, 144(4), 775–80.

[1161] Dakkak, M; Bennet, JR. A new dysphagia score withobjective validation. *J Clin Gastroenterol*, 1992, 14(2), 99–100.

[1162] Sebaratnam, D; Venugopal, S; Murrell, D. The development of an excel program to compare disease-specific instruments for assessing activity and the extent of autoimmune bullous disease. *Australas J Dermatol*, 2009, 50(Suppl2), A48.

[1163] Rapp, S; Feldman, S; Exum, M; et al. Psoriasis causes as much disability as other major medical diseases. *J Am Acad Dermatol*, 1999, 41, 401–7.

[1164] Sheffield, D; Biles, PL; Orom, H; Maixner, W; Sheps DS. Race and sex differences in cutaneous pain perception. *Psychosom Med*, 2000, 62, 517–23.

[1165] Ryan, TJ. Disability in dermatology. *Br J Hosp Med*, 1991, 46, 33–6.

[1166] Tabolli, S; Alessandroni, L; Gaido, J; Sampogna, F; Di Pietro, C; Abeni, D. Health-related quality of lifeand nail disorders. *Acta Derm Venereol*, 2007, 87, 255–9.

[1167] De Korte, J; Mombers, FM; Sprangers, MA; Bos, JD. The suitability of quality of life questionnaires for psoriasis research: a systematic literature review. *Arch Dermatol*, 2002, 138, 1221–7.

[1168] Ferrario, SR; Baiardi, P; Zotti, AM. Update on family strain questionnaire: a tool for the general screening of caregiving-related problems. *Qual Life Res*, 2004, 13, 1425–34.

[1169] Sampogna, F; Tabolli, S; Soderfeldt, B; et al. Measuring quality of life of patients with different clinical types of psoriasis using the SF-36. *Br J Dermatol*, 2006, 154, 844–9.

[1170] Masahiro, S; Shigaku, I; Yutaka, I; et al. An investigation of quality of life (QOL) of pemphigus patients in Japan (first report). *J Dermatol*, 2000, 110, 283–8.

[1171] Terrab, Z; Benchikhi, H; Maaroufi, A; et al. Quality of life and pemphigus. *Ann Dermatol Venereol*, 2005, 132, 321–8.

[1172] Mayrshofer, F; Hertl, M; Stinkraven, R; et al. Significant decrease in quality of life in patients with pemphigus vulgaris: results from the German bullous skin disease (BSD) study group. *J Dtsch Dermatol Ges*, 2005, 3, 431–5.

[1173] Kirtschig, G; Middleton, P; Bennett, C; et al. Interventions for bullous pemphigoid. *Cochrane Database Syst Rev*, 2010, (10), CD002292.

[1174] Sampogna, F; Picardi, A; Melchi, C; et al. The impact of skin diseases on patients: comparing dermatologist's opinions with research data collected on patients. *Br J Dermatol*, 2003, 148, 989–95.

[1175] Sampogna, F; Picardi, A; Chren, MM; et al. Association betweenpoorer quality of life and psychiatric morbidity inpatients with different dermatological conditions. *Psychosom Med*, 2004, 66, 620–4.

[1176] Tabolli, S; Mozzetta, A; Antinone, V; Alfani, S; Cianchini, G; Abeni, D. The health impact of pemphigus vulgaris and pemphigus foliaceus assessed usingthe medical outcomes study 36-item short form health survey questionnaire. *Br J Dermatol*, 2008, 158, 1029–34.

[1177] Paradisi, A; Sampogna, F; Di Pietro, C; et al. Quality of life assessment in patients with pemphigus using a minimum set of evaluation tools. *J Am Acad Dermatol*, 2009, 60(2), 261–9.

[1178] Apolone, G; Mosconi, P. The Italian SF-36 health survey: translation, validation and norming. *J Clin Epidemiol*, 1998, 51, 1025–36.

[1179] Darjani, A; Ghanbari, A; Sayadi Nejhad, A. Comparison of the health-related quality of life of patients suffering from pemphigus with healthy people. *J Guilan Univ Med Sci*, 2008, 17, 1–9.

[1180] Timóteo, P; Simões Marques, L; Bertoncello, D. Physiotherapy intervention promotes better quality of life for patients with pemphigus. *Rev Soc Bras Med Trop*, 2010, 43, 580–3.

[1181] Ghodsi, SZ; Chams-Davatchi, C; Daneshpazooh, M; et al. Quality of life and psychological status of patients with pemphigus vulgaris using DLQI and general health questionnaires. *J Dermatol*, 2012, 39(2), 141–4.

[1182] Tabolli, S; Pagliarello, C; Paradisi, A; et al. Burden of disease during quiescent periods in patients with pemphigus. *Br J Dermatol*, 2014, 170(5), 1087–91.

[1183] Tabolli, S; Sampogna, F; Di Pietro, C; et al. Quality of life in patients with epidermolysis bullosa. *Br J Dermatol*, 2009, 161, 869–77.

[1184] Paradisi, A; Cianchini, G; Lupi, F; et al. QoL in patients with pemphigus receiving adjuvant therapy. *Clin Exp Dermatol*, 2012, 37(6), 626–30.

[1185] Hanna, A; Sebaratnam, D; Chee, S; et al. A disease-specific quality of life instrument for autoimmune bullous diseases—the ABQOL. *Aust J Dermatol*, 2010, 52 Suppl 1, 27.

[1186] Sebaratnam, D; Chee, SN; Venugopal, S; et al. Advances in the clinical assessment of autoimmune bullous disease: the development of a disease-specific qualityof life instrument—the ABQOL. *J Invest Dermatol*, 2009, 129, 2908–23.

[1187] Sebaratnam, DF; McMillan, JR; Werth, VP; et al. Quality of life in patients with bullous dermatoses. *Clin Dermatol*, 2012, 30, 103–7.

[1188] Sampogna, F; Chren, MM; Melchi, CF; Pasquini, P;Tabolli, S; Abeni, D. Age, gender, quality of life and psychological distress in patients hospitalized with psoriasis. *Br J Dermatol*, 2006, 154, 325–31.

[1189] Sampogna, F; Sera, F; Abeni, D. IDI Multipurpose Psoriasis Research on Vital Experiences (IMPROVE) investigators. Measures of clinical severity, quality of life, and psychological distress in patients with psoriasis: a cluster analysis. *J Invest Dermatol*, 2004, 122, 602–7.

[1190] Kiebzak, G; Pierson, L; Campbell, M; et al. Use of the SF36 general health status survey to document health related quality of life in patients with coronary artery disease: effect of disease and response to coronary artery bypass graft surgery. *Heart Lung*, 2002, 31(3), 207–13.

[1191] Wiebe, S; Guyatt, G; Weaver, B; et al. Comparative responsiveness of generic and specific quality-of-life instruments. *J Clin Epidemiol*, 2003, 56, 52–60.

[1192] Ware Jr, J; Sherbourne, C. The MOS 36-item short form health survey (SF-36). Conceptual framework and item selection. *Med Care*, 1992, 30, 472–83.

[1193] Anderson, RT; Rajagopalan, R. Development and validation of a quality of life instrument for cutaneous disease. *J Am Acad Dermatol*, 1997, 37, 41–50.

[1194] Finlay, A; Khan, G. Dermatology Life Quality Index (DLQI)—a simple practical measure for routine clinical use. *Clin Exp Dermatol*, 1994, 19, 210–6.

[1195] Morgan, M; McCreedy, R; Simpson, J; Hay, RJ. Dermatology quality of life scales: a measure of impact of skin diseases. *Br J Dermatol*, 1997, 136, 202–6.

[1196] Chren, MM; Lasek, RJ; Flacke, SA; Zyzanski, SJ. Improved discriminative and evaluative capability of a refined version of Skindex, a quality of life instrument for patients with skin diseases. *Arch Dermatol*, 1997, 133, 1433–40.

[1197] Chren, MM; Lasek, RJ; Sahay, AP; Sands, LP. Measurement properties of Skindex-16: a brief quality-of-life measure for patients with skin disease. *J Cutan Med Surg*, 2001, 5, 105–10.

[1198] Nijsten, T; Sampogna, F; Chren, M; et al. Testing and reducing Skindex-29 using Rasch analysis: skindex-17. *J Invest Dermatol*, 2006, 126, 1244–50.

[1199] Abeni, D; Picardi, A; Pasquini, P; et al. Further evidence of the validity and reliability of the Skindex-29: an Italian study on 2, 242 dermatological outpatients. *Dermatology*, 2002, 204, 43–9.

[1200] Cohen, A; Ofek-Schlomai, A; Vardy, D; et al. Depression in dermatological patients identified by the mini international neuropsychiatric interview questionnaire. *J Am Acad Dermatol*, 2005, 54(1), 94–9.

[1201] Goldberg, D; Williams, P. A user's guide to the general health questionnaire. Windsor: NFER-Nelson, 1998.

[1202] Goldberg, D. The detection of psychiatric illness by questionnaire. London: Oxford University Press, 1972.

[1203] Picardi, A; Abeni, D; Pasquini, P. Assessing psychological distress in patients with skin diseases: reliability, validity and factor structure of the GHQ-12. *J Eur Acad Dermatol Venereol*, 2001, 15, 410–7.

[1204] Renzi, C; Tabolli, S; Picardi, A; et al. Effects of patient satisfaction with care on health-related quality of life: a prospective study. *J Eur Acad Dermatol Venereol*, 2005, 19, 712–8.

[1205] Chee, S; Martin, L; Murrell, D. The development of a quality of life instrument specific for pemphigus. *J Invest Dermatol*, 2009, 129, 2908–23.

[1206] Chen, S. Dermatology quality of life instruments: sorting out the quagmire. J Invest Dermatol, 2007, 127, 2726–39.

[1207] Frew, JW; Murrell, DF. Quality of life measurements inepidermolysis bullosa: tools for clinical research andpatient care. *Dermatol Clin*, 2010, 28, 185–90.

[1208] Frew, JW; Venugopal, SS; Murrell, DF. Quality of life outcomes of cultured allogeneic fibroblast therapy recipients with epidermolysis bullosa. *Aust J Dermatol*, 2011, 52 Suppl 1, 26.

[1209] Both, H; Essink-Bot, M; Busschbach, J; et al. Critical review of generic and dermatology-specific health related quality of life instruments. *J Invest Dermatol*, 2007, 127, 2726–39.

[1210] Horn, HM; Tidman, MJ. Quality of life in epidermolysis bullosa. *Clin Exp Dermatol*, 2002, 27, 707–10.

[1211] Maroti, M; Ulff, E; Wijma, B. Quality of life before and 6 weeks after treatment in a dermatological outpatient treatment unit. *J Eur Acad Dermatol Venereol*, 2006, 20(9), 1081–5.

[1212] VanBeek, M; Beach, S; Braslow, L; et al. Highlights from the report of the working group on "Core measures of the burden of skin diseases." *J Invest Dermatol*, 2007, 127, 2701–6.

[1213] Sampogna, F; Tabolli, S; Abeni, D. Impact of different skin conditions on quality of life. *G Ital Dermatol Venereol*, 2013, 148(3), 255-61.

[1214] Timóteo, RP; Marques, LS; Bertoncello, D. Physiotherapy intervention promotes better quality of life for individuals with pemphigus. *Rev Soc Bras Med Trop*, 2010, 43(5), 580-3.

[1215] Ghodsi, SZ; Chams-Davatchi, C; Daneshpazhooh, M; Valikhani, M; Esmaili, N. Quality of life and psychological status of patients with pemphigus vulgaris using Dermatology Life Quality Index and General Health Questionnaires. *J Dermatol*, 2012, 39(2), 141-4.

[1216] Rajan, B; Ahmed, J; Shenoy, N; Denny, C; Ongole, R; Binnal, A. Assessment of quality of life in patients with chronic oral mucosal diseases: a questionnaire-based study. *Perm J*, 2014, 18(1), e123-7.

About the Author

Andrés Tirado-Sánchez
Specialist in Dermatology-Autoimmune Bullous diseases.
Level 1 researcher at CONACYT
Hospital General de México, Instituto Mexicano del Seguro Social

Professor Tirado-Sánchez is a specialist in Dermatology, focusing in autoimmune bullous diseases like pemphigus and pemphigoid with nearly 20 years of experience in that area. He is a graduate professor at the University Anahuac and National Autonomous University of Mexico and the National Polytechnic Institute..

INDEX

A

B

C

D

E

F

G

H

I

J

K

L

M

N

O

P

Q

R

S

T

U

V

W

Y

Z